THE BIOLOGICAL BASIS OF RADIOTHERAPY

SECOND EDITION

The Biological Basis of Radiotherapy
Second Edition

Editors

G. Gordon Steel

Radiotherapy Research Unit, Institute of Cancer Research, Sutton, Surrey SM2 5NG, England

Gerald E. Adams

Radiobiology Unit, MRC, Chilton, Didcot, Oxfordshire OX11 0RD, England

and

Alan Horwich

Radiotherapy and Oncology Unit, The Royal Marsden Hospital, Downs Road, Sutton, Surrey SM2 5PT, England

1989

ELSEVIER

AMSTERDAM – NEW YORK – OXFORD

© 1989, Elsevier Science Publishers B.V. (Biomedical Division)

All rights reserved. No part of this publication may be reproduced, stored in a retrieval system, or transmitted in any form or by any means, electronic, mechanical, photocopying, recording or otherwise, without the prior written permission of the Publisher, Elsevier Science Publishers B.V. (Biomedical Division), P.O. Box 1527, 1000 BM Amsterdam, The Netherlands.

No responsibility is assumed by the Publisher for any injury and/or damage to persons or property as a matter of products liability, negligence or otherwise, or from any use or operation of any methods, products, instructions or ideas contained in the material herein. Because of the rapid advances in the medical sciences, the Publisher recommends that independent verification of diagnoses and drug dosages should be made.

Special regulations for readers in the USA.
This publication has been registered with the Copyright Clearance Center, Inc. (CCC), Salem, Massachusetts. Information can be obtained from the CCC about conditions under which the photocopying of parts of this publication may be made in the USA. All other copyright questions, including photocopying outside of the USA, should be referred to the Publisher.

ISBN 0–444–81099–4 (Hardback)
 0–444–81187–7 (Paperback)
This book is printed on acid-free paper.

Published by:
Elsevier Science Publishers B.V. (Biomedical Division)
P.O. Box 211
1000 AE Amsterdam
The Netherlands

Sole distributors for the USA and Canada:
Elsevier Science Publishing Company. Inc.
655 Avenue of the Americas
New York, NY 10010
USA

Library of Congress Cataloging-in-Publication Data

The Biological basis of radiotherapy / editors, G.G. Steel, G.E.
 Adams, and A. Horwich. – – 2nd ed.
  p. cm.
 Includes bibliographies and index.
 ISBN 0–444–81099–4 (U.S.)
 ISBN 0–444–81187–7 (pbk.)
  1. Tumors– –Radiotherapy. 2. Tumors– –Adjuvant treatment.
 3. Radiation– –Physiological effect. 4. Radiobiology. I. Steel, G.
 Gordon (George Gordon) II. Adams, Gerald E. III. Horwich, A (Alan)
  [DNLM: 1. Neoplasms– –radiotherapy. 2. Radiation Effects. QZ 269
 B6145]
 RC271.R3B565 1989
 616.99'40642– –dc20
 DNLM/DLC   89–16785
  for Library of Congress   CIP

Printed in The Netherlands

Preface

As a co-initiator of the successful British Council courses on the Biological Basis of Radiotherapy from which the first edition of this book arose, I am particularly pleased to have the opportunity of contributing a brief introductory note to the excellent second edition. I have always felt that the designation 'radiotherapy' is somewhat restrictive and tends not to do justice to the broadly based nature of the specialty. In recent years this has become increasingly true as the scope of radiotherapy extends to encompass advanced technological developments in physics, new concepts in biology and increased complexity in patient management. Indeed, over the past two decades the extent to which advances in biological and physical sciences have been brought to bear on this area of medicine is remarkable.

Whereas in the past radiotherapy was often practised at a routine technical level, today it is firmly based in internal medicine with a strong emphasis on clinical research. For the young clinician entering the specialty, the spectrum of possibilities is wide and it is particularly important that full advantage is taken of the opportunities to innovate and to maintain an awareness of developments in science that seem likely to impinge on the field.

Undoubtedly, the present volume will make an important contribution to this awareness; I am confident that it will whet the appetite of clinicians entering the specialty, nourish those in training and refresh senior clinicians in established practice.

Michael J. Peckham
Director
British Postgraduate
Medical Federation

Contributors

GERALD E. ADAMS   *MRC Radiobiology Unit, Chilton, Didcot, Oxfordshire OX11 0RD, England*
PETER E. BRYANT   *Department of Biology and Preclinical Medicine, University of St. Andrews, St. Andrews, Fife KY16 9TS, Scotland*
WENCESLAS CALVO   *Department of Clinical Physiology and Occupational Medicine, University of Ulm, Ulm, F.R.G.*
JULIANA DENEKAMP   *CRC Gray Laboratory, Mount Vernon Hospital, Northwood, Middlesex HA6 2RN, England*
STANLEY DISCHE   *Marie Curie Research Wing, Regional Centre for Radiotherapy and Oncology, Mount Vernon Hospital, Northwood, Middlesex HA6 2RN, England*
STANLEY B. FIELD   *MRC Cyclotron Unit, Hyperthermia Unit, Hammersmith Hospital, Ducane Road, London W12 0HS, England*
JACK F. FOWLER   *Department of Human Oncology K4/336, University of Wisconsin Clinical Cancer Center, 600 Highland Avenue, Madison, WI 53792, USA*
JOLYON H. HENDRY   *Department of Radiobiology, Paterson Institute for Cancer Research, Christie Hospital and Holt Radium Institute, Manchester M20 9BX, England*
JOHN H. HOPEWELL   *CRC Normal Tissue Radiobiology Research Group, Research Institute (University of Oxford), The Churchill Hospital, Headington, Oxford OX3 7LJ, England*
JEAN-CLAUDE HORIOT   *Centre G.F. Leclerc, Département de Radiothérapie, Rue du Prof. Marion, 21034 Dijon, France*
ALAN HORWICH   *Department of Radiotherapy and Oncology, The Royal Marsden Hospital, Downs Road, Sutton, Surrey SM2 5PT, England*
TREVOR J. McMILLAN   *Radiotherapy Research Unit, The Institute of Cancer Research, Cotswold Road, Sutton, Surrey SM2 5PT, England*
CHARLES S. PARKINS   *Radiotherapy Research Unit, The Institute of Cancer Research, Cotswold Road, Sutton, Surrey SM2 5NG, England*

HUIB S. REINHOLD *Department of Experimental Radiotherapy, Erasmus University, Rotterdam and Radiobiological Institute TNO, Rijswijk, The Netherlands*
G. GORDON STEEL *Radiotherapy Research Unit, The Institute of Cancer Research, Cotswold Road, Sutton, Surrey SM2 5NG, England*
IAN J. STRATFORD *MRC Radiobiology Unit, Chilton, Didcot, Oxfordshire OX11 0RD, England*
KLAUS-RUDIGER TROTT *Department of Radiotion Biology, Medical College of St. Bartholomew's Hospital, Charterhouse Square, London EC1M 6BQ, England*
WALTER VAN DEN BOGAERT *Department of Radiotherapy, University Hospital St. Rafaël, Kapucijnenvoer 33, 3000 Leuven, Belgium*
EMMANUEL VAN DER SCHUEREN *Department of Radiotherapy, University Hospital St. Rafaël, Kapucijnenvoer 33, 3000 Leuven, Belgium*

Contents

Preface v

Contributors vii

Chapter 1
Temporal stages of radiation action: free radical processes – *G.E. Adams* . 1

Chapter 2
Mechanisms of repair of DNA damage induced by ionising radiation –
P.E. Bryant 15

Chapter 3
The molecular basis of radiosensitivity – *T.J. McMillan* 29

Chapter 4
Survival of clonogenic cells: cell-survival curves – *G.G. Steel* 45

Chapter 5
Relation between cell survival and gross endpoints of tumour response and
tissue failure – *K.-R. Trott* 65

Chapter 6
Cell proliferation kinetics in tumours – *G.G. Steel* 77

Chapter 7
Radiation damage to early-reacting normal tissues – *J.H. Hendry* 89

Chapter 8
Radiation effects on blood vessels: role in late normal-tissue damage – *J.H. Hopewell, W. Calvo and H.S. Reinhold* 101

Chapter 9
Physiological hypoxia and its influence on radiotherapy – *J. Denekamp* . 115

Chapter 10
The clinical consequences of the oxygen effect – *S. Dische* 135

Chapter 11
Radiation sensitizers and bioreductive drugs – *I.J. Stratford and G.E. Adams* 145

Chapter 12
Radiobiology of human tumour cells – *G.G. Steel* 163

Chapter 13
Fractionation and therapeutic gain – *J.F. Fowler* 181

Chapter 14
Radiotherapy with multiple fractions per day – *W. van den Bogaert, J.-C. Horiot and E. van der Schueren* 209

Chapter 15
The dose-rate effect – *G.G. Steel* 223

Chapter 16
Clinical aspects of radiation dose rate – *A. Horwich* 237

Chapter 17
Heavy particles in radiotherapy – *J.F. Fowler* 249

Chapter 18
Combined radiotherapy–chemotherapy: principles – *G.G. Steel* 267

Chapter 19
Combined radiotherapy–chemotherapy in clinical practice – *A. Horwich* . 279

Chapter 20
Cellular and tissue effects of hyperthermia and radiation – *S.B. Field* . . 291

Chapter 21
Prediction of tumour response to treatment – *C.S. Parkins and A. Horwich* 305

Subject index 319

CHAPTER 1

Temporal stages of radiation action: free radical processes

GERALD E. ADAMS

MRC Radiobiology Unit, Chilton, Didcot, Oxfordshire OX11 ORD, England

---

1.1 Classification of time domains 1
    1.1.1   Introduction 1
    1.1.2   The physical stage 3
    1.1.3   The chemical stage 4
    1.1.4   The cellular stage 4
    1.1.5   The tissue stage 5

1.2 The radiation 'target' 6

1.3 The physical and chemical basis of radiation effects 8
    1.3.1   Energy deposition in DNA 8
    1.3.2   Influence of radiation quality 8
    1.3.3   Ultra-soft X-rays 9
    1.3.4   Radiation chemical effects 11

1.4 Modification of radiation response 12

1.1 Classification of time domains

1.1.1 Introduction

The energies of photon or particulate radiation emanating from natural and artificial radionuclides, X-ray sets and particle accelerators are vastly in excess of the energies of the various types of chemical bonds present in biological molecules. The process of ionisation, i.e., the ejection of electrons from the atoms with which the radiation interacts, is the major, though not the only, initial event in radiation action. The time-scale over which energy is imparted to an atom or small molecule during irradiation is extremely short and is governed by the velocity of the particle (at, or near, the

TABLE 1.1
Time domains of radiation action in biological systems

Physical stage:	
10^{-18} to 10^{-17} s	Fast particle traverses small atom or molecule
10^{-16}	Ionization $H_2O \rightarrow H_2O^+ + e^-$
10^{-15}	Electronic excitation $H_2O \rightarrow H_2O^*$
10^{-13}	Molecular vibrations and dissociation
10^{-12}	Rotation, relaxation and solvation of the electron in water
Chemical stage:	
10^{-10} to 10^{-7} s	Reactions of e^-_{aq} and other free radicals with solutes in radiation tracks and spurs
10^{-7}	Homogeneous distribution of free radicals
10^{-3}	Free-radical reactions largely complete
Seconds, minutes, hours	Biochemical changes (enzyme reactions)
Cellular and tissue stages:	
Hours	Cell division inhibited in microorganisms and mammalian cells; reproductive death
Days	Damage to gastrointestinal tract (and central nervous system at high doses)
Months	Haemopoietic death; acute damage to skin and other organs; late normal-tissue morbidity
Years	Carcinogenesis and expression of genetic damage in offspring.

velocity of light), the dimensions of the atom or molecule and the amount of energy lost, or transferred, in the process. A quantum of X or γ-radiation, or an energetic α-particle, will pass through a small atom or molecule (e.g. H_2O) and deliver energy to it, in a time between 10^{-17} and 10^{-18} seconds. The subsequent physical, chemical, biochemical and biological changes that follow these initial events cover a vast range and may not be expressed until months or even years later.

Some types of cancer may not appear until two to three decades after irradiation, as has been shown, for example, by the Life Span Study, an analysis of cancer incidence in survivors of the nuclear weapons dropped over Japan in 1945. Overall therefore, the time-scale of radiation action spans at least 26 orders of magnitude, extending from the earliest physical processes through to truly late effects such as cancer induction. It is not surprising therefore, that the interpretation of the biological effects of ionising radiation in terms of basic physical and chemical processes is complex and still far from fully understood.

It is convenient, though in no way rigorously precise, to classify the many identifiable processes of radiation action into four time-resolved domains. These represent the expression of damage, or change, at the physical, chemical, cellular and tissue levels (Table 1.1).

1.1.2 The physical stage

Ionising radiation transfers energy to molecular systems with which it interacts in discrete quanta or 'packages'. The magnitude of these energy transfers and their spatial distributions depends on various factors, including the energy of the radiation, the nature and constitution of the absorbing medium and particularly the type of radiation. The damaging effects of different types, or 'qualities', of radiation vary considerably and depend to a large extent upon their 'density of ionisation'. The densely ionising radiations (i.e., α-particles, protons, neutrons and heavier particles produced by certain types of high-energy accelerators), lose energy over a much shorter distance than do the so-called sparsely ionising radiation such as X or γ-rays. For a given radiation dose, the biological effectiveness of the particulate radiations in causing cell inactivation, mutation, cell transformation and frank malignancy in mammalian species including man are substantially greater than the effectiveness of sparsely ionising or 'low LET' radiations. LET or 'Linear Energy Transfer' is a measure of the rate at which energy is imparted to the absorbing medium per unit distance of track length. The absorbed dose, normally defined in terms of energy absorbed per unit mass, is convenient and usually quite applicable for most purposes in radiation biology. The quantity becomes increasingly inappropriate, however, when applied to very small heterogeneous systems such as subcellular volumes, or for constructing certain types of models used for describing quantitatively radiobiological phenomena at the sub-cellular level.

Interaction of radiation with an atom causes ejection of one or more extra-nuclear electrons in times of the order of 10^{-16} seconds. Initially, these ejected electrons have energies greatly in excess of atomic ionisation potentials and therefore cause many more 'secondary' ionisations which are themselves almost entirely responsible for the subsequent chemical changes which lead to biological damage. During their energy degradation process, the secondary electrons undergo collisions with neighbouring atoms and molecules, causing further ionisations and particularly electronic and vibrational excitations. Eventually their excess energy is lost and they undergo dipole interaction with the medium. If, for example, the medium is water, this involves electrostatic interactions between the negative charges of the secondary (or tertiary electrons) and the slight positive polarisation of charge associated with the hydrogen atoms in water. In aqueous media, this interaction is complete in about 10^{-12} seconds. This period of interactions is called the dielectric relaxation time. The trapped electron, or, as it is called in water, 'the hydrated electron' (e^-_{aq}), has the properties of a free radical. It can diffuse considerable distances and undergo reactions with a wide range of chemical structures including those present in many biological systems. Its formation marks the transition to the chemical stage of radiation action.

1.1.3 The chemical stage

The chemical stage of radiation action concerns in the main, the formation and subsequent reactions of molecular fragments such as free radicals, radical-ions and energetically excited molecules. In approximate terms, the energy deposited in a multi-component chemical system is partitioned primarily according to the relative proportions of the constituent atoms. Strictly speaking, this energy partitioning is also dependent to some extent upon atomic volume or 'electron fraction' but for elements of low atomic number (appropriate therefore for biological tissue) the approximation is acceptable. This is known as 'The Principle of Equipartition of Energy' and, because of the high proportion of water in the mammalian cell ($\sim$80%) it implies that most of the energy absorbed in irradiated cells will occur in the aqueous component. This is the reason why so much attention has been devoted in the past to the study of the radiation chemistry of water and dilute aqueous solutions.

Water dissociates rapidly following absorption of radiation. The ionised water molecule, H_2O^+ interacts with neighbouring water molecules to form OH radicals, which are very strongly oxidising species of very high reactivity. They are also formed by dissociation of 'excited' water molecules. Both these processes occur over timescales usually shorter than that for dielectric relaxation. Overall, the radiation-induced dissociation of water, i.e.,

$$H_2O \rightarrow (H + e^-_{aq}) + OH$$

gives rise to both oxidising species (OH) and highly reactive reducing species ($H + e^-_{aq}$). In some situations, a proportion of the radicals react together to reform water or to produce molecular hydrogen (H_2) and hydrogen peroxide (H_2O_2). The remaining reactive radicals diffuse away from the regions of the radiation tracks where they are formed and react with neighbouring molecules in the environment. Eventually, the spatial distribution of free radicals becomes homogeneous (in $\sim 10^{-7}$ seconds). Depending upon the chemical nature of the environment, free-radical reactions are usually largely complete in times of milliseconds or less. There is abundant evidence that damage to biological molecules caused by reactions with free radicals contributes to loss, or change, of cellular function following irradiation. A major unsolved problem in molecular radiation biology is concerned with identifying and characterising those early chemical reactions that are relevant to the important cellular and sub-cellular responses to radiation. These processes are almost always complete within times much less than a millisecond. Some, however, may take somewhat longer.

1.1.4 The cellular stage

Change in structure, function or emergence from quiescence in cellular macromolecules, including some types of repair systems, may occur very early following irradiation. Changes *observable* at the cellular level do not appear until later, although ultrastructural changes in some cells can be observed quite early. For example, local protrusions of the plasma membrane can be detected within minutes of exposure of cells to a relatively high dose of radiation. These changes are followed within a few hours by membrane distention and invagination of the nuclear membrane. These changes are accompanied by modifications in membrane permeability and loss of some essential enzymes. Actual loss of cellular function, which can occur at lower radiation doses, cannot be observed immediately. Loss of reproductive capacity, or cell death, can only be observed and measured quantitatively when the cell fails to divide. Further, changes in the chromosomal content, configuration or morphology, or development of mutations, only appear after a sufficient number of cell divisions have taken place in order to allow the analyses of aberrant cells in the total population.

Measurements of changes in the efficiency, or capacity, for repair of radiation damage usually require cell-cloning techniques. While fast free-radical repair (by sulphydryl compounds for example) can occur in sub-second times, other repair processes can take much longer. Enzymic repair of sub-lethal radiation damage in mammalian cells is usually complete in 2–3 hours. The so-called 'repair of potentially lethal damage' may occur over longer times and usually requires delayed plating for its observation in cells in vitro.

Despite the limitations often imposed by the time-scale of experimental processes required for demonstration of some intra-cellular processes, the stages in the cell's mitotic cycle when radiation damage appears to be most critical are now known with some precision. Mammalian cells are usually at their most radiation-sensitive during mitosis and during the G_2-phase. They are usually most resistant in the early S-phase, although such variations in inter-mitotic sensitivity are highly dependent on radiation quality. Cellular sensitivity to low LET radiation is usually much more variable than it is to more densely ionising radiation.

1.1.5 The tissue stage

In view of the correlation just referred to between radiosensitivity and phase within the cell cycle, it is not surprising that the manifestation of damage to biological tissues in vivo also depends upon their proliferation rate. As will be discussed in Chapters 7 and 8, the extent of radiation damage (and especially its time of appearance) depends upon the rate of cellular turnover. Tissues with a rapid turnover exhibit their damage early after irradiation; those with a very low rate of cell turnover exhibit their damage much later. For example, damage to the intestines becomes apparent within 2 weeks of irradiation, damage to the lung appears after 3 to 4 months, damage to cells of the central nervous system that proliferate only during embryogenesis requires higher radiation doses and appears later still. Sub-lethal effects of radiation, including mutation and oncogenesis, occur even after doses of radiation that are relatively low compared with those required for cytotoxic effects in vivo. The latency period for induction of cancer varies widely, depending on the dose, radiation quality, and the particular type of tumour induced. In the low-dose range, low LET radiation is less effective per unit dose in inducing cancer than the densely ionising high LET radiation. Thus neutrons, which are 5-times more effective than γ-rays for a given radiation dose may be relatively even more effective at low radiation doses. Population studies, including follow-up of the survivors of the nuclear weapons used in Japan, show that leukaemias tend to have the shortest induction period, 5–15 years. Some other tumours, multiple myeloma for example, may not appear until 25–30 years after exposure.

1.2 The radiation 'target'

The evidence that damage to the genomic material of the cell is the *principal* cause of radiation-induced cell death and various sub-cellular changes such as mutation, chromosomal fragment exchanges and malignant transformation, is now overwhelming (Figure 1.1). Radiation damage to other cellular constituents may, however, also contribute to radiation effects.

Early indications that DNA is the major target came from various ingenious laboratory experiments. Microdissection studies with sea urchin eggs showed that the cytoplasmic materials of the cell could withstand large doses of radiation without greatly affecting the viability of the cell, *provided* the nucleus was temporarily removed by microdissection during irradiation of the remaining material. Many studies revealed, for several cellular species, a strong correlation between radiation sensitivity and chromosomal volume. Similarly, inverse relationships between radiation sensitivity and ploidy have been observed in various yeast cells.

Direct evidence pointing specifically to the critical role of DNA damage came with the discovery of the BUdR effect (Djordevic and Szybalski, 1960). The thymi-

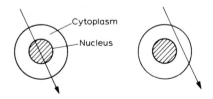

Radiation must pass through the nucleus of the cell to cause

mutation, cell death, cancer

Figure 1.1. Importance of the cell nucleus as a radiation target.

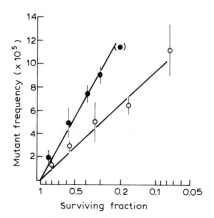

Figure 1.2. Relationship between mutation and survival for X-ray induction of thioguanine resistance in Chinese hamster cells irradiated with X-rays (o) and plutonium α-particles ($\bullet$) (data from Thacker et al., 1982).

dine analogue 5-bromodeoxyuridine (BUdR) can easily be incorporated into the DNA of proliferating cells in culture by supplementing the culture medium with 5-bromodeoxyuridine. Uptake and incorporation occurs because of similarities in molecular structure and topography between thymidine and the analogue. The fact that BUdR incorporation substantially enhances the *cellular* sensitivity to ionising radiation directly demonstrates the importance of intracellular DNA damage. The mechanism of the BUdR effect is complex, but the evidence is strong that fast free-radical processes are involved.

More recently, strong quantitative inter-relationships for radiation-induced cell lethality, chromosomal changes and mutation efficiency have been observed. Thacker and colleagues have observed for example, a log–linear relationship between the frequency of radiation-induced mutations at the HGPRT locus and radiation lethality (Thacker, 1979; Thacker et al., 1982). This relationship has been observed for several cell lines and does not appear to be affected by variation in the shapes of the individual radiation dose-response curves. It also holds for high LET α-particle irradiation (Figure 1.2). It has been argued that the processes used by the cell for dealing with the initial radiation damage are not entirely error-free. If for any radiation quality the probability of the repair system for *changing* the genetic material relative to that for *elimination* of the lesion in order to give non-mutant survivors is fixed, this would explain the constancy of the relationship in Figure 1.2.

8   G.E. Adams

1.3 The physical and chemical basis for radiation effects

1.3.1 Energy deposition in DNA

The deposition of energy in intracellular DNA during irradiation is rapid, heterogeneous and highly dependent on radiation quality. A radiation dose of 1 Gy (1 J/kg, 100 rads in the old units), will cause on average about $2 \cdot 10^5$ ionisations in a mammalian cell, of which approximately 1% will occur in the genomic material. A major consequence is breakage of DNA strands (Section 2.1). Of the 1000 or so that occur, almost all will be repaired by cellular defence mechanisms and are of no consequence. Some, mainly double-strand breaks, are not repaired however, and lead directly to cell death or other irreversible changes.

The quantity 'absorbed radiation dose', defined in terms of energy deposited per unit mass, becomes increasingly inappropriate when considering the spatial distribution of energy deposition in minute volumes – in regions of the chromosome for example. This is because of the essentially heterogeneous nature of energy deposition within 'tracks' of secondary particles. The energy absorption process in such small volumes is best described using the terminology and concepts of 'microdosimetry' originally introduced by Rossi and co-workers. A detailed and rigorous treatment of this subject, including key references, is given in Report No. 36 of the International Commission on Radiological Units and Measurements (ICRU, 1983).

1.3.2 Influence of radiation quality

High LET radiation is relatively more damaging than low LET radiation. Figure 1.3 compares simplistically the energy deposition within tracks of a high LET particle and a low energy particle traversing a segment of the DNA helix. Some α-particles will initially deposit energy at an average rate of about 100 keV per micron track length. Many ionisations will therefore be caused in or near the DNA molecule. The deposition rate is substantially less for high-energy electons. There is therefore a much greater probability of double-strand breakage from a single α-particle track than there is from a single electron track. The probability of two electron tracks coinciding to produce two aligned single-strand breaks is even lower. Various physical models of these processes have been proposed, often involving concepts derived from microdosimetry. The hypothesis of interactions of sub-lesions is frequently invoked to explain the production of various sub-cellular effects, including exchange aberrations in the chromosomes of irradiated cells.

Figure 1.4 compares the efficiencies for the formation of asymmetrical interchanges (dicentric aberrations) in human lymphocytes irradiated with single doses either of γ-rays or fission neutrons (Lloyd et al., 1975; 1976). As is the case for cell inactivation, the high LET neutrons are more effective than the low LET γ-rays. The linearity

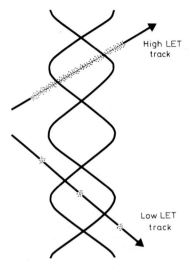

Figure 1.3. Spatial representation of low and high LET radiation traversing a section of the DNA helix.

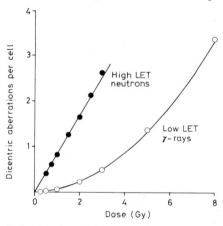

Figure 1.4. The different efficiencies of high LET fission neutrons and low LET γ-rays in causing dicentric chromosome aberrations in human lymphocytes (data from Lloyd et al., 1975; 1976).

of the neutron curve implies single-hit events; the curved form of the γ-ray curve implies interaction between sub-lesions.

1.3.3 Ultra-soft X-rays

Goodhead and collaborators (Goodhead et al., 1979; 1981) have carried out various experiments using ultra-soft X-rays to examine biophysical models of radiation action. Electrons produced by absorption of approximately 1 keV X-rays deposit their energy in small volumes. This is analogous to the energy deposition in electron track-ends,

TABLE 1.2
Range of secondary particles from ultra-soft X-rays

	Energy (keV)	Range of secondary particles (nm)
Carbon K	0.28	< 7
Aluminium K	1.49	< 70
Titanium	4.55	< 550
Hard-X-rays	250	Up to 500 000

From Goodhead and Nikjoo (1989).

structures that are produced in the slowing-down spectrum of energetic electrons from 'hard' X-rays. The dimensions of these track-ends are of the same order as those sub-cellular structures likely to be sites of critical radiation-induced damage. The interpretation of the mechanisms involved in cellular radiation damage is considerably helped by knowledge of the spatial pattern of energy depositions. For 'hard' X-rays, energy deposition occurs over track distances that are long compared with the dimensions of the critical sub-structures, and this complicates interpretation of the inactivation process in terms of interaction distances and the parameters of radiation absorption. However, the use of ultra-soft X-rays can simplify analysis because they give rise to electrons of well-defined energies and very short track lengths.

An important area of enquiry has concerned the theory of dual radiation action (Kellerer and Rossi, 1972; 1978). Critical intracellular damage is assumed to arise as a consequence of the interaction of two separate sub-lesions caused by the radiations. The interactions, which may occur over large distances, could involve sub-lesions formed in the *same* radiation track or in two separate tracks. The dose-response relationships observed are presumed to reflect the track origins of the sub-lesions as indicated in Figure 1.5. Various attempts have been made to interpret dose-response relationships in terms of this model, and both linear and quadratic responses have been observed (Section 4.2). However, other factors, repair for example, can confound the interpretation of such dose-response relationships.

One rationale for using soft X-rays is that if long-range interactions of sub-lesions are necessary to produce chromosomal exchange aberrations, then the soft X-rays should be much less efficient than hard X-rays. Experiments have shown that the reverse is the case. The efficiency of dicentric formation in irradiated human lymphocytes and V79 cells is actually increased relative to that for 250 kV X-rays (Virsik et al., 1980; Thacker et al., 1983). It was concluded that dicentrics could only be formed if a *single* secondary track traversed segments of two chromosomes that were very close together, or that dicentric aberrations could arise from interaction of a chromosome fragment with an *undamaged* chromosome. The latter mechanism has implications in interpreting the origin of chromosomal damage caused by agents other than radiation.

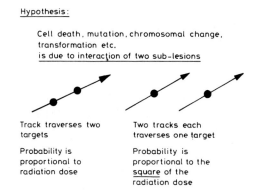

Figure 1.5. Illustrating the theory of dual radiation action.

1.3.4 Radiation chemical effects

Problems posed for the interpretation of early effects in irradiated cellular systems include the following: the chemical nature of DNA damage and the mechanisms of its formation; the role of free radicals and their classification according to abstraction, addition and elimination reactions; the relevance of long-range energy migration processes; and the free radical basis for various dose-modification phenomena including cellular radiation sensitisation by oxygen and other electron-affinic agents.

The radiation chemistry of DNA, even in aqueous solution, is too complex to review here (for a detailed discussion, see von Sonntag (1987)). However, some comments are appropriate. Many attempts have been made to classify intracellular radiation damage to DNA in terms of 'direct' and 'indirect' mechanisms. The indirect mechanism assumes that damage to DNA does not arise from energy deposited directly in the molecule itself but is caused rather by reactive entities formed by radiolysis of nearby water molecules. There is evidence that reactions of the hydroxyl radical, a major product of water radiolysis, contributes to radiation-induced cell kill. For example, various chemical agents that react rapidly with OH radicals protect against radiation damage, although high concentrations are usually required.

However, the distinction between direct and indirect mechanisms may not be clear-cut. It is generally thought that only those free radicals generated in water located close to the DNA molecule are able to diffuse and react with the constituent base and sugar moieties and initiate the chain of processes that leads ultimately to irreversible damage. It is unlikely that the maximum diffusion distance exceeds 2 to 3 nm. Water located close to DNA will be strongly influenced structurally by electrostatic and other interactions which means that the dielectric relaxation times in this region may be extended by orders of magnitude compared with those in very dilute solutions. Electrons liberated in radiolysis of DNA-associated water may never go through even the hydration stage and may interact with the DNA directly, possibly at a site in DNA remote from the point of origin. The generation of OH radicals by dissociative reactions of H_2O^+ ions may also be much slower than in free water. It has been suggested that negative charge transfer *from* the neighbouring DNA to the water ion may occur under these conditions, thereby transporting the damage to the DNA. Overall, therefore, the implications of this model are that ionic centres may be generated in the DNA that are similar to those arising from *direct* energy absorption in DNA, even though the initiating processes occur elsewhere.

1.4 Modification of radiation response

The phenomenon of response modification is considered in more detail in Chapter 11. Many substances that alone have little or no effect on cell viability can radically change cellular radiation sensitivity either positively or negatively. Since some of these substances act by fast free-radical processes, some comment is appropriate in this introductory chapter.

The oxygen effect (Chapter 10) is almost universal in radiobiology and despite large differences in absolute radiation sensitivity between some cell types the magnitude of the effect does not vary greatly. For the vast majority of cell types investigated, the values of the oxygen enhancement ratio (OER) usually lie between 2 and 3.5. Further, the range of sensitizing efficiencies, defined in terms of the concentration range of oxygen required for sensitization, is also small. This, together with the fact that the oxygen effect can be mimicked by many other chemical substances of diverse structures is consistent with the free radical nature of the oxygen effect.

An early proposal for the mechanism of the oxygen effect, and one for which there is still much evidence in support, is the oxygen fixation hypothesis (for a full discussion and relevant references see Alper, 1979). In this model, free radicals formed in a critical target molecule (e.g. DNA) react rapidly with oxygen to form peroxyradicals. An essential feature of the model is that this irreversible reaction which leads to cell damage competes with a 'healing' or 'repair' reaction in which hydrogen atoms are transferred from SH-containing compounds (or other hydrogen-donating molecules) endogenous to the cell.

	radiation	
Target molecule	——>	free radical ($R^{\bullet}$)
$R^{\bullet} + O_2$	——>	$RO_2^{\bullet}$ (fixation)
$R^{\bullet} + XSH$	——>	$RH + XS^{\bullet}$ (chemical repair)

In model chemical systems, both peroxyl radical formation and the chemical repair reaction have been observed directly using fast-response pulse radiolysis techniques. Michael and co-workers (1986) have also obtained direct evidence for the fast time scale of this competition mechanism in mammalian cells, from experiments using a fast oxygen-explosion technique.

Radiation sensitization by many electron-affinic agents also involve fast free-radical reactions, although some of these compounds can also sensitize by various non-radical processes including suppression of intracellular thiol compounds, inhibition of repair processes and bioreductive activation.

References

Alper, T. (1979) Cellular Radiobiology, Cambridge University Press, Cambridge.
Djordevic, B. and Szybalski, W. (1960) Genetics of human cell lines: III, Incorporation of 5-bromo and 5-iododeoxyuridine into the deoxyribonucleic acid of human cells and its effect on radiation sensitivity. J. Exp. Med. 112, 509–518.
Goodhead, D.T., Thacker, J. and Cox, R. (1979) Effectiveness of 0.3 keV Carbon Ultrasoft X-rays for the inactivation and mutation of cultured mammalian cells. Int. J. Radiat. Biol. 36, 101–114.
Goodhead, D.T., Cox, R. and Thacker, J. (1981) Do ultrasoft X-rays produce lesions characteristic of high LET and low LET or neither), in: Proceedings VII Symposium, Microdosimetry Oxford U.K., 8–12 September 1980 [EUR7147] (Booz, J., Ebert, H.G. and Hartfield, H.D., eds.), pp. 929–939, Harwood Academic Publishers for the CEC.
Goodhead, D.T. and Nikjoo, H. (1989) Track structure analysis of ultrasoft X-rays compared to high and low LET radiations. Int. J. Radiat. Biol., in press.
ICRU Report No. 36: (1983) Microdosimetry; International Commission on Radiation Units and Measurements.
Lloyd, D.C., Purrott, H.R.J., Dolphin, G.W., Bolton, D., Edwards, A.A. and Corp, M.J. (1975) The relationship between chromosome aberrations and low LET radiation dose to human lymphocytes. Int. J. Radiat. Biol. 28, 75–90.
Lloyd, D.C., Purrott, R.J., Dolphin, G.W. and Edwards, A.A. (1976) Chromosome aberrations induced in human lymphocytes by neutron irradiation. Int. J. Radiat. Biol. 29, 169–182.
Michael, B.D., Davies, S. and Held, K.D. (1986) Ultrafast chemical repair of DNA single and double-strand break precursors in irradiated V79 cells, in: Mechanisms of DNA Damage and Repair. (Simic, M.G., Grossman, L. and Upton, A.C., eds.), pp. 89–100, Plenum Press, New York.
Thacker, J. (1979) The involvement of repair processes in radiation-induced mutation of cultured mammalian cells, in: Proceedings 6th International Congress of Radiation Research, Tokyo, pp. 612–620, Japanese Association for Radiation Research, Tokyo.
Thacker, J., Stretch, A. and Goodhead, D.T. (1982) The mutagenicity of α-particles from plutonium-238. Radiat. Res. 92, 343–352.
Thacker, J., Goodhead, D.T. and Wilkinson, R.E. (1983) The role of localised single-track events in the formation of chromosome aberrations in cultured mammalian cells, in: Radiation Protection, VIII Symposium Microdosimetry, Jülich, F.R.G., 27 Sept – 1 Oct 1982. [EUR8395] (Booz, J. and Ebert, H.G. eds.), pp. 587–595, Commission of the European Communities, Luxembourg.
Virsik, R.P., Goodhead, D.T., Cox, R., Thacker, J., Schafer, C.H. and Harder, D. (1980) Chromosome aberrations induced in human lymphocytes by ultrasoft Al_k and C_k X-rays. Int. J. Radiat. Biol. 38, 545–557.
Von Sonntag, C. (1987) The Chemical Basis of Radiation Biology, Taylor and Francis, London.

CHAPTER 2

Mechanisms of repair of DNA damage induced by ionising radiation

PETER E. BRYANT

Department of Biology and Preclinical Medicine, University of St. Andrews, St. Andrews, Fife KY16 9TS, Scotland

---

2.1	Types of damage induced in DNA	15
	2.1.1 Strand breakage	16
	2.1.2 Base damage	17
	2.1.3 Cross-links	17
2.2	Methods of detecting DNA damage	18
	2.2.1 Detection of base damage	18
	2.2.2 Detection of strand breaks	18
2.3	Repair of DNA damage in irradiated cells	21
	2.3.1 Repair of single-strand breaks	21
	2.3.2 Repair of base damage	22
	2.3.3 Repair of double-strand breaks	22
2.4	Biological consequences of DNA damage and misrepair	23
	2.4.1 The role of double-strand breaks	23
	2.4.2 Induction of chromosomal aberrations by restriction endonuclease dsb	24
	2.4.3 The relationship between dsb and chromosomal aberrations in irradiated cells	24
	2.4.4 Possible consequences of misrepair of dsb in ataxia-telangiectasia cells	25
2.5	Conclusions	25

2.1 Types of damage induced in DNA

It is now generally recognised that the damage caused to cells by ionising radiation is a result of induction of lesions in the nuclear DNA. This damage to DNA may result in the observed biological end-points of mutation, oncogenic transformation, chromosomal aberrations and cell death.

In order to understand the relationship between DNA damage and these end-points it is necessary to consider : (a) the types and frequencies of DNA lesions induced;

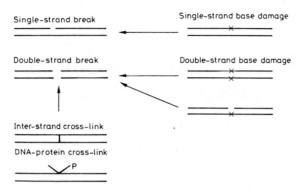

Figure 2.1. Types of damage occurring in DNA of cells exposed to ionising radiation. Protein indicated by P. Arrows indicate possible enzymatic conversion of base damage or interstrand cross-links into single- or double-strand breaks.

(b) which of these are critical in causing the biological effects; and (c) how the cell repairs or misrepairs these lesions.

What then are the types of damage occurring in cells exposed to ionising radiations? They can be divided into three main categories: direct strand breakage, base damage and cross-links (Figure 2.1).

2.1.1 Strand breakage

Strand breaks can be divided into those which affect only one strand of the double-helix (single-strand breaks, ssb) and those affecting both strands of the double helix (double-strand breaks, dsb). The cleavage of the phosphodiester bonds which form the DNA backbone may leave 3'-hydroxyl and 5'-phosphoryl groups at the break ends. This is thought to be a relatively infrequent event, occurring in not more than about 30% of the breaks. This type of break has been termed 'clean' because it may be ligated, using a single enzymic step. Note that the term 'clean' should not be confused with the terms 'blunt-' and 'cohesive-ended' as applied to restriction endonuclease-induced dsb. Clean breaks may be of single or double-stranded types and can have, in the case of dsb, either a blunt or cohesive-ended structure. Thus, restriction endonuclease-induced dsb are all of the 'clean' type. Most radiation-induced breaks will, however, have a more complex ('dirty') end structure, and therefore require some enzymic cleaning prior to subsequent repair steps. The mechanisms of this repair will be considered later. Single-strand breaks are one of the most frequent lesions occurring in DNA: at approximately 1000 ssb/diploid genome/gray. They are induced as a linear function of the radiation dose, implying that they occur as a result of single ionising events. Breakage of the DNA may be non-random, actively transcribing DNA suffering more breakage than inactive DNA (Chiu and Oleinick, 1982).

Double-strand breaks comprise essentially two ssb, either exactly opposite to one another or in close proximity (probably not more than four bases apart, see below). Double-strand breaks are also found in several instances to be induced linearly with dose (although recent controversy, discussed below, has challenged this view), showing that they too arise from single events, probably of much higher energy (100–1000 eV) in the form of large clusters of ionisations. Probably as a result of this large energy requirement dsb are induced much less frequently than ssb; at a frequency of approximately 40 dsb/G_1 diploid genome/gray (Blöcher, 1982). Dsb may not be evenly distributed throughout the genome in irradiated cells, some non-random clustering of damage has been reported (Baverstock, 1985). The implications of this are not yet clear. However, in general dsb are thought to be the most important group of lesions that cause biological damage.

2.1.2 Base damage

Base damage involves chemical alteration of the bases of DNA without frank breakage of a strand. The damage to the base may involve severance of a side group from the base or damage to the ring structure itself. The frequency of base damage is thought to be equal or similar to the frequency of strand breakage. There also is evidence for non-random distribution of base damage: DNA which is undergoing active gene expression appears to be more susceptible to damage than suppressed DNA, although the repair of damage in active DNA is found to be more rapid than in suppressed DNA (Patil et al., 1985). Base-damaged sites can be cleaved by specific enzymes which may result in breakage of the phosphodiester backbone of DNA. It is also known that double-stranded base damage sites occur and that cleavage of these leads to dsb (Ahnström and Bryant, 1982). Similarly, cleavage of a base-damaged site opposite an ssb would lead to a dsb (Figure 2.1).

2.1.3 Cross-links

Two sorts of cross-links are known to occur in irradiated DNA. The first is the interstrand cross-link (Lett et al., 1961; Bohne et al., 1970) and their frequency in cells can be estimated to be approximately 0.5 cross-links/G_1 diploid genome per gray, a low frequency when compared to other lesions. These lesions may also be converted into dsb during repair (Figure 2.1). It has for example been shown that during repair, interstrand cross-links induced in yeast cells by psoralen-UVA treatment, lead to dsb (Magana-Schwencke et al., 1982).

The second type is the DNA-protein cross-link. The presence of these lesions can be detected using a filter elution assay in which the DNA is treated with a protease enzyme which releases the DNA from the covalently linked protein. This is then observed as an increased elution of the DNA from the filter (Kohn et al., 1981). The absolute frequency of these lesions in cells cannot be determined from filter elution data. However, we can estimate the frequency from data for bacteriophage to be approximately $1/G_1$ diploid genome per gray (Bohne et al., 1970).

2.2 Methods of detecting DNA damage

The following sections deal with a few of the currently used methods, especially those used to obtain estimates of absolute frequencies of lesions in irradiated cells. Only methods that measure base damage and frank strand-breakage will be considered.

2.2.1 Detection of base damage

Absolute numbers of base alterations of specific kinds in DNA (e.g., altered thymine) have been obtained using chemical analysis of the base moieties in DNA from irradiated cells (Cerutti, 1974; Patil et al., 1985). These assays involve radioactive labelling of a base in DNA, for example the methyl group in thymine, and analysis of the hydrolysis products of the DNA from irradiated cells treated with either sodium borohydride or strong acid and alkali. The damaged thymine is thus converted to 2-methyl glycerol or acetol, respectively, which can be separated by ion-exchange chromatography and counted for radioactivity. Alteration of the methyl side-group of thymine may also be observed as hydrogen abstraction from the methyl group. This can be monitored by the measurement of the amount of tritiated water formed from irradiated DNA (Cerutti, 1974).

Another popular but less specific method of detecting and measuring base damage in DNA is by conversion of damaged sites to strand breaks, using crude or purified enzyme extracts from bacteria, e.g. *Micrococcus luteus* (Paterson, 1976). In this type of assay the isolated DNA is subjected to digestion by the mixture of enzymes which are assumed to incise the DNA at sites of base damage. The result of incision is a strand break which can be detected using any of the methods currently available for measuring strand breakage (see below). A modification of this assay was used to show that double-stranded base-damaged sites occur in irradiated cells (Ahnström and Bryant, 1982). In this case a purified enzyme extract of *M. luteus* was introduced into cells that had been permeabilised by a mild non-ionic detergent and the dsb measured using neutral velocity sedimentation.

2.2.2 Detection of strand breaks

The frequency of strand breaks can be measured by the classical method of velocity sedimentation. This involves releasing DNA by detergent lysis, then centrifuging through a linear sucrose gradient (Figure 2.2) which ensures a constant rate of

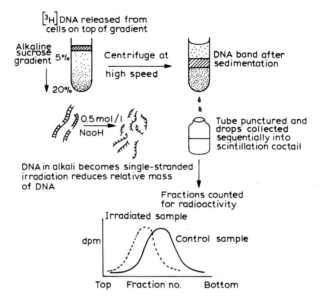

Figure 2.2. Diagram illustrating the principles of alkaline velocity sedimentation to determine relative molecular mass.

sedimentation with time (McGrath and Williams, 1966). Ssb are determined by centrifugation under strongly alkaline conditions, which allow the two strands of DNA to separate. The relative molecular mass of the irradiated DNA can be determined by the rate of sedimentation under a given set of conditions, relative to known standards in order to obtain a 'sedimentation coefficient' (s). From the change in the s value with radiation dose the relative molecular mass of the DNA can be determined and from this the frequency of strand breaks (Lohman, 1968).

Dsb can be measured by a similar procedure but involving centrifugation under neutral conditions so that DNA remains double-stranded. Blöcher (1982) used this technique to measure dsb in high molecular mass DNA released from irradiated mouse ascites tumour cells by detergent and enzyme digestion of the proteins associated with the DNA. He also used a computer to simulate breakage of control (unirradiated DNA) and compare the 'broken' profile with that of the irradiated one, thereby obtaining values of the change in relative molecular mass.

Recently, alternative methods have been devised, notable among them, filter elution involving lysis of radioactively labelled cells on plastic filters, and elution of the DNA during very slow pumping over many hours. Under alkaline conditions a mixture of both ssb and dsb are detected, as in the case of alkaline elution (Kohn et al., 1981). The basis of the method is that cells are lysed with detergent on a filter and the smaller DNA fragments, generated when cells are irradiated, eluted. From the extent of elution a relative measure of the frequency of strand breaks can be obtained. The

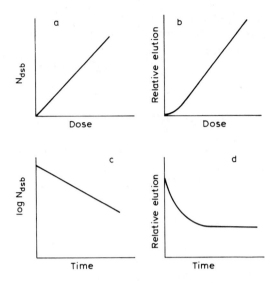

Figure 2.3. Dose-effect relationships for induction of DNA double-strand breaks (dsb), using (a) neutral velocity sedimentation or (b) neutral filter elution. Also shown are repair kinetics of dsb, using (c) neutral velocity sedimentation or (d) neutral filter elution. The diagrams are not drawn to scale.

disadvantage of this method is that the absolute frequencies of breaks cannot be obtained. The advantage of filter elution is the ease with which large numbers of samples can be processed and kinetics of repair of breaks monitored.

Dsb can be monitored using filter elution under 'neutral' conditions, usually pH 9.6 (Bradley and Kohn, 1979). This is currently the most widely used method of measuring the relative frequency of dsb. It should be mentioned, however, that there is controversy regarding the validity of the neutral filter elution (NFE) method in measuring dsb. Briefly, the controversy centres around the shape of the dose-effect curve for induction of dsb at low doses and the repair kinetics obtained with this method when compared with results of the neutral velocity sedimentation method (NVS) which requires high doses to be given to cells before reliable measurements can be made. The NFE method shows non-linear induction kinetics with a threshold occurring at low doses (Figure 2.3), whereas linear induction kinetics are obtained with the NVS method. Another difference in the results obtained with the two methods is the kinetics of dsb repair. With NFE the kinetics of dsb repair in mammalian cells are rapid, with a half-time of some 10–20 minutes (Weibezahn and Coquerelle, 1981) and repair is complete in 1–2 hours (Figure 2.3). In contrast, the repair of dsb observed with NVS is slower in mammalian cells, with a half-time of some 1.5–4 h (Blöcher and Pohlit, 1982).

At this time it is not known what are the reasons for the discrepancies between these two methods. It seems likely that the non-linear induction kinetics (Figure 2.3b) may result from incomplete separation of the DNA from other molecules (Okayasu et al.,

1988); however, other explanations are possible (Radford, 1987). Further work clearly needs to be done to solve this problem. It is very important that this controversy is resolved because of the already widespread use of the NFE method. We shall return to this problem later when considering the biological effects of dsb.

2.3 Repair of DNA damage in irradiated cells

All types of radiation-induced DNA damage appear to be repaired; however, the rates of the repair of different types of lesion are found to vary. This difference in kinetics immediately indicates that several mechanisms may occur.

2.3.1 Repair of single-strand breaks

Ssb are repaired very rapidly with a half-time for an initial component of 2–5 minutes (Körner et al., 1978). Similar rates of repair are observed with a variety of methods, including alkaline velocity sedimentation and alkaline filter elution. The kinetics of repair of ssb indicate that there may be more than one component present and that the conversion of base-damaged sites into ssb could also be involved (Bryant et al., 1984). Since alkaline methods of measuring breaks cannot distinguish between

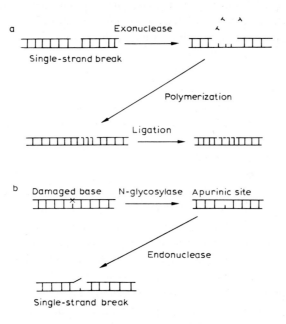

Figure 2.4. Diagram illustrating the probable steps in the repair of (a) a single-strand break and (b) a base-damaged site.

ssb and dsb, a slow component in the repair kinetics (representing repair of dsb) would be expected, based on data for NVS. This was indeed the case when the repair of ssb and dsb were compared in the same system (Bryant and Blöcher, 1980).

The precise details of the mechanism of repair of ssb are unknown but probably involve excision of damaged bases, where these exist, from the ends of ssb by an 'exonuclease' (a trimming enzyme which acts on free ends of DNA) and subsequent repolymerisation of the gap, ending in a ligation step joining the ends of the break (Figure 2.4a).

Some ssb may have 'clean' ends, with 3'-hydroxyl and 5'-phosphoryl groups, which only require simple ligation for repair. These are thought not to be more than 30% of the total ssb (Bryant and Blöcher, 1982).

In the case of repair of 'dirty' breaks, evidence indicates that the gap produced by the exonuclease-cleaning of an ssb is very short; of the order of only 1–3 bases (Painter and Young, 1972; Fox and Fox, 1973).

2.3.2 Repair of base damage

Base-damage repair may be slower than that of ssb (Cerutti, 1974) and is thought, like the repair of UV-induced pyrimidine dimers, to involve the removal of the damaged base from the sugar (Figure 2.4b) by an N-glycosylase (Breimer and Lindahl, 1980) prior to the induction of a ssb by an endonuclease (Gates and Linn, 1977). The ssb thus enzymatically induced would then presumably be repaired in the same way as a frank ssb. The slower repair kinetics for base damage may thus reflect the additional steps required to complete the repair.

As mentioned above, the work of Patil et al. (1985) shows that the distribution of base damage in DNA is non-random and that transcribing DNA may be more heavily damaged than non-transcribing regions of the genome although the rate of repair in the transcribing regions may be more rapid than in non-transcribing DNA.

2.3.3 Repair of double-strand breaks

As mentioned above, the dsb is probably the most important lesion induced in irradiated cells, but we probably know least about its mode of repair. As outlined above, the kinetics of dsb repair reported are controversial, although the only absolute method (neutral velocity sedimentation) shows that the dsb are repaired with a half-time of 1.5–4 hours (Bryant and Blöcher, 1980; Blöcher and Pohlit, 1982). This slow repair indicates a more complex mechanism. The repair of dsb in yeast is dependent on the *RAD* 52 gene which also facilitates recombination. A connection has been made between these two processes and a model for repair of dsb based on recombination has been proposed (Resnick, 1976). On this model a dsb (where sequence information is lost at the site) can be repaired by using the corresponding specific sequence on the homologous (undamaged) chromosome. Evidence supporting this model is that recombination negative (rec⁻) strains of bacteria (Krasin and Hutchinson, 1977) and RAD 52 strains of yeast (Ho, 1975) are deficient in the repair of dsb. Haploid wild-type RAD 52 yeast in the G_1 phase of the cell cycle are also observed to be dsb-repair negative (Brunborg et al., 1980) as are WT bacteria when only one copy of the genome is present (Krasin and Hutchinson, 1977).

In mammalian cells, assuming this model applies, it is possible that non-homologous chromosomes may be used providing that local homology exists, since even highly aneuploid cells (e.g. immortalised Chinese hamster ovary cells) where no pairs of homologous chromosomes exist, are well able to repair dsb. The evidence for recombinational repair in mammalian cells is circumstantial. Recombinational intermediates (hybrid regions of the DNA, indicating pairing of DNA strands) has been observed (Moore and Holliday, 1976; Fonck et al., 1984). Also extracts of Chinese hamster cells have been shown to induce recombination between cut plasmid (pSV2Neo) fragments in a cell-free system (Moore et al., 1986).

We know that the repair of dsb involves DNA synthesis, since at high concentrations of the nucleoside analogue 9-β-D-arabinofuranosyladenine (ara A) repair of dsb is completely inhibited (Bryant and Blöcher, 1982). This indicates that a polymerisation step is involved so that a simple blunt-end ligation mechanism (Weibezahn and Coquerelle, 1981) cannot be operative.

Several radiosensitive genetic mutants of Chinese hamster cells called 'xrs' (X-ray sensitive) have been isolated (Jeggo et al., 1983) which are apparently dsb-repair negative (Kemp et al., 1984; Costa and Bryant, 1988). The function of the xrs gene product has not yet been identified although in vitro recombinant DNA experiments (see above) have indicated an absence of recombinational activity in the extracts from xrs cells (Moore et al., 1986).

2.4 Biological consequences of DNA damage and misrepair

2.4.1 The role of double-strand breaks

Evidence suggests that ssb and base damage are not critical lesions for cellular and genetic damage, possibly because of very efficient and accurate repair of these lesions where homology on the strand opposite the break of base-damaged lesion is always present. Certain lines of ataxia-telangiectasia cells deficient in base-damage repair appear to have a similar radiation sensitivity to those in which repair of base damage is present (Van der Schans, 1980). Dsb are, however, thought to be a critical lesion leading to cellular and genetic damage. It has been shown that dsb can lead to the induction of chromosomal aberrations (Natarajan et al., 1980; Bryant, 1984a), mutation (Obe et al., 1986) and cell death (Bryant, 1985). These end-points may

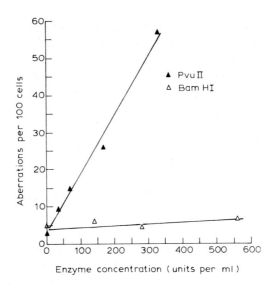

Figure 2.5. Chromosome aberration frequency as a function of either *Pvu*II (inducing blunt-ended double-strand breaks) or *Bam*HI (inducing cohesive-ended double-strand breaks). (Redrawn from Bryant, 1984a).

be related in that mutations and cell death may both be caused by the presence of chromosomal aberrations (Joshi et al., 1981; Bryant, 1984b; Thacker, 1986).

2.4.2 Induction of chromosomal aberrations by restriction endonuclease dsb

Treatment of permeabilised Chinese hamster cells with restriction enzymes (which cut DNA at specific base sequences leading to dsb with either 'blunt' or 'cohesive' ends) has been shown (Bryant, 1984a) to induce chromosomal aberrations. As illustrated in Figure 2.5, it was also shown that dsb with cohesive ends overlapping by four bases (e.g. *Bam*HI which cuts at the specific sequence: GG'ATCC) were much less effective in causing aberrations than dsb with blunt ends (e.g. *Pvu*II which cuts at the specific sequence: CAG'CTG).

2.4.3 The relationship between dsb and chromosomal aberrations in irradiated cells

Natarajan and his co-workers (Natarajan et al., 1980) showed that when the frequency of dsb was increased in irradiated and permeabilised cells by treatment with the endonuclease from the fungus *Neurospora crassa* (some of the ssb are converted to dsb by this treatment) both the frequency of dsb and the frequency of induced chromosomal aberrations approximately doubled. Chromosome deletions or fragments may represent unrepaired dsb and a technique involving the premature condensation of chromosomes by fusion of an interphase (test) cell with a blocked mitotic cell

(Premature Chromosome Condensation, PCC) shows that the frequency of PCC fragments present soon after irradiation (in practice 0.5–1 hour, since this is the minimum time for condensation to take place) decreases with time between irradiation and fixing the cells. The half-time for rejoining was found to be very similar to that for the repair of dsb (Cornforth and Bedford, 1983).

Chromosomal aberrations of the 'exchange' type (involving illegitimate joining between two chromosomes) also result from dsb (Bryant, 1984a). Those exchanges which result in translocation could in somatic cells act as initiating events in oncogenic transformation (Klein and Klein, 1984; Rowley, 1980).

2.4.4 Possible consequences of misrepair of dsb in ataxia-telangiectasia cells

The human autosomal recessive condition ataxia-telangiectasia (AT) shows a 2 to 3-fold increased intrinsic cellular radiosensitivity to ionising radiation (Section 3.2.1). AT cells also show higher than normal levels of chromosomal aberrations and in particular high numbers of breaks or deletions in the G_2 phase of the cell cycle, which can result from irradiation of cells in the G_1 phase of the cycle (Taylor, 1978; Parshad et al., 1985). However, the repair of dsb in these cells appears normal (Lehmann and Stevens, 1977). Recent work using recombinant DNA methods (Cox et al., 1984, 1986; Debenham et al., 1987) has shown that AT cells may suffer from a higher degree of molecular misrepair of dsb than normal cells. This was shown by a technique in which a restriction endonuclease dsb was induced into a plasmid vector carrying a dominant selectable genetic marker: the bacterial guanine phosphoribosyltransferase (GPT) gene which is not present in mammalian cells. The dsb was induced either in the coding frame for GPT or outside in some non-essential sequence, and the plasmid transfected into either normal human or AT cells. It was found that when the dsb was made outside the GPT coding frame, AT cells were just as able as normal cells to join the dsb. However, when the survival of the cells in selective medium depended on correct repair of the GPT coding sequence, AT cells were found to be deficient in correct repair of this dsb. This result for AT cells was interpreted as an imbalance between the exonuclease cleaning of the ends of dsb (resulting in loss of vital sequence) and the rejoining of the dsb. In AT cells the exonuclease trimming occurred at a faster rate than the rejoining step, resulting in severe loss of base sequence.

It is not yet known what contribution this type of misjoining and the occurrence of high levels of chromosomal aberrations make to the overall increased sensitivity of AT cells, or whether there is a link between these two apparent defects.

2.5 Conclusions

Ionising radiation induces a variety of types of damage in the DNA of cells (ssb, dsb, base damage, cross-links) amongst which dsb are thought to be the most significant. Dsb may exert their effect via the intermediate step of sequence deletion or misrepair, leading to chromosomal aberrations of the deletion or exchange types. Current research is aimed at understanding both the modes of repair and misrepair of dsb and their relationship to the cellular and genetic end-points described above.

References

Ahnström, G. and Bryant, P.E. (1982) DNA double-strand breaks generated by the repair of X-ray damage in Chinese hamster cells. Int. J. Radiat. Biol. 41, 671–676.
Baverstock, K.F. (1985) Abnormal distribution of double-strand breaks in DNA after direct action of ionising radiation. Int. J. Radiat. Biol. 47, 369–374.
Blöcher, D. (1982) DNA double-strand breaks in Ehrlich ascites tumour cells at low doses of X-rays. I. Determination of induced breaks by centrifugation at low speed. Int. J. Radiat. Biol. 42, 317–328.
Blöcher, D. and Pohlit, W. (1982) DNA double-strand breaks in Ehrlich ascites tumour cells at low doses of X-rays. II. Can cell death be attributed to double-strand breaks? Int. J. Radiat. Biol. 42, 329–338.
Bohne, L., Coquerelle, T. and Hagen, U. (1970) Radiation sensitivity of bacteriophage DNA. II. Breaks and cross-links after irradiation in vivo. Int. J. Radiat. Biol. 17, 205–215.
Bradley, M.O. and Kohn, K.W. (1979) X-ray induced double-strand breaks produced and repaired in mammalian cells as measured by neutral elution. Nucl. Acids Res. 7, 793–804.
Breimer, L. and Lindahl, T. (1980) A DNA-glycosylase from *E. coli* that releases free urea from a polydeoxyribonucleotide-containing fragment of base residues. Nucl. Acids Res. 8, 6199–6205.
Brunborg, G., Resnick, M.A. and Williamson, D.H. (1980) Cell-cycle specific repair of DNA double-strand breaks in *Saccharomyces cerevisiae*. Radiat. Res. 82, 547–558.
Bryant, P.E. (1984a) Enzymatic restriction of mammalian cell DNA using *Pvu*II and *Bam*H1: evidence for the double-strand break origin of chromosomal aberrations. Int. J. Radiat. Biol. 46, 52–65.
Bryant, P.E. (1984b) Effect of ara A and fresh medium on chromosome damage and DNA double-strand break repair in X-irradiated stationary cells. Brit. J. Radiol. 49 (Suppl. VI), 61–65.
Bryant, P.E. (1985) Enzymatic restriction of mammalian cell DNA: evidence for double-strand breaks as potentially lethal lesions. Int. J. Radiat. Biol. 48, 55–60.
Bryant, P.E. and Blöcher, D. (1980) Measurement of the kinetics of DNA double-strand break repair in Ehrlich ascites tumour cells using the unwinding method. Int. J. Radiat. Biol. 38, 335–347.
Bryant, P.E. and Blöcher, D. (1982) The effects of 9-β-D-arabinofuranosyladenine on the repair of DNA strand breaks in Ehrlich ascites tumour cells. Int. J. Radiat. Biol. 42, 385–394.
Bryant, P.E., Warring, R. and Ahnström, G. (1984) DNA repair kinetics after low doses of X-rays: a comparison of results obtained with the unwinding and nucleoid sedimentation methods. Mutat. Res. 131, 19–26.
Cerutti, P.A. (1974) Effects of ionising radiation on mammalian cells. Naturwissenschaften 61, 51–59.
Chiu, S.M. and Oleinick, N.L. (1982) Sensitivity of active and inactive chromatin to ionising radiation-induced DNA strand breakage. Int. J. Radiat. Biol. 41, 71–77.
Cornforth, M.N. and Bedford, J.S. (1983) X-ray induced breakage and rejoining of human interphase chromosomes. Sciences 222, 1141–1143.
Costa, N. and Bryant, P.E. (1988) Repair of DNA single-strand and double-strand breaks in the Chinese hamster xrs 5 mutant cell line as determined by DNA unwinding. Mutat. Res. DNA Repair Rep. 194, 93–99.
Cox, R., Masson, W.K., Debenham, P.G. and Webb, M.B.T. (1984) The use of recombinant plasmids

for the detection of DNA repair and recombination in cultured mammalian cells. Brit. J. Radiol. 49 (Suppl. VI), 67–72.
Cox, R., Debenham, P.G., Masson, W.K. and Webb, M.B.T. (1986) Ataxia-telangiectasia: a mutation giving a high frequency of misrepair of DNA double-strand scissions. Mol. Biol. Med. 3, 229–244.
Debenham, P.G., Webb, M.B.T., Jones, N.J. and Cox, R. (1987) Molecular studies on the nature of the repair defect in ataxia-telangiectasia and their implications for cellular radiobiology. J. Cell Sci. (Suppl. 6), 177–189.
Fonck, K., Barthel, R. and Bryant, P.E. (1984) Kinetics of recombinational hybrid formation in X-irradiated mammalian cells: a possible first step in the repair of DNA double-strand breaks. Mutat. Res. 132, 113–118.
Fox, M. and Fox, B.W. (1973) Repair replication in X-irradiated lymphoma cells in vitro. Int. J. Radiat. Biol. 23, 333–338.
Gates, F.T., II and Linn, S. (1977) Endonuclease from *E. coli* that acts specifically upon duplex DNA damaged by ultraviolet light, osmium tetroxide or X-rays. J. Biol. Chem. 252, 2802–2807.
Ho, K. (1985) Induction of DNA double-strand breaks by X-rays in a radioresistant strain of the yeast *Saccharomyces cerevisiae*. Mutat. Res. 30, 327–334.
Jeggo, P.A., Kemp, L.M. and Holliday, R. (1983) The application of the microbial tooth-pick techniques to somatic cell genetics and its use in the isolation of X-ray sensitive mutants of Chinese hamster ovary cells. Biochemie 64, 713–715.
Joshi, G.P., Nelson, W.J., Revell, S.H. and Shaw, C.A. (1981) X-ray-induced chromosome damage in live mammalian cells, and improved measurement of its effect on their colony forming ability. Int. J. Radiat. Biol. 41, 161–181.
Kemp, L.M., Sedgewick, S.G. and Jeggo, P.A. (1984) X-ray sensitive mutants of Chinese hamster ovary cells defective in double-strand break rejoining. Mutat. Res. 132, 189–196.
Klein, G. and Klein, E. (1984) Oncogene activation and tumour progression. Carcinogenesis 5, 429–435.
Korner, I.J., Geunter, K. and Malz, W. (1978) Kinetics of single-strand break rejoining in X-ray and neutron-irradiated Chinese hamster cells. Stud. Biophys. 70, 175–182.
Kohn, K.W., Ewig, R.A.G., Erickson, L.C. and Zwelling, L.A. (1981) Measurement of strand breaks and cross-links by alkaline elution, in DNA Repair: A Laboratory Manual of Research Procedures (Friedberg, E.C. and Hanawalt, P.C., eds.) Vol. 1B, pp. 379–401, Marcel Dekker, New York.
Krasin, F. and Hutchinson, F. (1977) Repair of DNA double-strand breaks in *Escherichia coli* which require *rec* A function in the presence of a duplicate genome. J. Mol. Biol. 116, 81–98.
Lehmann, A.R. and Stevens, S. (1977) The production and repair of double-strand breaks in cells from normal humans and from patients with ataxia-telangiectasia. Biochim. Biophys. Acta 474, 49–60.
Lett, J.J., Stacey, K.A. and Alexander, P. (1961) Cross-linking of dry DNA by electrons. Radiat. Res. 14, 349–362.
Lohman, P.H.M. (1968) Induction and rejoining of breaks in the DNA of human cells irradiated at various phases of the cell cycle. Mutat. Res. 6, 449–458.
McGrath, R.A. and Williams, R.W. (1966) Reconstruction in vivo of irradiated *E. coli* DNA: the rejoining of broken pieces. Nature 212, 53 4–535.
Magana-Schwenke, N., Henriques, J.-A.P., Chanet, R. and Moustacchi, E. (1982) The fate of 8-methoxypsoralen photo-induced cross-links in nuclear and mitochondrial DNA: comparison of wild-type and repair-deficient strains. Proc. Natl. Acad. Sci. USA 79, 1722–1726.
Moore, P.D. and Holliday, R. (1976) Evidence for the formation of hybrid DNA during mitotic recombination in Chinese hamster cells. Cell. 8, 573–579.
Moore, P.D., Song, K.Y., Chekuri, L., Wallace, L. and Kucherlapati, R.S. (1986) Homologous recombination in a Chinese hamster X-ray sensitive mutant. Mutat. Res. 160, 149–155.
Natarajan, A.T., Obe, G., Van Zeeland, A.A., Palitti, F., Meijers, M. and Verdegaal-Immerzeel, E.A.M. (1980) Molecular mechanisms involved in the production of chromosomal aberrations. II. Utilization

of neurospora endonuclease for the study of aberration production by X-rays in G_1 and G_2 stages of the cell cycle. Mutat. Res. 69, 293–305.

Obe, G., Von der Hude, W., Scheutwinkel-Reich, M. and Baseler, A. (1986) The restriction endonuclease AluI induces chromosomal aberrations and mutations in the hypoxanthine phosphoribosyltransferase locus but not in the Na^+/K^+-ATPase locus in V79 hamster cells. Mutat. Res. 174, 71–74.

Okayasu, R., Blöcher, D. and Iliakis, G. (1988) Variation through the cell cycle of DNA neutral filter elution dose-response in X-irradiated synchronous Chinese hamster ovary cells. Int. J. Radiat. Biol. 53, 729–748.

Painter, R.B. and Young, B.R. (1972) Repair replication in mammalian cells after X-irradiation. Mutat. Res. 14, 225–235.

Parshad, R., Sanford, K.K., Jones, G.M. and Tarone, R.E. (1985) G_2 chromosomal radiosensitivity of ataxia-telangiectasia heterozygotes. Cancer Genet. Cytogenet. 14, 163–168.

Paterson, M.C. (1976) Use of purified lesion recognising enzymes to monitor DNA repair in vivo. Adv. Radiat. Biol. 7, 1–53.

Patil, M.S., Locher, S.E. and Harihan, P.V. (1985) Radiation-induced thymine base damage and its excision-repair in inactive and inactive chromatin of HeLa cells. Int. J. Radiat. Biol. 48, 691–700.

Radford, I.R. (1987) Use of nuclear monolayers to identify factors influencing DNA double-strand breakage by X-rays. Int. J. Radiat. Biol. 52, 853–858.

Resnick, M.A. (1976) The repair of double-strand breaks in DNA: a model involving recombination. J. Theoret. Biol. 59, 97–106.

Rowley, J.D. (1980) Chromosome abnormalities in cancer. Cancer Genet. Cytogenet. 2, 175–198.

Taylor, A.M.R. (1978) Unrepaired DNA strand breaks in irradiated ataxia telangiectasia lymphocytes suggested from cytogenetic observations. Mutat. Res. 50, 407–418.

Thacker, J. (1986) The use of recombinant DNA technology to study radiation-induced damage and genetic change in mammalian cells. Int. J. Radiat. Biol. 50, 1–30.

Van der Schans, G.P., Centen, H.B. and Lohman, P.H.M. (1980) Studies on the repair defects of ataxia-telangiectasia cells, in: Proceedings of NATO Advanced Study Institute. (Seeburg, E. and Kleppe, K.K., eds.) June 1980, Bergen, Norway.

Weibezahn, K.F. and Coquerelle, T. (1981) Radiation-induced DNA double-strand breaks are rejoined by ligation and recombinational processes. Nucl. Acids Res. 9, 3139–3150.

CHAPTER 3

The molecular basis of radiosensitivity

TREVOR J. McMILLAN

Radiotherapy Research Unit, The Institute of Cancer Research, Cotswold Road, Sutton, Surrey SM2 5PT, England

3.1 Introduction 30

3.2 Cells with extreme sensitivity or resistance to ionising radiation 30
    3.2.1 Inherited diseases 30
    3.2.2 Variation among tumour and normal tissue cells 31
    3.2.3 Laboratory-derived variants 32
    3.2.4 Biological modification of sensitivity 32

3.3 Parallel alterations in sensitivity to other cytotoxic agents 33

3.4 The amount of damage induced 34
    3.4.1 The induction of damage in DNA 34
    3.4.2 Cellular thiols 34

3.5 The role of repair 35
    3.5.1 Cellular studies of recovery 35
    3.5.2 Repair of specific lesions 37

3.6 Molecular features which may affect the induction and processing of radiation-induced damage . 38
    3.6.1 Chromatin structure 38
    3.6.2 Membrane structure 39
    3.6.3 Topoisomerase type II 39
    3.6.4 Precursor pools 40

3.7 The search for the genes 40
    3.7.1 The number of genes 40
    3.7.2 Specific known genes 40
    3.7.3 Random searches 41

3.8 Conclusions 41

3.1 Introduction

The previous chapter dealt with the DNA damage induced by ionising radiation. We now turn to consider how the initial damage is processed within the cell. The current view of radiobiology (Chapter 12) is that human tumour cells differ in their inherent sensitivity to ionising radiation and the extent of these differences seems large enough to be a significant determinant of the success of radiotherapy. What molecular processes underlie these differences in radiosensitivity?

3.2 Cells with extreme sensitivity or resistance to ionising radiation

The search for the molecular basis of radiosensitivity depends critically on the availability of cell systems with defined and very different sensitivity. These have become available in the following ways:

3.2.1 Inherited diseases

Among the most widely used cells for radiation sensitivity studies are those derived from people with diseases or syndromes that make them inherently more sensitive than normal to radiation. The list of such syndromes is large and increasing (Table 3.1). Best-known and most extensively studied is ataxia-telangiectasia (AT, for overview see Bridges and Harnden, 1982).

AT is an autosomal recessive syndrome which presents clinically as oculocutaneous telangiectasia and progressive cerebellar ataxia. In addition immunodeficiency, high levels of serum α-foetoprotein and high frequency of neoplasia are associated features. The peculiarity of the radiation response of AT patients became evident when they suffered an excessive degree of normal tissue reaction following radiotherapy (Gotoff et al., 1967). Subsequently, lymphocytes and fibroblasts from these patients when assessed in vitro have demonstrated a marked hypersensitivity to ionising radiation (Figure 3.1A). Clonogenic assays on fibroblasts produce survival curves with D_o in the

TABLE 3.1
Human syndromes which can exhibit radiosensitivity

Ataxia-telangiectasia	Bridges and Harnden, 1982
Huntington's chorea	Arlett, 1979
Nijmegen Breakage syndrome	Taalman et al., 1983
Inherited retinoblastoma	Arlett, 1979
Homocystinuria	Sinelshichikova et al., 1987
Fanconi's anaemia	Arlett, 1979
Cockayne's syndrome	Deschavanne et al., 1984
Gardner's syndrome	Little et al., 1980

range 0.35–0.6 Gy for AT patients compared with 1.0 to 1.6 Gy for normal subjects (Cox, 1982; Lehmann, 1982).

3.2.2 Variation among tumour and normal tissue cells

Normal tissues vary widely in their sensitivity to radiation (Chapter 7). The magnitude and speed of development of radiation damage is largely related to the tissue organization but some variation in cellular radiosensitivity has been observed in cell lines removed from normal tissues (Potten and Hendry, 1987; Figure 3.1B). It could be that in the normal process of cellular differentiation the expression of genes that affect cellular sensitivity is altered.

Tumour cells from different tissues of origin can vary considerably in their in vitro sensitivity (Figure 3.1C) in a way that is consistent with the radiocurability of the

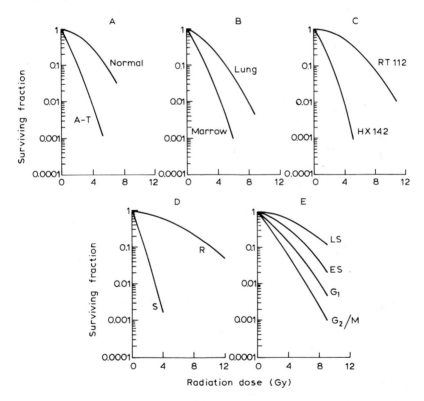

Figure 3.1. Representative cell-survival curves for various cell types which are useful in investigations of the molecular basis of radiosensitivity. (A) Ataxia-telangiectasia and normal human fibroblasts. (B) Murine lung and bone marrow cells. (C) Human neuroblastoma (HX142) and bladder carcinoma cells (RT112). (D) Murine L5178 Y lymphoma cells: the sensitive parent and a resistant subline. (E) Cell survival in different phases of the cell cycle. (See text for references.)

tumour types in the clinic (see Chapter 12). Thus, cell lines from human tumours can also provide a source of material for mechanistic studies.

3.2.3 Laboratory-derived variants

The isolation of radio-resistant variants from mammalian cell lines has rarely been achieved, in contrast to the situation with drugs where it is comparatively easy to select chemo-resistant variants. Quite drastic radiation treatment has usually been required. Rhynas and Newcombe (1960) gave repeated high-dose treatment (10 or 20 Gy) to obtain resistance in murine fibroblasts. Courtenay (1969) treated the L5178Y murine lymphoma continuously for 50–100 days by incorporating tritium in the culture medium and eventually a number of resistant sublines grew out (Figure 3.1D). Some of these had an increased D_o, others an increased extrapolation number. There are also a few reports of clonal variation in radiosensitivity within a particular tumour (Brouwer et al., 1983; Leith et al., 1982; Welch et al., 1983) but where this does occur the differences appear to be relatively small.

In an early study Dittrich et al. (1956) noted a reduction in radiosensitivity in a line of Ehrlich carcinoma treated in vivo with X-rays in a number of consecutive passages. Subsequent studies by other investigators, including some in which radiation was given continuously for many months (Conger and Luippold, 1957; Peacock and Shipley, unpublished data) have not confirmed the development of radioresistance. The difficulty of inducing radioresistance in the laboratory suggests that this is unlikely to be a significant problem in the clinical setting.

Resistant variants have consequently been fairly limited in their usefulness as far as mechanistic studies are concerned. Investigators have therefore turned to hypersensitive variants. Many sensitive variants have been produced in various mammalian cell systems during the last few years and these have been well summarised by Collins and Johnson (1987). Two of the most widely used are those that were derived in the L5178Y murine lymphoma by Beer et al. (1963), and more recently those by Jeggo and Kemp (1983) in Chinese hamster ovary cells (CHO). An analysis of 9000 clones was required in CHO cells in order to obtain 12 X-ray sensitive mutants, 6 of which were appreciably more sensitive than the parent line (Jeggo and Kemp, 1983). These clones have been called xrs mutants and they have been widely studied. Two of the lines in particular, xrs-5 and xrs-6, are highly sensitive with apparently exponential survival curves and a surviving fraction at 2 Gy of less than 0.01, compared with over 0.95 in the parent line.

3.2.4 Biological modification of sensitivity

An alternative to using different cell lines or sublines is to utilize the fact that the radiosensitivity of cells can vary through the cell cycle (Terasima and Tolmach, 1963).

Cells in G_2 and mitosis usually give steep and almost shoulderless survival curves. This is shown by the classic studies of Sinclair (1968) on Chinese hamster cells (shown schematically in Figure 3.1E). Although these observations have been repeated on a few other cell lines, the amount of information of this type is not large, especially on cells of human origin. An essential objective of the molecular approach to radiobiology is to explain the cell-cycle variations.

3.3 Parallel alterations in sensitivity to other cytotoxic agents

There are important mechanistic implications in studies of the profile of resistance or sensitivity with other cytotoxic agents.

The search for parallel sensitivities to UV and ionising radiation has been quite exhaustive, largely because the nature of induced lesions and the mechanisms of repair after UV are better understood. Unfortunately few such general parallels have been found. In AT cell lines, no general hypersensitivity to UV has been observed (Paterson and Smith, 1981; Lehmann et al., 1977). A sensitive mutant of L5178Y showed an increased resistance to UV, as also did a resistant subline (Beer et al., 1983; McMillan, unpublished data). Most of the CHO xrs mutants do show an increased sensitivity to UV light, but the effect is quite small and certainly not to the same extent as the change in X-ray sensitivity (Jeggo and Kemp, 1983).

The most common cytotoxic drug that shows increased sensitivity in radiosensitive cells is bleomycin (Jeggo and Kemp, 1983). In addition, cells selected for their sensitivity to bleomycin are also often sensitive to ionising radiation (Stamato et al., 1987). This is an agent which induces single- and double-strand breaks in DNA in a similar way to ionising radiation. AT cells show an increased sensitivity to novobiocin and VP16 (Debenham et al., 1987; Henner and Blazka, 1986) both of which are influenced by the level of topoisomerase II. It could be, therefore, that differences in topoisomerase II may be involved in the AT phenotype. Other drugs, such as actinomycin D and mitomycin C have been found to be more effective against AT cells and the CHO xrs mutants but these findings are not universal. Ethylmethane sulphonate (EMS) is another agent to which some of the CHO xrs mutants have increased sensitivity.

Overall, these studies of sensitivity to other cytotoxic agents support the view that hypersensitivity may be the result of several possible alterations. The processing of DNA strand breaks is likely to be an important determinant of radiosensitivity due to the fact that bleomycin sensitivity often parallels X-ray sensitivity. The excision repair processes that predominate for UV probably have a minor role in the case of ionising radiation.

3.4 The amount of damage induced

Ionising radiation induces a wide variety of lesions in DNA: base damage, single and double-strand breaks, multiple lesions, etc. One of the fundamental problems in radiobiology is to identify the relative roles of such lesions in radiation cell killing. Studies in lower organisms, especially yeast, suggest that a double-strand break (dsb) can be lethal, hence many studies in mammalian cells have also concentrated on this lesion (Chapter 2).

3.4.1 The induction of damage in DNA

It has been suggested by some authors that the level of damage induced in DNA by radiation (rather than its repair) is the primary determinant of radiosensitivity. Central to this argument are measurements of dsb using the neutral filter elution technique (Bradley and Kohn, 1979) in which the extent and rate of passage of double-stranded DNA through a filter at relatively neutral pH is taken as an indicator of the number of dsb present. In a series of recent studies Radford (1986a,b) has shown that the level of dsb induced by radiation correlated well with radiosensitivity under a variety of radiomodifying conditions, in different phases of the cell cycle and in different cell lines. In addition, we have produced data in a series of human tumour cells which show that although the level of induced damage is not the same in all cell lines, in broad terms the more sensitive cells do have higher levels of induced damage than resistant cells (unpublished data). Wlodek and Hittelman (1987) also demonstrated a difference in induction of dsb in two lines of the L5178Y murine lymphoma which differed in their radiosensitivity.

The idea that it is the level of initial damage that determines radiosensitivity has met with much opposition from those who believe it is the processing of such damage that is important. It has been argued that the curvi-linear dose response curves for neutral filter elution, which are a feature of the studies above, could be an artifact of this technique. Other measures of DNA strand breakage such as sucrose sedimentation do not seem to produce this sort of pattern, and since these measure damage at much lower doses than neutral elution they are thought by some to be more comparable with cell survival studies. Cases where no difference in induction of damage (dsb and other) has been observed include the CHO-xrs5 (Iliakis et al., 1988), and AT cells (Cornforth and Bedford, 1985).

3.4.2 Cellular thiols

One possible mechanism by which the amount of damage might be modified is by the neutralization of free radicals before they produce irreversible damage. Cellular thiols play an important role in this process.

It has been well established that compounds such as buthionine sulphoximine (BSO) which deplete thiols, in particular glutathione, can increase the cell kill caused by radiation; also the addition of sulphydryl compounds such as cysteamine can protect cells from the induction of damage and the killing of cells by radiation (Radford, 1986b). It has, however, been more difficult to establish whether different inherent levels of thiols are responsible for differences in radiosensitivity. While there are several candidate molecules, most studies have concentrated on glutathione and related enzymes, but generally no correlations have been found with radiosensitivity. For example, Carmichael et al. (1988) found a wide range of total cell content of glutathione, glutathione reductase, and γ-glutamyl transpeptidase in a series of thirteen human colo-rectal cancer cell lines but no correlation with radiation sensitivity. Shea and Henner (1987) reported levels of GSH transferase activity ranging from 40 mU/mg protein in a carcinoid tumour of the lung to 1010 mU/mg for a malignant melanoma, again with no correlation. AT cells have been shown to be deficient in cysteine transport, which limits glutathione resynthesis after irradiation (Meredith and Dodson, 1987) but it is unclear how this relates to the radiosensitivity of AT cells.

3.5 The role of repair

To what extent are differences in radiation sensitivity the result of different repair capacities among mammalian cells? On the multi-target model of cell killing the sensitivity of cells to low radiation doses is greatly influenced by the shoulder on the cell survival curve, which is reconstituted after each radiation dose. The response to a series of dose fractions is thus very much determined by recovery.

It is essential at this point to define our terms carefully. 'Recovery' will be used for evidence for an increase in cell survival. 'Repair' will be used for the correction of damage in biologically important molecules. 'Rejoining' is the disappearance of DNA breaks. 'Misrepair' or 'fixation' is where the processing of lesions terminates with a product that differs from the original molecule.

3.5.1 Cellular studies of recovery

The ability of cells to recover from the effects of irradiation has been measured by allowing time for cells to recover between two doses of radiation (SLD recovery), by reducing the dose rate and thus allowing recovery during treatment, or by holding the cells in a resting state for a period of time after treatment (PLD recovery). While there are those who believe that these are different manifestations of the same process, Thacker and Stretch (1983) have separated recovery during low dose rate and that during a holding period in plateau phase on the basis of their influence on mutation frequency. Lowering the dose rate resulted in a decrease in mutation frequency while holding in plateau phase had no effect on mutation frequency. One interpretation of this could be that low dose-rate recovery reflects an error-free repair process, while potentially lethal damage repair is error-prone, but this requires further investigation.

The classical interpretations of recovery experiments have led to the suggestion that recovery (and by inference, repair) capacity is a major determinant of cellular sensitivity. AT cells, for example, have been demonstrated to be deficient in PLD recovery and they have a survival curve with little if any shoulder. This has been taken to indicate a low capacity for SLD recovery. However, a recent reanalysis of split-dose experiments on human tumour cells by Peacock et al. (1988) has shown that if the survival curve is continuously bending then split-dose recovery may be masked in steep survival curves (see Section 12.4.2). The inability to demonstrate SLD recovery in radiosensitive cells may in fact be a consequence of the large amount of damage that is non-recoverable. Paradoxically, the extent of SLD recovery is greatest in the most radiosensitive human tumour cell lines. It would therefore appear that although recovery deficient cells may exist, radiosensitive cells may still have a significant capacity for recovery of SLD.

The use of repair inhibitors demonstrates that by altering repair one can modify the response of cells to radiation. Altering the production of DNA precursors (e.g., with hydroxyurea), inhibiting DNA polymerases (e.g., with aphidicolin) or modifying

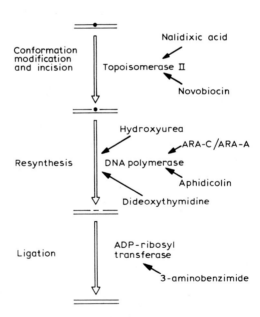

Figure 3.2. The inhibition of a simple excision repair pathway. Excision repair can be split into three steps with a number of enzymes involved at each stage. Inhibitors of enzymes known to be directly involved in this process can stop repair, as can agents which interfere with the production of precursors needed for resynthesis.

ligation (e.g., with 3-aminobenzamide) have led to successful inhibition of repair (Figure 3.2) and to modified radiation response in some cells. The inability of these compounds to affect all cells may be an indicator of the relative importance of the repair processes in different cells.

3.5.2 Repair of specific lesions

The insensitivity of detection techniques for DNA lesions is a limiting factor in studies of their repair. Neutral filter elution, for example, usually requires doses up to 30–100 Gy in order to measure damage in human cells. The fraction of cells that survive such a dose is very small, thus the DNA damage is being studied within cells that mostly will go on to die. In recent years this has been overcome by looking at the ability of cells to repair a piece of DNA which has been damaged prior to its incorporation into the cells. In the plasmid reactivation assay a specific lesion is placed within a drug resistance gene in a plasmid (a small, circular piece of DNA)

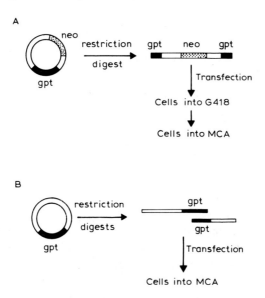

Figure 3.3. The use of plasmids in the study of DNA repair. (A) Plasmids containing two genes which confer drug resistance (*neo* and *gpt*) can be linearized by a specific cut, using a restriction endonuclease. If the cut is within the *gpt* gene this renders the gene inactive in cells into which it is transfected. Growth in the drug G418 selects for cells that have taken up the plasmid (i.e., contain the *neo* gene). Subsequent growth in mycophenolic acid (MCA) selects for cells that have been able to rejoin the two halves of the *gpt* gene to produce a functional unit. The relative proportion of cells growing in MCA gives an indication of the repair capacity of the cells. (B) Using appropriate restriction endonucleases, a plasmid containing *gpt* can be cut to give two independent fragments, neither with the complete gene but containing overlapping sequences. In order to produce an intact *gpt* gene, the cell, once transfected with the two fragments, has to perform a recombination process between the fragments. The ability to do this is assessed by growth in MCA.

and the ability of cells to repair that break is detected by the occurrence of drug-resistance following transfection of the plasmid into target cells (Figure 3.3). The big advantage of this technique is that it measures the fidelity of repair and not just the physical rejoining of the two ends of the DNA. This technique has been used in at least two studies using AT and normal fibroblasts. Both Cox et al. (1986) and Green and Lowe (1987) have demonstrated that the number of resistant colonies from transfection of cut plasmid can be lower in AT cells than normal cells. Cox et al. (1986) have shown that this is likely to be due to inaccurate break rejoining in AT cells, but Green and Lowe (1987) suggest that these two observations may not be directly related. Methodological problems seem to be at the centre of this discordance and thus need to be resolved.

In an extension of this technique, Hoy et al. (1987) used two sectors of the plasmid which were inactive by themselves but which contained a homologous region (Figure 3.3). A recombination process was required to restore gene function and the capacity to do this was found to be reduced in a radiosensitive mutant of CHO cells.

3.6 Molecular features which may affect the induction and processing of radiation-induced damage

In addition to the processes directly involved in the induction and repair of damage following irradiation there are features of cells which can indirectly alter these processes.

3.6.1 Chromatin structure

Within the cell, DNA takes up a complex multi-coiled structure in association with considerable amounts of protein. The compactness of the DNA varies throughout the genome and also through the intermitotic cycle. DNA conformation within the cell is a vital factor in its function and as such is likely to influence its response to radiation-induced damage. One of the first hints that this may be so came from the work of Philbrick (1976) who found that radiosensitivity increased as the cell volume per chromosome decreased, i.e., the tighter the chromatin packing the more sensitive were the cells. One possible explanation of this is that repair enzymes can gain better access to the less compact regions, usually the regions that are undergoing transcription. Indeed Mellon et al. (1987) have suggested that the transcribing strand of the DNA may be more repairable than its opposite DNA strand.

The structure of the DNA may also influence the nature of the induced damage, either by altering the proximity of sublesions within the chromatin or by influencing the interaction of DNA with other molecules. The interaction of lesions (not necessarily a physical interaction) is an important aspect of some models of radiation action. Oleinick et al. (1986) have shown that DNA-protein cross-links (DPC) are more abundant in transcribing regions of the DNA. While the importance of DPC in cell death is not clear, it is a further suggestion that chromatin structure might modify the effects of ionising radiation.

3.6.2 Membrane structure

While it is generally accepted that the main critical target for radiation within the cell is DNA there is also a body of experimental data that does not fit with the idea of a simple direct action on DNA itself. This evidence has been reviewed in detail by Alper (1979). It relates mainly to the observation that the oxygen-enhancement ratio for the irradiation of some bacteria depends on physiological factors in a way that is unlikely to be the case with DNA itself. Alper was led to postulate that free-radical damage causes two types of lesion: primary lesions in DNA ('N' lesions), and lesions that are responsible for sensitization by oxygen ('O' lesions). It is envisaged that type O lesions are associated with damage to cell membranes or with the points of attachment between DNA and the nuclear membrane. More recently Szumiel (1981) has argued that there may be an indirect influence of membrane damage on repair of DNA. Therefore, while it is unlikely that membrane damage is directly responsible for cell death following irradiation, its influence on other functions may be important.

3.6.3 Topoisomerase type II

Topoisomerase type II is an enzyme that has the ability to pass a DNA duplex through a second duplex by making and sealing a double-strand break. As such it has an essential function in controlling DNA conformation in a wide variety of species. Collins and Johnson (1979) demonstrated that novobiocin, which inhibits topoisomerase II appears to inhibit endonuclease recognition of UV-induced DNA damage. It has subsequently been proposed that this action may be due to a requirement for a topological change in the DNA, involving topoisomerase II, prior to the incision event (Collins et al., 1984; Figure 3.2), although the specificity of this effect is now in doubt (Downes et al., 1985).

The possibility that topoisomerase II might be influential in the determination of radiosensitivity is raised by the finding that AT cells can be hypersensitive to etoposide, an agent which exerts its cytotoxic effect via topoisomerase II (Henner and Blazka, 1986). It would appear, however, that the enzyme is not altered in these cells and there is no change in its activity so the mechanism underlying this sensitivity is not known. Debenham et al. (1987) have suggested that it may play a role in the continued DNA synthesis after irradiation which is a feature of AT cells, in contrast to normal cells which stop synthesis for a while after treatment (Painter, 1981). A defective interaction between topoisomerase II and the factor involved in its double-strand break repair activity would leave the topoisomerase II available for its role in unwinding DNA prior to synthesis. In normal cells, topoisomerase II interacts normally and is thus heavily involved in its double-strand break repair activity which reduces its availability for its role in DNA synthesis. Thus, in normal cells DNA synthesis is reduced after irradiation. As yet this scenario is purely theoretical, but it provides an interesting possibility for a factor involved in the determination of radiosensitivity.

3.6.4 Precursor pools

The levels of deoxyribonucleoside triphosphates (dNTP) in *E. coli* and lower eucaryotes have been shown to affect DNA repair and other closely related processes. The SOS response and mitotic recombination have both been shown to be altered by pool imbalances. In mammalian cell mutants with an altered pool balance the accuracy with which a DNA polymerase incorporates nucleosides during replication is reduced and this can lead to an increased rate of mutation (Meuth, 1984). These imbalances have been shown to alter the response to EMS but not to UV or ionizing radiation. However, Booth et al. (1987) have linked the radiation sensitivity of a series of cell lines with differences in the level of dNTPs and enzymes associated with their production either before or after irradiation. How common this association is remains to be determined.

3.7 The search for the genes

3.7.1 The number of genes

In view of the many factors involved in the determination of radiosensitivity it is likely that many genes are involved. An estimate can be obtained by complementation analysis in which two sensitive cells are fused together. If the resulting hybrid is also sensitive then this suggests that the two lines are deficient in the same gene. On the other hand, if the hybrid is resistant then the two lines have complemented each other, implying that at least two genes are involved. This has been done with a number of cell lines. In particular AT cells have been analysed in this way and have been separated into at least five complementation groups (McKinnon, 1987). Therefore, even in a phenotype which is relatively constant there are likely to be a number of genes involved.

3.7.2 Specific known genes

One way of identifying critical genes in the determination of radiosensitivity is by utilising genes that have been isolated in mammalian cells in a different context or which have been seen to be important in the radiosensitivity of lower organisms. To do this, known genes can either be inserted into mammalian cells to establish their effect on radiosensitivity or they can be used as probes for closely related genes in higher organisms. This approach has not received much attention in the study of ionising radiation, but the feasibility of such studies has been well shown in the work on UV sensitivity. For example, Bootsma et al. (1987) have shown that the *Rad10* gene in yeast hybridises with a sequence in *Drosophila* which in turn shows homology with a piece of DNA in human cells which can complement a UV repair defect in CHO cells. In this case, the yeast and human genes had been isolated independently, but they demonstrate the feasibility of using known genes from lower organisms to probe for human counterparts.

3.7.3 Random searches

While providing useful information, the technique just described does not give the opportunity for isolating totally new genes. For this, the more random approach of inserting new DNA into radiosensitive cells and selecting for radioresistance is required. This can be done in a number of ways, including the addition of whole chromosomes and by DNA transfection techniques.

This approach has to date been very limited in its success. One of the more promising reports is that from Spiro et al. (1986) who have reversed the sensitive phenotype of the EM9-CHO cells by transfection of human DNA into cells, and this was associated with an increased ability to repair DNA single-strand breaks. In a similar way Green et al. (1987) have published initial findings on a clone of AT cells which were transfected with DNA from normal human cells. This clone is radioresistant but interestingly still exhibits the abnormal synthesis response of AT cells (Lehmann et al., 1986). Studies such as these are likely to lead to the isolation of genes that are important in controlling radiosensitivity.

3.8 Conclusions

The fact that ionising radiation produces such a wide variety of lesions in cells means that elucidating the molecular processes which control the response of cells to irradiation is a difficult task. We can postulate that the cell might modify the amount of damage induced in its DNA by neutralising free radicals, and, indeed, this process can be manipulated artificially. Similarly, there is no doubt that cells can repair most of the damage that is induced by radiation and, again, cell kill can be altered by inhibiting these pathways. Unfortunately it has not been possible to relate any one of these functions consistently to radiosensitivity.

Perhaps we are expecting too much to imagine that a unified hypothesis to explain the response of all cells to ionising radiation can be established. All of the mechanisms mentioned here, and probably many more, may be important in different cells at different times. This is a relatively new field, and, in view of the power of the techniques available, it will be surprising if a much clearer picture does not emerge within the next decade.

References

Alper, T. (1979) Cellular Radiobiology. Cambridge University Press, Cambridge.
Arlett, C.F. (1979) Survival and mutation in gamma irradiated human cell strains from normal or cancer-prone individuals, in: Proceedings 6th International Congress of Radiation Research (Okada, S., Imamura, M., Terasima, T. and Yamaguchi, H., eds.), pp. 596–602, Japanese Association of Radiation Research, Tokyo.
Beer, J.Z., Lett, J.T. and Alexander, P. (1963) Influence of temperature and medium on the X-ray sensitivities of leukaemia cells in vitro. Nature 199, 193–194.
Beer, J.Z. et al. (1983) Loss of tumorigenicity with simultaneous changes in radiosensitivity and photosensitivity during in vitro growth of L5178Y murine lymphoma cells. Cancer Res. 43, 4736–4742.
Booth, J.D., Ockey, C.H. and Saffhill, R. (1987) The sizes of cellular deoxynucleoside 5-triphosphate pools in relation to sensitivity to electron irradiation, using sensitive and resistant cell lines. Carcinogenesis 8, 409–414.
Bootsma, D., Koken, M.H.M., Van Duin, M., Westerveld, A., Yasui, A., Prakash, S. and Hoeijmakers, J.H.J. (1987) Homology of mammalian, *Drosophila*, yeast and *E. coli* repair genes, in: Proceedings 8th International Congress of Radiation Research (Fielden, E.M., Fowler, J.F., Hendry, J.H. and Scott, D., eds.), pp. 412–417, Taylor and Francis, London.
Bradley, M.O. and Kohn, K.W. (1979) X-ray induced double-strand break production and repair in mammalian cells as measured by neutral filter elution. Nucleic Acids Res. 7, 793–804.
Bridges, B.A. and Harnden, D.G. (1982) Ataxia-Telangiectasia: A Molecular Link Between Cancer, Neuropathology and Immune Deficiency (Bridges, B.A. and Harnden, D.G., eds.), John Wiley, Chichester.
Brouwer, M., Smets, L.A. and Jongsma, A.P.M. (1983) Isolation and characterisation of subclones of L1210 murine leukemia with different sensitivities to various cytotoxic agents. Cancer Res. 43, 2884–2888.
Carmichael, J., Park, J.G., Degraff, W.G., Gamson, J., Gazdar, A.F. and Mitchell, J.B. (1988) Radiation sensitivity and study of glutathione and related enzymes in human colorectal cancer cell lines. Eur. J. Cancer Clin. Oncol. 24, 1219–1224.
Collins, A. and Johnson, R. (1979) Novobiocin; an inhibitor of the repair of UV-induced but not X-ray-induced damage in mammalian cells. Nucleic Acids Res. 7, 1311–1320.
Collins, A.R.S., Downes, C.S. and Johnson, R.T. (1984) Introduction: an integrated view of repair, in: DNA Repair and Its Inhibition (Collins, A., Downes, C.S. and Johnson, R.T., eds.), pp. 1–11, IRL Press, Oxford.
Collins, A. and Johnson, R.T. (1987) DNA repair mutants in higher eukaryotes. J. Cell Sci. (Suppl. 6), 61–82.
Conger, A.D. and Luippold, H.J. (1957) Studies on the mechanism of acquired radioresistance in cancer. Cancer Res. 17, 897–903.
Cornforth, M.N. and Bedford, J.S. (1985) On the nature of the defect in cells from individuals with ataxia-telangiectasia. Science 227, 1589–1591.
Courtenay, V.D. (1969) Radioresistant mutants of L5178Y cells. Radiat. Res. 38, 186–203.

Cox, R. (1982) A cellular description of the repair defect in ataxia-telangiectasia, *in*: Ataxia-Telangiectasia: A Molecular Link Between Cancer, Neuropathology and Immune Deficiency (Bridges, B.A. and Harnden, D.G., eds.), pp. 141–154, John Wiley, Chichester.

Cox, R., Debenham, P.G., Masson, W.K. and Webb, M.B.T. (1986) Ataxia-telangiectasia: a human mutation giving high-frequency misrepair of DNA double-stranded scissions. Mol. Biol. Med. 3, 229–244.

Debenham, P.G., Webb, M.B.T., Jones, N.J. and Cox, R. (1987) Molecular studies on the nature of the repair defect in ataxia-telangiectasia and their implications for cellular radiobiology. J. Cell Sci. (Suppl. 6), 177–189.

Deschavanne, P.J., Chavaudra, N., Fertil, B. and Malaise, E.P. (1984) Abnormal sensitivity of some Cockaynes syndrome cell strains to UV and γ-rays. Mutat. Res. 131, 61–70.

Dittrich, W., Hohne, G. and Schubert, G. (1956) Development of a radio-resistant strain of Ehrlich carcinoma in mice, *in*: Progress in Radiobiology (Mitchel, J.S., Holmes, B.E. and Smith, C.L., eds.), pp. 381–385, Oliver and Boyd, London.

Downes, C.S., Ord, M.J., Mullinger, A.M., Collins, A.R.S. and Johnson, R.T. (1985) Novobiocin inhibition of DNA excision repair may occur through effects on mitochondrial structure and ATP metabolism, not on repair topoisomerases. Carcinogenesis 6, 1343–1352.

Gotoff, S.P., Amirokri, E. and Liebrer, E.J. (1967) Ataxia-telangiectasia. Am. J. Dis. Child 114, 617–625.

Green, M.H.L. and Lowe, J.E. (1987) Failure to detect a DNA repair-related defect in the transfection of ataxia-telangiectasia by enzymatically restricted plasmid. Int. J. Radiat. Biol. 52, 437–446.

Green, M.H.L. et al. (1987) A γ-ray-resistant derivative of an ataxia-telangiectasia cell line obtained following DNA mediated gene transfer. J. Cell. Sci. (Suppl. 6), 127–137.

Henner, W.D. and Blazka, M.E. (1986) Hypersensitivity of cultured ataxia-telangiectasia cells to etoposide. J. Natl. Cancer Inst. 76, 1007–1011.

Hoy, C.A., James, J.C. and Thompson, L.H. (1987) Recombination and ligation of transfected DNA in CHO mutant EM9, which has high levels of sister chromatid exchange. Mol. Cell Biol. 7, 2007–2011.

Iliakis, G., Okayasu, R. and Seaner, R. (1988) Radiosensitive xrs-5 and parental CHO cells show identical DNA neutral filter elution dose-response: implications for a relationship between cell radiosensitivity and induction of DNA double-strand breaks. Int. J. Radiat. Biol. 54, 55–62.

Jeggo, P.A. and Kemp, L.M. (1983) X-ray sensitive mutants of Chinese hamster ovary cell line. Isolation and cross-sensitivity to other DNA-damaging agents. Mutat. Res. 112, 313–327.

Lehmann, A.R., Kirk-Bell, S., Arlett, C.F., Harcourt, S.A., De Weerd-Kastelelein, E.A., Keijzer, W. and Hall-Smith, P. (1977) Repair of ultraviolet-light damage in a variety of human fibroblast cell strains. Cancer Res. 37, 904–910.

Lehmann, A.R. (1982) The cellular and molecular response of ataxia-telangiectasia to DNA damage, *in*: Ataxia-Telangiectasia: A Molecular Link Between Cancer, Neuropathology and Immune Deficiency (Bridges, B.A. and Harnden, D.G., eds.), pp. 141–154, John Wiley, Chichester.

Lehmann, A.R., Arlett, C.F., Burke, J.F., Green, M.H.L., James, M.R. and Iowe, J.B. (1986) A derivative of an ataxia-telangiectasia (AT) cell line with normal radiosensitivity but AST-like inhibition of DNA synthesis. Int. J. Radiat. Biol. 49, 639–643.

Leith, J.T., Dexter, D.L., DeWyngaert, J.K., Zeman, E.M., Chu, M.Y., Calabresi, P. and Glicksman, A.S. (1982) Differential responses to X-irradiation of sub-populations of two heterogeneous human carcinoma in vitro. Cancer Res. 42, 2556–2561.

Little, J.B., Nove, J. and Weichselbaum, R.R. (1980) Abnormal sensitivity of diploid skin fibroblasts from a family with Gardners syndrome to the lethal effects of X-irradiation, ultra violet and mitomycin-C. Mutat. Res. 70, 241–250.

McKinnon, P.J. (1987) Ataxia-telangiectasia: an inherited disorder of ionizing-radiation sensitivity in man. Human Genet. 75, 197–208.

Mellon, I., Spivak, G. and Hanawatt, P.C. (1987) Selective removal of transcription-blocking DNA damage from the transcribed strand of the mammalian *DHFR* gene. Cell 51, 241–249.

Meredith, M.J. and Dodson, M.L. (1987) Impaired glutathione biosynthesis in cultured human ataxia-telangiectasia cells. Cancer Res. 47, 4576–4581.

Meuth, M. (1984) The Relevance of DNA Precursor Pools to Repair in DNA Repair and its Inhibition (Collins, A., Downes, C.S. and Johnson, R.T., eds.), pp. 217–229, IRL Press, Oxford.

Oleinick, N.L., Chiu, S.-M., Friedman, L.R., Xue, L.-Y. and Ramakrishnan, N. (1986) DNA-protein cross-links: new insights into their formation and repair in irradiated mammalian cells, in: Mechanisms of DNA Damage and Repair (Simic, M.G., Grossman, L. and Upton, A.C., eds.), pp. 181–192, Plenum Press, New York.

Painter, R.B. (1981) Radioresistant DNA synthesis: an intrinsic feature of ataxia-telangiectasia. Mutat. Res. 84, 183–190.

Peacock, J.H., Cassoni, A.M., McMillan, T.J. and Steel, G.G. (1988) Radiosensitive human tumour cell lines may not be recovery deficient. Int. J. Radiat. Biol. 54, 945–953.

Philbrick, D.A. (1976) Radiation-induced reproductive death as a function of mammalian cell ploidy. Lawrence Berkley Laboratory Reports IBI–4783.

Potten, C.S. and Hendry, J.H. (1985) Cell Clones. Manual of Mammalian Cell Techniques. Churchill Livingstone, Edinburgh.

Radford, I.R. (1985) The level of induced DNA double-strand breakage correlates with cell killing after X-irradiation. Int. J. Radiat. Biol. 48, 45–54.

Radford, I.R. (1986a) Evidence for a general relationship between the induced level of DNA double-strand breakage and cell killing after X-irradiation of mammalian cells. Int. J. Radiat. Biol. 49, 611–620.

Radford, I.R. (1986b) Effect of radiomodifying agents on the ratios of X-ray-induced lesions in cellular DNA: use in lethal lesion determination. Int. J. Radiat. Biol. 49, 621–637.

Rhynas, P.O.W. and Newcombe, H.B. (1960) A heritable change in radiation resistance of strain L mouse cells. Exp. Cell Res. 21, 326–331.

Shea, T.C. and Henner, W.D. (1987) Glutathione transferase II in human tumors, in: Glutathione S-Transferase and Carcinogenesis (Mantle, T.J., Pickett, C.B. and Haynes, J.D., eds.), Taylor and Francis, London.

Sinclair, W.K. (1968) Cyclic X-ray responses in mammalian cells in vitro. Radiat. Res. 33, 620–643.

Sinelshchikova, T.A., Lvova, G.N., Shoniya, N.N. and Zasukhina, G.D. (1987) Defective DNA excision repair in cells of patients with homocystinuria. Mutat. Res. 184, 265–270.

Smith, P. and Paterson, M.C. (1981) Abnormal responses to mid-ultraviolet light of cultured fibroblasts from patients with disorders featuring sunlight sensitivity. Cancer Res. 41, 511–518.

Spiro, I.J., Barrows, L.R., Kennedy, K.A. and Ling, C.C. (1986) Transfection of a human gene for the repair of X-ray and EMS-induced DNA damage. Radiat. Res. 108, 146–157.

Stamato, T.D., Peters, B., Patil, P., Denko, N., Weinstem, R. and Giaccia, A. (1987) Isolation and characterization of bleomycin-sensitive Chinese hamster ovary cells. Cancer Res. 47, 1588–1592.

Szumiel, I. (1981) Intrinsic radiosensitivity of proliferating mammalian cells. Adv. Radiat. Biol. 9, 281–317.

Taalman, R.D.F.M., Jaspers, N.G.J., Shenes, J.M.J.C., De Wit, J. and Hustine, T.W.J. (1983) Hypersensitivity to ionizing radiation, in vitro, in a new chromosomal breakage disorder, the Nijmegen Breakage Syndrome. Mutat. Res. 112, 23–32.

Terasima, T. and Tolmach, L.J. (1963) Variations in several responses of HeLa cells to X-irradiation during the division cycle. Biophys. J. 3, 11–33.

Thacker, J. and Stretch, A. (1983) Recovery from lethal and mutagenic damage during post-irradiation holding and low-dose-rate irradiations of cultured hamster cells. Radiat. Res. 96, 380–392.

Welch, D.R., Milas, L., Tomasovic, S.P. and Nicolson, G.L. (1983) Heterogeneous response and clonal drift of sensitivities metastatic 13762NF mammary adenocarcinoma clones to γ-radiation in vitro. Cancer Res. 43, 6–10.

Wlodek, D. and Hittelman, W.N. (1987) The repair of double-strand DNA breaks correlates with radiosensitivity of L5178Y-S and L5178Y-R cells. Radiat. Res. 112, 146–155.

G.G. Steel, G.A. Adams & A. Horwich (Eds.)
The Biological Basis of Radiotherapy, Second Edition
© 1989 Elsevier Science Publishers B.V. (Biomedical Division)

CHAPTER 4

Survival of clonogenic cells: cell-survival curves

G. GORDON STEEL

Radiotherapy Research Unit, The Institute of Cancer Research, Cotswold Road, Sutton, Surrey SM2 5NG, England

4.1	Cell survival	46
	4.1.1 Concept of clonogenic cells	46
	4.1.2 Basic idea of a clonogenic cell-survival assay	47
4.2	Models of cell survival	48
	4.2.1 The multitarget model	48
	4.2.2 The multitarget model with single-hit component	48
	4.2.3 The linear-quadratic model	49
	4.2.4 Repair saturation models	50
	4.2.5 The Lethal-Potentially Lethal (LPL) model	52
	4.2.6 The 'incomplete repair' model	53
	4.2.7 Overview of cell-survival models	54
4.3	The measurement of cell survival	54
	4.3.1 Assays for tumour-cell survival	54
	4.3.2 Assays for cell survival in normal tissues	55
	4.3.3 Cell survival following in vivo irradiation of tumours	55
4.4	Cell survival following chemotherapy	56
	4.4.1 Classification of cytotoxic agents	57
	4.4.2 Drug resistance	58
	4.4.3 Tumour-size dependence	58
4.5	Cell survival and gross response to treatment	59
	4.5.1 Duration of remission and tumour growth delay	59
	4.5.2 Local tumour control	60
	4.5.3 Cell survival and the failure of normal tissues	61

4.1 Cell survival

4.1.1 Concept of clonogenic cells

A tumour is a complex biological structure consisting not only of cells that are frankly neoplastic or malignant but also of a variety of types of normal non-neoplastic cell and descendents of malignant cells that have lost their proliferative capacity as the result of differentiation (see Chapter 6). Not all the cells in a tumour are therefore dangerous. We envisage that within the tumour there is a sub-group of neoplastic cells that have the capacity to produce a large family of descendents. These are the cells that have the ability to regrow the tumour if left intact at the end of treatment. We call these cells 'clonogenic', in other words, 'colony-producing' cells. It may be useful to draw a distinction between:

Clonogenic cells: Cells that under defined experimental circumstances have the ability to produce a colony of descendents (usually more than 50 cells).

Tumour stem cells: Cells that within the tumour, treated or untreated, can produce a large family of descendents.

It is widely assumed that these two concepts can be equated but it may be wise to keep them separate for the following reasons: making a cell suspension may destroy cellular interactions that are essential to stem-cell capacity; stem cells may be damaged during separation and thus fail to be clonogenic; the test environment may be worse (or conceivably better) than the in situ environment within the tumour.

At the present time it is usually impossible to detect colony-forming cells in situ within a tumour; we can only do this in defined environments in tissue-culture or in transplantation sites. Clonogenic cells are thus the cells that we study: we envisage that they may be similar to but perhaps not identical to the cells that have high proliferative capacity within the tumour.

A remarkable exception is the murine AT17 adenocarcinoma studied by Kummermehr (1985). After high doses of irradiation this tumour does not shrink rapidly and repopulation is found to occur in discrete foci. It is possible to count these, to calculate the number of repopulating clones per tumour, and thus to quantify in situ cell survival. By extrapolating survival up to the tumour control dose (i.e., the 'TCD_{50}') Kummermehr was able to calculate the average number of stem cells in an untreated tumour.

When a clonogenic cell proliferates to produce a colony of descendents it does so as shown in Figure 4.1. Every division gives two daughter cells, but some cells may die or disappear (A) and others may fail to divide (B and C). As a result of these retarding processes the colony may not grow at its ultimate rate, but provided it keeps

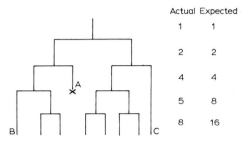

Figure 4.1. The expansion of a proliferating clone of cells by binary division may not take place at the full exponential rate. Some may die or disappear (A), others may fail to divide (B and C).

expanding and surpass the arbitrary limit of 50 cells (about six full generations of descendents) we would call it a viable clonogenic cell.

After treatment with radiation or cytotoxic drugs, some clonogenic cells fail to divide and subsequently die, others may produce a small number of descendents all of which die, and others again may produce an expanding colony of descendents but within which cell death and sterility (A, B and C) are commoner than normal. It is important therefore to distinguish between the death of a treated cell and impairment of its colony-forming ability. Tumour shrinkage requires cell death and resorption; tumour cure (i.e., the prevention of tumour regrowth), results from the abolition of colony-forming ability in all tumour stem cells.

4.1.2 Basic idea of a clonogenic cell-survival assay

We take a fixed number (say 100) untreated tumour cells and a fixed number (say 1000) identical tumour cells which have been irradiated. Both are plated out in tissue culture under conditions that give a high efficiency of colony formation. At the end of the period of incubation we might find an average of 10 colonies in each 'treated' dish and 30 in each 'control' dish. We then say:

$$\text{plating efficiency of untreated cells} = \frac{30}{100} = 0.3$$

$$\text{plating efficiency of treated cells} = \frac{10}{1000} = 0.01$$

Then the surviving fraction of clonogenic cells is given by:

$$S = \frac{PE_{\text{treated}}}{PE_{\text{control}}} = \frac{0.01}{0.30} = 0.033$$

This is the basic idea of a clonogenic cell-survival assay. A plot of surviving fraction (usually on a logarithmic scale) against dose yields a 'cell-survival curve'.

4.2. Models of cell survival

Many mathematical models have been described which aim to simulate actual cell-survival data. The underlying belief is that if such a model is successful, and if it is based upon plausible cellular mechanisms, then the modelling procedure may help us to understand radiation cell killing better. This approach has not been as successful as might be hoped. Some experimental data are best fitted by one model, others by a different model; the scatter of the data also often frustrates discrimination between models. As a result, there are a number of models that currently are of interest.

4.2.1 The multitarget model

An early idea in radiobiology was that the shoulder on cell-survival curves could be explained on the basis that each mammalian cell contains a fixed number of targets, all of which have to be inactivated before the reproductive integrity of the cell is abolished.

At low radiation doses some targets may be hit, but the likelihood of them all being inactivated will be low. At higher radiation doses most of the targets will be hit and the average number of intact targets per cell may be one or less; thereafter, cell survival will decrease steeply with increasing dose. This model therefore leads to a simple explanation of the shoulder on the cell-survival curve.

This 'single-hit multitarget model' leads to the following equation for the shape of the cell-survival curve:

$$S = 1 - (1 - e^{-D/D_o})^n \qquad \text{(Eqn. 4.1)}$$

Here D is the dose, n is the extrapolation number, and D_o is the dose required (on the exponential part of the curve) to reduce survival to e^{-1} (i.e., to 0.37). When $n = 1$, we have a simple exponential survival curve, linear on the semi-logarithmic plot.

This equation always produces survival curves that are flat at the origin and when n is fairly high this plateau is quite distinct (Figure 4.2). For radiation dose fractions in the therapeutic range (around 2 Gy per fraction) very little cell kill would be predicted. The survival curves predicted by this model have a shoulder that is largely within the first decade of survival: below a survival of about 0.1 the curves are approximately exponential. Cell-survival curves for human tumours often do not conform to these characteristics (see Chapter 12). It has therefore been necessary to invoke alternative models.

4.2.2 The multitarget model with single-hit component

The flexibility of the multitarget model can be increased by adding an exponential

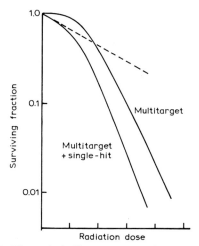

Figure 4.2. Effect of adding a single-hit component to the multitarget survival equation.

term, e^{-D/D_s}:

$$S = e^{-D/D_s} [1 - (1 - e^{-D/D_o})^n] \quad \text{(Eqn. 4.2)}$$

The effect of this term on the shape of the survival curves is to bend the whole curve down and thus to increase the initial slope (Fig. 4.2). The mechanistic interpretation might be that in addition to n targets all of which must be inactivated to kill the cell, it can also be killed by a hit on a single target that is critical for cell viability. This 'single hit' target must be rather small, in keeping with the fact that D_s values are often large. Not everyone would accept this mechanistic interpretation of the model, but use it rather as a flexible equation that fits most data very well. All models based on target theory suffer from the drawback that the shoulder on the cell-survival curve varies considerably through the cell cycle, and it is difficult to envisage how the number of targets could do this.

4.2.3 The linear-quadratic model

This simple and widely useful cell-survival relationship has the following form:

$$S = e^{-\alpha D - \beta D^2}$$

or $\log S = -\alpha D - \beta D^2$ (Eqn. 4.3)

When plotted as log S against dose (D), this curve has two components: a straight line (log $S = -\alpha D$) and a quadratic term or parabola (log $S = -\beta D^2$). As indicated in

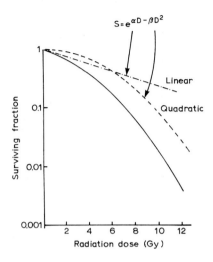

Figure 4.3. The linear-quadratic equation results from the summation of two components: the linear and quadratic terms.

Figure 4.3, it has an initial slope at low dose that is determined by the α-component and the rest of the curve bends continuously; there is no exponential asymptote at high dose. This relationship was proposed by Chadwick and Leenhouts (1981) on the basis of a molecular model of cell inactivation. They supposed that double-strand breaks in DNA could arise either by a single particle track damaging both strands (the probability of which would be proportional to dose) or by random ionisations producing lesions on opposite strands that by chance are close enough to give rise to a double-strand break (an event that would be proportional to the square of the dose). This mechanistic interpretation is not now widely accepted and the linear-quadratic equation is simply regarded as an empirical relationship that successfully fits a wide range of actual cell-survival data.

The importance of the linear-quadratic relationship has greatly increased as a result of the new approach in recent years to the analysis of time-dose relationships for the effect of fractionated irradiation on normal tissues. Analysis of such data is consistent with the assumption of an underlying linear-quadratic dose-effect relationship and, as described in Chapter 13, it leads to the use of the α/β ratio as a way of specifying the steepness of isoeffect plots of total dose against fraction number.

4.2.4 Repair saturation models

A number of cell-survival models have been described that incorporate processes of radiation damage repair. As an illustration of this approach, we describe the Q-factor model of Alper (1979).

The model assumes that cell killing is by single-hit events and that cell survival in

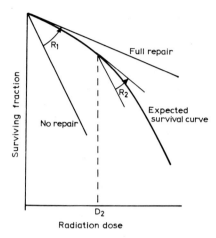

Figure 4.4. Illustrating the way in which the Q-factor model leads to a shouldered cell-survival curve.

the absence of repair is a simple exponential function of dose with an extrapolation number of 1.0.

It is then assumed that within the cell there exists a substance ('Q-factor') that is essential to the repair of radiation damage. Furthermore, the substance is *consumed* during the process of repair. Low radiation doses produce little damage, and during the ensuing recovery process a full quantity of Q-factor will be available; recovery will therefore be maximally efficient and will reduce the apparent radiosensitivity by a ratio R_1 (Figure 4.4). Greater radiation doses lead to more damage and also to a reduced capacity for repair. The extent of repair at dose D_2 (i.e., R_2) is therefore less. The model predicts a shouldered cell-survival curve that at high dose becomes exponential; the existence of the shoulder derives from the assumption that repair is a dose-dependent saturable process.

The nature of Q-factor has not been elucidated. If all damage is repairable, this model leads to a survival curve that has zero initial slope. To simulate a finite initial slope it must be assumed that there is a component of non-repairable damage (Figure 4.4), as is the case with the linear-quadratic model.

An important advantage of repair models is that they allow a straightforward explanation of variation in the shape of survival curves for cells in different parts of the cell cycle: the availability of Q-factor is not constant through the cell cycle. Durand and Sutherland (1972) found that when V79 cells were removed from multicell spheroids, the shoulder size decreased over a period of 8 h; this could be attributed to a loss of Q-factor from separated cells. Further evidence in support of this concept is the observation that the half-time for repair of DNA damage increases with radiation dose (Wheeler and Nelson, 1987).

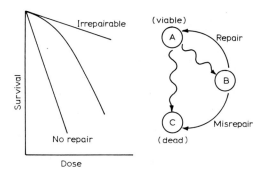

Figure 4.5. The basic form of the lethal–potentially lethal model (right) and the range of survival curves that it generates.

4.2.5 The lethal–potentially lethal (LPL) model

Most models of radiation cell killing generate dose-response curves without reference to dose rate. A significant advance was the description by Curtis (1986) of a dynamic model which is capable of simulating radiation cell killing as a function of dose rate. The model (Figure 4.5), which was in part based on the earlier Repair–Misrepair (RMR) model of Tobias and the work of Pohlit and his colleagues, envisages that viable cells (A) as a result of irradiation suffer two types of lesion: lethal (unrepairable) lesions that directly produce death (C), and potentially lethal lesions. The fate of cells (B) that have acquired potentially lethal lesions depends on competing processes of repair (B→A) and fixation (B→C). The fixation process is conceived as one of binary interaction of potentially lethal lesions. The model is described by four basic parameters: two sensitivity parameters (A→B and A→C) and two rate constants (repair, fixation). Finite values of the four parameters describe shouldered cell-survival curves at high-radiation dose rate, and the model successfully simulates the dose-rate effect in mammalian cells. In principle it therefore leads to a prediction about the relative extent of repair/fixation, but these are seldom very precisely defined by experimental data. More reliably, it allows calculation of the half-time for repair.

An attractive feature of the LPL model is that it provides a unified theory of repair in radiobiology. It simultaneously predicts four manifestations of repair:
  (i) The shoulder on the acute radiation survival curve. This is seen as being due to 'unstoppable repair', i.e., repair that occurs prior to and during the cell-cloning procedure itself.
  (ii) Split-dose recovery, due to repair of potentially lethal lesions during the split interval.
  (iii) Delayed-plating recovery, due to repair of potentially lethal lesions.
  (iv) The dose-rate effect, due to repair of potentially lethal lesions during irradiation.
   It also predicts that there is an underlying exponential (i.e., single-hit) survival

curve in the total absence of repair. The D_o value of this curve is low (often in the range 0.3–0.8 Gy) and is the steepest curve theoretically attainable with perfect repair inhibitors. At the other extreme, where repair is complete and there is no fixation of damage, the model again predicts an exponential survival curve, the slope of which reflects the amount of killing associated with the A→C transition alone.

4.2.6 The 'incomplete repair' model

By comparison with the LPL model, the 'incomplete repair' model is an empirical attempt to simulate time-dependent cell-survival proces. As described by Thames (1985) it follows earlier work by Lajtha and Oliver in assuming that reconstitution of the shoulder of the cell-survival curve can be described in terms of exponential decline in the 'dose equivalent' of damage. The model assumes that the acute cell-survival curve conforms to the linear-quadratic equation, and it adds only one further parameter: the time-constant for the decay of dose-equivalent of damage (further described in Section 15.3). The model is also applicable to fractionated exposures with any interfraction interval; if this interval is insufficient to allow full repair, then response will be greater than for longer intervals (hence the name 'incomplete repair' model).

Figure 4.6 shows a family of cell-survival curves calculated on the incomplete repair model for a range of radiation dose rates. An identical set of curves could be calculated by the LPL model. Note how the curves come together at very low dose rates (where repair is very nearly complete) and also at high dose rates (where repair during irradiation is negligible).

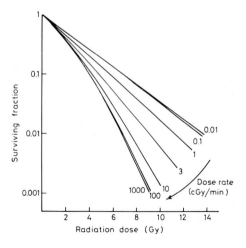

Figure 4.6. Cell-survival curves produced by the 'incomplete repair' model at a range of dose-rates.

4.2.7 Overview of cell-survival models

There is still no agreed explanation for the shoulders or curvature of radiation cell-survival curves. That the data usually indicate a finite initial slope is clear, and the models that simulate this have the common feature of incorporating two components: one that is exponential with dose (i.e., a 'linear' or 'single-hit' component), the other being non-linear. The explanation of the non-linear component is thought to lie either in the idea that potentially repairable lesions may interact to produce fixation of damage (the probability of interaction increasing with a power of the dose), or in the idea that as the amount of damage increases repair processes may become progressively less capable of dealing with it (i.e., they become 'saturated').

The thought that damage can usually be separated into two components and that recovery is associated with the non-linear component has important implications for understanding of differences in radiosensitivity among human tumours (see Sections 12.4 and 12.5).

4.3 The measurement of cell survival

4.3.1 Assays for tumour-cell survival

There are a variety of methods by which the clonal growth of tumour cells taken directly from an animal can be detected. Growth can be evaluated in tissue culture or by transfer to another animal. An essential first step is to prepare a single-cell suspension. The ease by which this can be done varies widely from one tumour type to another. Some, such as lymphomas, may fall apart under gentle agitation of chopped fragments. Others require protracted digestion with enzymes such as trypsin, pronase, or collagenase, to the point where cell viability may be compromised. The commonest approach is then to culture the disaggregated cells in vitro. Some cloning techniques involve growth as monolayers on plastic dishes; the drawback is often the overgrowth of fibroblasts that are also present in the cell suspension. A common alternative is to make the culture medium semi-solid with agar or methyl-cellulose. This inhibits the growth of connective-tissue cells; it may also inhibit the growth of some tumour cells and the proportion of cells that grow (the 'plating efficiency') is often low. But some animal and human tumours give plating efficiencies in excess of 1%, and for these the soft agar assay is useful (see Potten, 1985, for practical details).

A variety of other assays have been developed for rodent tumour cells, including the spleen colony assay, lung colony assay and limiting dilution assay. More details of these can be found in Steel (1977).

Human tumour cells are more difficult to grow than cells taken from established lines of transplanted mouse or rat tumour; they are also more difficult to disaggregate successfully. The method developed by Courtenay (1984) has been used widely. A variety of other cell-survival assays have been used for human tumours, aiming to provide data within a time-scale that can be of use to the patient. Some of these short-term assays are referred to in Section 21.2.

4.3.2 Assays for cell survival in normal tissues

Radiobiological studies on normal tissues are often performed by fixing endpoints of gross tissue damage and on this basis seeking to identify treatments that are isoeffective. The results are then interpreted in terms of the response of the stem cells of the tissue (Potten and Hendry, 1983). But in some normal tissues of the mouse it is possible to observe focal regeneration after irradiation which is attributed to clonal regrowth from small numbers of surviving stem cells. Cloning assays have been widely used in studies on bone marrow, intestinal epithelium, skin and testis. These are described in detail in the books by Potten and Hendry (1983, 1985).

4.3.3 Cell survival following in vivo irradiation of tumours

As a result of spatial variation in oxygen tension the clonogenic cells within a tumour usually vary considerably in radiosensitivity. There will be cells close to blood vessels that have an oxygen tension near to the arteriolar levels and which therefore will have almost the radiosensitivity of fully oxic cells. At the other extreme, there will be cells distant from blood vessels and on the verge of necrosis which will have a low oxygen tension and will have the radiosensitivity of hypoxic cells (a factor of perhaps 2.5 less sensitive than oxic cells – see Chapter 9). Between these extremes there will be cells

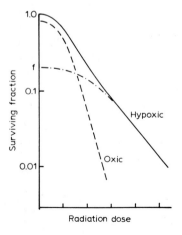

Figure 4.7. In vivo cell-survival curve for a mixed population of oxic and hypoxic cells. f is the hypoxic fraction.

56 G.G. Steel

of intermediate oxygen tension and radiosensitivity. Because of the steep dependence of radiosensitivity on oxygen tension (Figure 9.3) in vivo cell populations often appear as though they consist of mixtures of fully oxic and fully hypoxic cells. This is shown diagrammatically in Figure 4.7 where it can be seen that:
(i) The slope (i.e., D_o value) at high dose is that of the hypoxic cells.
(ii) The cell kill at low doses is dominated by the radiosensitivity of oxic cells

If the hypoxic fraction is sufficiently low (say below about 0.2) the survival curve for the whole cell population can sometimes be seen to be biphasic, but this change of slope is often hard to distinguish.

4.4 Cell survival following chemotherapy

Precisely the same methodology can be used to document the survival of clonogenic tumour cells after in vivo treatment with chemotherapeutic agents. The steepness of the survival curve is a good measure of the effectiveness of a cytotoxic drug. It will usually be plotted as a function of the drug dose to the animal (say in mg/kg body weight) and the observed response will be the result of two main factors: the actual sensitivity of the clonogenic cells to the drug, and the level of drug access to clonogenic cells. Access could be defined as the ratio of the levels of drug or active metabolites to which clonogenic cells are exposed, in relation to the levels in the systemic circulation. If access is poor, then even highly chemosensitive cells will

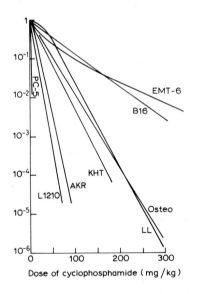 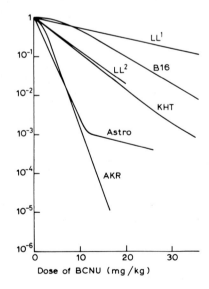

Figure 4.8. Cell-survival curves for various transplanted tumours in rodents, treated either with cyclophosphamide or BCNU. For the original sources, see Steel (1977), p. 258.

give shallow in vivo cell-survival curves.

The steepness and shape of in vivo cell-survival curves for cytotoxic drugs are much more variable than for radiation. Figure 4.8 shows a collection of survival curves for various mouse and rat tumours exposed to cyclophosphamide or BCNU. The curves are roughly exponential, although some show evidence of a shoulder and others are concave upwards. But it is the difference in slope that is the most obvious feature of these data. The cyclophosphamide doses required to give a fixed level of cell survival, say 10^{-2}, differ by a factor of 50. For BCNU the factor is about 10. This is evidence that drugs are more selective in their killing action than is radiation, and the therapeutic implication is that the success of chemotherapy depends to a large extent on correct drug selection.

4.4.1 Classification of cytotoxic drugs

The best-known classification of cytotoxic drugs in terms of the steepness and shape of cell-survival curves is that of Bruce, Meeker and Valeriote (1966). They compared the survival curves for normal unstimulated mouse bone-marrow stem cells with curves for a rapidly proliferating mouse lymphoma, treated over a period of 24 h. The differences were considered to reflect the relative effects of the drugs on rapidly and slowly proliferating cells. On this basis they described three main categories of agent:

Class I:	Cell-survival curves exponential and similarly steep for rapidly and slowly proliferating cells.	'Proliferation-independent' agents.
Class II:	Cell-survival curves decrease to a plateau, the level of which is lower in the more rapidly proliferating cells.	'Cycle phase-specific' agents.
Class III:	Survival curves exponential and steeper for the more rapidly proliferating cells.	'Proliferation-dependent' agents.

Subsequent research has shown that this classification is not as clear-cut as was originally supposed. It is, for instance, doubtful whether there are any truly proliferation-independent agents. Nevertheless, the underlying concepts are important in the consideration of dose-response relationships and in the formulation of drug combinations for chemotherapy.

4.4.2 Drug resistance

The ability to demonstrate resistant subpopulations is a particular advantage of the cell-survival approach. If a cell population contains a small proportion of cells that is markedly less sensitive to drug treatment, then the overall survival curve will show a change of slope, much as is seen with hypoxic cells resistant to radiation (Figure 4.7). The size of the resistant fraction can be judged from the level of cell survival at which the break occurs, and the relative degree of resistance is indicated by the slope ratio. Subpopulations resistant to drugs are often present in much lower proportions than are hypoxic cells and their degree of resistance can be considerable. As a result, there are many published examples of survival curves for chemotherapy that clearly show two components of cell killing. An example is shown in Figure 4.8, the curve for the astrocytoma treated with BCNU. It is to be expected that treatment of a tumour cell population that contains two such disparate subpopulations will lead to a relative reduction in the sensitive component and an increase in the resistant. This is probably an important mechanism underlying the phenomenon of treatment-induced drug resistance.

4.4.3 Tumour-size dependence

Large tumours are more difficult to control than small tumours, but this is mainly because they contain a greater number of stem cells. Is it also true that cells within large tumours are less *sensitive* to drug treatment? To answer this question using

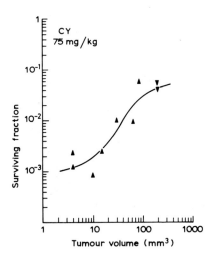

Figure 4.9. Cell survival in subcutaneous Lewis lung tumours treated at various sizes with a dose of 75 mg/kg cyclophosphamide. (From Stanley et al. (1977), with permission.)

measurements of tumour regrowth after treatment is difficult, because the end-point itself is size-dependent. But cell-survival studies in tumours of different size allow a direct basis for comparison of sensitivity. Figure 4.9 shows the results of studies on the Lewis lung tumour in mice in which the surviving fraction following a fixed dose of 75 mg/kg cyclophosphamide was determined in subcutaneous tumours over a wide range of sizes (Stanley et al., 1977). In terms of log cell-kill, the smallest tumours were twice as sensitive as the largest. A similar size dependency has been found with other drugs and other tumour types.

As tumours grow up through a diameter of a few millimetres it may often be that the vascular supply begins to be less adequate and as a consequence both drug access and cellular sensitivity decrease. This also is the size range at which radiobiological hypoxia often appears. Unfortunately, tumours of millimetre size are usually undetectable in patients and therefore these important mechanisms of therapeutic resistance are usually established well before treatment can be started.

4.5 Cell survival and gross response to treatment

4.5.1 Duration of remission and tumour growth delay

Careful measurement of tumours following irradiation or cytotoxic drug treatment often shows three phases:

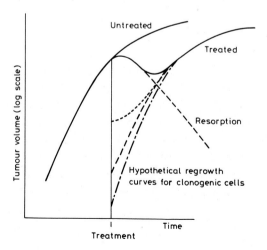

Figure 4.10. The volume response of a treated tumour is the composite result of two components: resorption and regrowth.

(i) A transient period in which the tumour continues to grow. This could be due to cell division continuing even in cells that are doomed to die (Section 5.2), or to oedema.
(ii) A period of tumour shrinkage which may continue to the point where the tumour is no longer detectable (i.e., complete regression). This phase involves the resorption of dead tissue and the disappearance by natural cell turnover of cells whose existence depends upon replacement by the products of tumour stem cells. It has been well emphasized by Thomlinson (1980) that tumour regression is a biological process that depends upon the *tumour*, not on the way it was treated. The rate of regression tends to be constant for a given tumour but vary widely between tumours, even of the same type.
(iii) A period of recurrence or tumour regrowth. Often the speed of regrowth is similar to that of an untreated tumour of the same size. Sometimes regrowth is slowed down, a phenomenon that has come to be known as the 'tumour-bed effect'.

This composite response to treatment is illustrated in Figure 4.10. The growth curve for untreated tumours is non-exponential, as is typical of tumours in experimental animals. The point of this diagram is that although regrowth is the result of repopulation by stem cells that survive treatment, the time at which regrowth begins will depend upon the time course of repopulation: this will influence the relation between cell survival and tumour-growth delay.

A revealing example of this is shown in Figure 4.11. B16 melanomas were treated in vivo either with cyclophosphamide or CCNU (Stephens and Peacock, 1977). Cell survival was measured by an in vitro assay, and the results compared with the time tumours took to grow to a fixed size. For a surviving fraction of 10^{-2} the tumours treated with cyclophosphamide were delayed by 4 days; those treated with CCNU by 14 days. Studies of tumour-cell repopulation showed that this difference was due to much slower regrowth after CCNU.

How much cell kill do we have to produce in order to obtain a good tumour response? The curve shown for cyclophosphamide in Figure 4.11 is typical of other data on experimental tumours in being concave upwards. Killing 99% of clonogenic cells only produced a growth delay of 4 days, a little over one volume-doubling time of the untreated tumours, and there was only slight tumour regression. It is the regression component (Fig. 4.10) that prevents tumour volume from responding quickly to clonogenic cell kill; as a result, it is necessary to achieve some decades of cell kill for the volume response to be marked. Conversely, when a complete regression is achieved, treatment must have reduced the surviving fraction of clonogenic cells by several decades.

4.5.2 Local tumour control

It is widely believed that regrowth will occur if one tumour stem cell is left intact

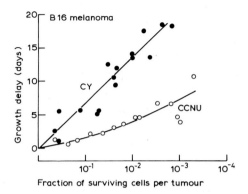

Figure 4.11. The relationship between cell survival and tumour growth delay in the B16 mouse melanoma. (o) treatment with cyclophosphamide; (•) treatment with CCNU. (From Stephens and Peacock, 1977, with permission.)

at the end of treatment. This follows from the definition of a stem cell, and it is supported by the evidence that some mouse tumours can be transplanted by very small numbers of cells (Hewitt, 1958; Steel and Adams, 1975). Direct evidence that tumours do regrow after treatment from very small numbers of surviving stem cells is available but not universal. Skipper and his co-workers using the L1210 leukaemia were convinced that the last surviving clonogenic cell had to be eradicated (Schabel, 1968). As cited above, Kummermehr (1985), using the AT17 mouse adenocarcinoma and in situ cloning, has obtained data that support the idea that regrowth only occurs from a very small number of surviving stem cells.

However, other investigators have found that some mouse tumours are controlled by radiation doses that are lower than would be expected from the slope of in vivo cell-survival curves. This is usually explained on the basis that many transplanted animal tumours are not truly syngeneic, and therefore are subject to host rejection. The big question, therefore, is whether human tumours also are subject to rejection processes and as a result may be more curable than we anticipate. Careful studies on truly syngeneic mouse tumours (Hewitt et al., 1976) and the general failure of immunotherapy in man argue against immunological helper mechanisms.

Further discussion of the relation between cell survival and the gross response of tumours is given in Chapter 5.

4.5.3 Cell survival and the failure of normal tissues

Not all of the effects of radiation on normal tissues are attributable to the sterilisation of stem cells (Chapters 7 and 8). In contrast to the situation in tumours where regrowth from subcurative therapy *must* depend on cells with extensive proliferative capacity, some normal tissue effects may result from non-stem-cell damage. Examples are:

erythema of the skin, brain oedema, haemopoietic damage resulting from proliferation-specific drugs (e.g., methotrexate), perhaps also late tissue fibrosis. On the other hand, a wide range of normal tissue reactions, particularly those that involve gross tissue failure, probably are the result of damage to stem cells, reducing them to numbers that are inadequate to maintain the integrity of the tissue. Examples are: desquamation of the skin, early radiation damage to the bowel, haemopoietic failure resulting from stem-cell damaging drugs (e.g., busulphan).

References

Alper, T. (1979) Cellular Radiobiology, Cambridge University Press.
Bruce, W.R., Meeker, B.E. and Valeriote, F.A. (1966) Comparison of the sensitivity of normal hematopoietic and transplanted lymphoma colony-forming cells to chemotherapeutic agents administered in vivo. J. Natl. Cancer Inst. 37, 233–245.
Chadwick, K.H. and Leenhouts, H.P. (1981) The Molecular Theory of Radiation Biology, Springer-Verlag, Berlin.
Courtenay, V.D. (1984) A replenishable soft agar colony assay for human tumour sensitivity testing, in: Predictive Drug Testing on Human Tumour Cells (Hofmann, V., Berens, M.E. and Martz, G., eds.), Springer-Verlag, Berlin.
Curtis, S.B. (1986) Lethal and potentially lethal lesions induced by radiation – a unified repair model. Radiat. Res. 106, 252–270.
Durand, R.E. and Sutherland, R.M. (1972) Effects of intercellular contact on repair of radiation damage. Expl. Cell Res. 71, 75–80.
Hewitt, H.B. (1958) Studies of the dissemination and quantitative transplantation of a lymphocytic leukaemia of CBA mice. Br. J. Cancer 12, 378–401.
Hewitt, H.B., Blake, E.R. and Walder, A.S. (1976) A critique of the evidence for host defence against cancer, based on personal studies of 27 murine tumours of spontaneous origin. Br. J. Cancer 33, 241–259.
Kummermehr, J. (1985) Measurement of tumour clonogens in situ, in: Cell Clones (Potten, C.S. and Hendry, J.H., eds.), pp. 215–222, Churchill-Livingstone, Edinburgh.
Potten, C.S. and Hendry, J.H. (1983) Cytotoxic Insult to Tissues, Churchill-Livingstone, Edinburgh.
Potten, C.S. and Hendry, J.H. (1985) Cell Clones: A Manual of Mammalian Cell Techniques, Churchill Livingstone, Edinburgh.
Schabel, F.M. (1968) In vivo leukemic cell-kill kinetics and 'curability' in experimental systems, in: Proliferation and Spread of Neoplastic Cells. Williams and Wilkins, Baltimore. University of Texas and M.D. Anderson Hospital, Houston, TX.
Shipley, W.U., Stanley, J.A. and Steel, G.G. (1975) Tumor-size dependency in the radiation response of the Lewis lung carcinoma. Cancer Res. 35, 2488–2493.
Stanley, J.A., Shipley, W.U. and Steel, G.G. (1977) Influence of tumour size on hypoxic fraction and therapeutic sensitivity of Lewis lung tumour. Br. J. Cancer 36, 105–113.
Steel, G.G. (1977) Growth Kinetics of Tumours. Clarendon Press, Oxford.
Steel, G.G. and Adams, K. (1975) Stem-cell survival and tumor control in the Lewis lung carcinoma. Cancer Res. 35, 1530–1535.
Stephens, T.C. and Peacock, J.H. (1977) Tumour volume response, initial cell kill and cellular repopulation in B16 melanoma treated with cyclophosphamide and BCNU. Br. J. Cancer 36, 313.
Thames, H.D. (1985) An 'incomplete-repair' model for survival after fractionated and continuous irradiations. Int. J. Radiat. Biol. 47, 319–339.

Thomlinson, R.H. (1982) Measurement and management of carcinoma of the breast. Clin. Radiol. 33, 481–493.

Wheeler, K.T. and Nelson, G.B. (1987) Saturation of a DNA repair process in dividing and non-dividing mammalian cells. Radiat. Res. 109, 109–17.

CHAPTER 5

Relation between cell survival and gross endpoints of tumour response and tissue failure

KLAUS-RUDIGER TROTT

Department of Radiation Biology, Medical College of St. Bartholomew's Hospital, Charterhouse Square, London EC1M 6BQ, England

---

5.1	Introduction	65
5.2	Radiation effects on cells in vitro	66
5.3	Tumour response	68
5.4	Normal tissue responses	72
5.5	Conclusions	75

5.1. Introduction

The various responses of tumours and normal tissues to irradiation can be explained to some degree by the radiation responses of their constituent cells as they can be observed and quantitated in vitro (Chapter 4). However, different types of cellular radiation effects contribute to the different observed clinical responses. The goal of this chapter is to discuss the relationship between the various types of radiation effects seen in cell culture and the development and progression of different types of radiation response in tumours and normal tissues. A brief description of cellular radiation effects is given first followed by a separate analysis of their importance for the radiation responses of tumours and normal tissues.

5.2 Radiation effects on cells in vitro

Cells grown in vitro respond to irradiation with a variety of changes, all of which may also occur in irradiated tissues in vivo and which contribute to a greater or lesser degree to the development of clinical radiation response. Loss of the ability to form colonies, first described by Puck and Marcus (1956) and discussed in some detail in Chapter 4, is by no means the only cellular radiation effect and for some types of radiation injury to tissues it may not even be the most important.

Time-lapse cinephotography of cells growing and irradiated under the microscope gives the most direct insight into the variety of cellular radiation responses (Thompson and Suit, 1972; Hurwitz and Tolmach, 1975). Typically, pedigrees of irradiated cells are constructed from these films as shown in Figure 5.1, which shows the growth history of a single cell. The longitudinal lines indicate cell life-span. After the second division, the four grand-daughter cells which are genetically identical (a clone) are irradiated at exactly the same stage in their life cycle with exactly the same dose, and their further development is followed. Various changes have been recorded:

(*a*) *Clonogenic survival.* One of the four cells irradiated with 5 Gy continued to grow as if it was completely unharmed. After six successful divisions the cell number of this clone would exceed the commonly set limit of 50 progeny for colony formation and it would be counted as a survivor with unlimited proliferative potential, comparable to a stem cell in vivo. However, very often, surviving cells may show severe proliferative injury (delayed mitosis, cell death among some progeny, loss of whole sectors of the pedigree, etc.) yet still qualify as 'surviving cells'. By counting the number of offspring in surviving colonies, qualitative changes in the viability of surviving clonogenic cells can be demonstrated. The mean number of offspring per

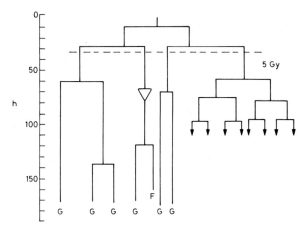

Figure 5.1. Pedigree of the progeny of a single clonogenic cell which was irradiated with 5 Gy at the 4-cell stage, in the G_1 phase of the cell cycle. G = giant cell; F = cell fragmentation. The progeny of the cell on the right exceeded 50 cells at the end of the recording period.

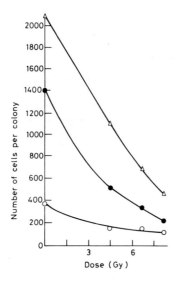

Figure 5.2. The dependence of the mean number of progeny per surviving colony in irradiated HeLa cells after various incubation times (○ = 210 h; ● = 270 h; ▲ = 320 h). (Data from Puck and Marcus 1956.)

surviving clone counted 10 days after irradiation decreases as the dose increases, as shown in Figure 5.2. Although clonogenic survival is an all-or-nothing effect, there are also qualitative alterations in the surviving clonogenic cells after irradiation to be considered. Conversely, a sterilised cell, though not able to form a colony, may still go through a number of cell divisions until all its progeny are extinct. After doses in the clinical range, many abortive divisions may occur and increase the total number of cells which, although carrying proliferative injury, may still be perfectly able to differentiate into functioning cells. For a considerable time after doses in excess of 3–5 Gy, mitoses are visible and an increase in total cell number arises from abortive divisions of these sterilised 'inactivated cells'.

(b) *Cell death.* In vitro, pyknosis, nuclear fragmentation and giant-cell formation (with or without endomitosis) are observed after irradiation. Cell death may occur at any time after irradiation, in sterilised as well as in surviving clones, yet most often it is related to an attempted mitosis in the sterilised clone. Nearly all cells irradiated with doses up to about 10 Gy proceed to the next mitosis, although this is usually delayed. Failure to progress through mitosis in the normal orderly fashion is a common mechanism of radiation-induced cell death. This mitotic death is usually due to severe chromosomal injury which in histological slides is seen as anaphase or telophase bridges or micronuclei in daughter cells after cell division. In some slowly proliferating tissues, however, morphological signs of cell death are not seen after irradiation, unless cells are stimulated into proliferation, e.g., the liver. In other cell lines, cells which cannot pass through subsequent mitoses may persist for prolonged periods, not proliferating but morphologically and metabolically intact. These cells usually grow in volume and, in vivo, may even differentiate. If cytolysis occurs before attempted mitosis it is called 'interphase death'. In tissue culture, this is rarely seen at doses below 10 Gy. In vivo, however, it may be more common at low doses and is well documented in oocytes, lymphocytes and some glandular cells, especially in the salivary glands.

(c) *Cell function*. Very little is known about the effects of radiation on cell function. Various effects of radiations on membranes have been documented, some of them at rather low doses, but no consistent picture has emerged which helps to interpret clinical responses in irradiated tissues. However, in our attempt to interpret such tissue responses in terms of cellular responses we should be aware that present radiobiological knowledge only deals with cell numbers and cell proliferation which, as we shall see, can explain some but not all effects of radiation on tissues and tumours.

5.3 Tumour response

The close quantitative relationship between tumour recurrence after radiotherapy and clonogenic survival of tumour stem cells was realised as soon as the first radiation survival curves of tumour cells in vitro and in vivo had been published (Wilson, 1961; Suit and Shalek, 1963). The basic assumption is that a tumour recurrence represents the progeny of just one or several independent tumour stem cells which survived irradiation. This concept that a tumour recurrence is analogous to a colony in vitro and, after high radiation doses, may indeed derive from a single surviving tumour stem cell, is supported by experimental evidence in mouse tumours.

Transplantation of non-immunogenic tumours in rodents can be performed by injecting a suspension of tumour cells into the host. The proportion of successful

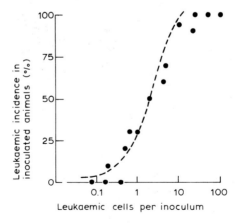

Figure 5.3. Relationship between the number of leukaemic cells in the inoculum and the take rate, i.e., the incidence of successfully transplanted leukaemia. (Data from Hewitt, 1958.)

tumour-takes increases as the number of transplanted cells increases (Figure 5.3). This sigmoid curve corresponds to a cumulative Poisson distribution of the probability that the inoculum contained one or more tumour transplanting units, i.e., tumour stem cells. A great number of similar studies supports the conclusion that most spontaneous (and thus non-immunogenic) mouse tumours can indeed be transplanted by one tumour stem cell acting independently from all other cells which may be present in the inoculum. The concentration of tumour stem cells varies considerably among different tumours. In the tumour analysed in Figure 5.3, one out of two tumour cells was a stem cell; in others it may be as low as one in 10 000.

By analogy with these tumour transplantation studies, a tumour recurrence may arise from a single surviving tumour stem cell. Consequently, the probability of tumour recurrence increases according to Poisson statistics with increasing mean number of surviving tumour stem cells. In theory, a decrease in recurrence rate of an irradiated tumour from 90 to 10%, i.e., an increase in local control rate from 10 to 90%, corresponds to a decrease in the mean number of surviving tumour stem cells from 2.3 to 0.1 and thus, roughly to 3-times the D_o of an exponential survival curve (D_o reduces survival to 0.37, hence 3 D_o reduces it to $(0.37)^3 = 0.05$). However, even in very well-controlled animal experiments, this relationship is never as close as in theory, since heterogeneity between individual tumours tends to make the dose–cure relationship flatter than is expected for a Poisson distribution (Figure 5.3). Therefore it is impossible to derive the parameters of cellular radiosensitivity (such as D_o and the number of tumour stem cells) from dose–cure curves in experimental or in human tumours by the analysis of their steepness.

However, some information about these parameters can be derived by comparing the dose–cure relationships of tumours of different sizes (Suit et al., 1965). The radiation dose needed for local control of 37% of tumours (i.e., to leave on average

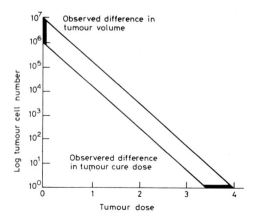

Figure 5.4. Schematic representation of the quantitative relation of tumour control dose to tumour size.

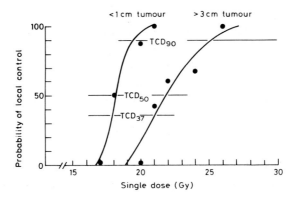

Figure 5.5. The dependence of local tumour control on radiation dose after single-dose radiotherapy of skin cancers of 0.5–1 cm diameter or 3–4 cm diameter. (Data from Trott et al., 1984.)

one surviving tumour stem cell per tumour) depends on two parameters: the slope of the survival curve and the initial number of tumour stem cells (Figure 5.4). A tumour containing 10-times the number of tumour stem cells compared to a smaller tumour thus requires a radiation dose which gives an additional cell kill of a factor of 10, i.e., 2.3-times the D_o. From the data in Figure 5.5 for human skin cancer treated with single doses one arrives at a D_o of 1.3 Gy. Further, by dividing the mean curative dose of 22 Gy for the 3–4 cm diameter skin cancer by the D_o of 1.3 Gy, one arrives at the conclusion that this large skin cancer is controlled if the surviving fraction is decreased to 10^{-7} and conversely that the total number of tumour stem cells within this tumour is less than 10^7. The remainder of the tumour cells, at least 100-times more, are viable tumour cells, many of them proliferating, but not tumour stem cells.

In view of these data, tumour control by radiotherapy can be described as the stepwise dilution of the concentration of tumour stem cells within the total tumour mass as the total dose accumulates. Each successive 2 Gy fraction will dilute the concentration of tumour stem cells by approximately a factor of 2 (Section 12.3.2) until there is a realistic probability that not a single stem cell is left within the total tumour mass. There is no proof that any other mechanism, be it specific immunological response against tumour stem cells or radiation injury to the tumour stroma, contributes significantly to this process of direct stem cell inactivation by radiation.

Tumour regression varies enormously between different tumours but is largely independent of the amount of sterilisation of tumour stem cells by radiation. In general, the mechanisms of tumour regression are poorly understood and no close relationship can be demonstrated to any of the above-mentioned cellular radiation effects.

In experimental cancer therapy, the delay in tumour growth imposed by treatment with a subcurative dose is taken as a quantitative indicator of the decrease in the surviving fraction of tumour stem cells (Figure 5.6). Yet regrowth delay depends as

Cell survival and tissue response 71

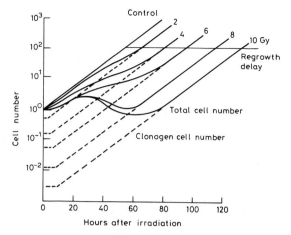

Figure 5.6. Schematic representation of the changes in cell number in vitro after irradiation with different doses. Derived experimentally by Elkind et al. (1963) to demonstrate the principle of the relation between cell survival and regrowth delay.

much on regrowth *rate* as it does on the fraction of surviving tumour cells – and both may change with dose and fractionation. Often, irradiated tumours regrow slower than the original growth rate. Therefore, it is usually impossible to relate directly regrowth delay to level of clonogenic survival. However, one may assume that the same growth delay under different treatment conditions corresponds to the same level of clonogenic survival. No reliable method is available to compare the regrowth delay of different tumours in different patients in order to compare stem-cell survival. Therefore, experimental protocols in human cancer usually rely on a comparison of the responses of multiple metastases in the same patient which are given different treatments (Figure 5.7).

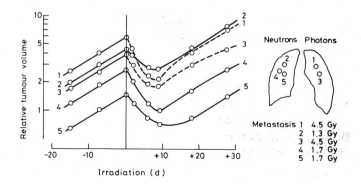

Figure 5.7. Growth curves of five lung metastases within one patient assessed by repeated chest X-rays before and after single doses of neutrons (right lung, solid lines) or X-rays (left lung, dotted lines). (Data by van Peperzeel, 1972.)

5.4 Normal tissue responses

Whereas local tumour control can be interpreted in terms of cellular radiobiology, local recurrence being analogous to survival of one or more tumour stem cells, this simple relationship does not hold for normal tissue responses.

The acute radiation responses of the bone marrow and the small bowel were related to the proliferative organization of these tissues and the various cellular radiation effects by Bond et al. (1968). A general pathogenic mechanism for tissues with a steady-state cell turnover was described and based on the identification of different cell compartments (Chapter 7). The stem-cell compartment is small, proliferating slowly to maintain its size but able to respond to perturbations by feed-back mechanisms. After irradiation, the number of stem cells decreases according to the dose-response curves described in Chapter 4. Methods for the identification and quantitation of stem cells have been developed in various tissues of the mouse, e.g. bone marrow, gut mucosa and skin epithelium. The proliferative or transit compartment consists of cells supplied by the stem-cell compartment and performing a rapid succession of cell divisions to multiply the number of cells available for differentiation. Most mitotic figures observed in any tissue belong to cells of this compartment. The number of successive cell divisions, i.e., the multiplication factor of the transit compartment, may be regulated by demand. After irradiation mitosis-linked cell death and a dose-dependent decrease in the number of offspring, i.e., of the multiplication factor, occur as described above.

The differentiating and functional compartments consist of non-proliferating, post-mitotic cells with a defined life span which is unaltered by the radiation doses used in radiotherapy. Also cell differentiation is assumed not to be detectably influenced by irradiation with such doses.

This model is very useful for describing the typical response pattern not only of the bone marrow and the mucosal epithelia of the bowel but also of other tissues with a continuous cell turnover. Acute radiation effects develop as cells in the proliferative compartment die and the number of progeny from the transit compartment decreases. As long as a normal supply of cells from the stem-cell compartment is available for cell differentiation and for the duration of the normal life span of functional end cells, no signs of acute radiation injury will be apparent. The number of functional cells starts to decrease when the supply from the transit compartment fails to compensate for the natural loss of differentiated cells which have passed their normal life span. Many specific signs of acute radiation injury to tissues are directly related to the decrease in number of functional cells. This hypoplasia is progressive – as is the severity of the acute radiation injury – until, by stimulated proliferation of the surviving stem cells, the stem-cell compartment and the other compartment are gradually restored to their normal size. It is especially during this phase of regeneration that various regulatory mechanisms play an important role and modify the primary radiation response.

In this pathogenic model, the level of stem-cell survival has little or no influence on the development of the acute radiation response but it is crucially important for its duration. However, the severity of any acute radiation injury increases with its duration as the risk of secondary infection and other complications increase.

Michalowski (1981) and Wheldon et al. (1982) further developed this model of radiation injury in normal tissues in an attempt to make it applicable even to tissues lacking an identifiable hierarchy of proliferative and differentiating compartments such as liver and kidney. The authors used the term 'hierarchical tissues' (H-type tissues) for tissues with structured organisation of the various cell compartments (see Chapter 7). In other tissues, termed F-type for flexible tissues, functional parenchymal cells are assumed to have some proliferative potential as well. Upon demand, cell production can be considerably accelerated by recruiting non-cycling cells into the proliferating compartment. This triggering of radiation-damaged cells into proliferation will lead to their mitotic death and hence to an increased rate of cell loss from the population which, in turn, recruits even more functioning cells into cycle. This 'avalanche' effect results in a pronounced dose-dependence of the rate of decline in cell number and thus of latency time to clinical injury. For both H and F types of tissue the changes in cell number after irradiation have been computed, taking into account stem-cell inactivation, abortive cell divisions, stimulated proliferation and mitosis-related cell death. Characteristic differences in the time-course and dose-dependence of cell depletion between F-type tissues and H-type tissues were found. The main differences between the radiation responses are listed in Table 5.1.

TABLE 5.1
General properties of alternative models of proliferative normal tissues (from Wheldon et al., 1986)

Property	H-type model	F-type model
Proliferative capacity of functional cells	Zero	Infinite
Physiological rate of turnover of functional cells	Fast	Slow
Time-scale of expression of radiation injury	Early	Late
Rate of radiation-induced depopulation of functional cells	Constant; largely dose-independent	Accelerating with time: faster after higher doses (Avalanche effect)
Time to reach a given level of functional cell depletion	Dose-independent: predictable from steady-state kinetics	Dose-dependent: shorter than expected from steady-state kinetics
Dose-response curve for impairment of tissue function	Approximates the shape of clonogenic cell survival curve (from stem cells)	Differs from clonogenic cell survival curve (increased curvature)
Effect of deliberate stimulation of cell proliferation following irradiation	Protective (promotes stem cell repopulation and truncates run-down of functional cells)	Damaging: precipitates synchronous death of functional cells

It should be realised that this pathogenic model involves only one particular cell type in any one tissue and does not allow for effects of interaction of damage to different cell populations within a tissue or organ, as for example between stroma and parenchyma. Moreover, the basic assumption of the model is the direct relationship of clinical signs and symptoms of radiation injury to parenchymal cell depletion beyond a threshold for early as well as for chronic radiation effects. These assumptions are controversial and may only apply to some responses in some tissues.

A further development of this pathogenic model was presented by Thames and Hendry (1987) who suggested that radiation injury occurs by the sterilisation of 'targets' in a tissue, each of which may consist of more than one cell but each target responds independently to irradiation. The survival of a single one of these targets is assumed to prevent the manifestation of radiation injury (Chapter 7). Therefore these targets are analogous to the recurrence-forming units in tumours, i.e., the tumour stem cells, and to spleen colony-forming units of the bone marrow, the bone marrow stem cells. They are therefore called tissue-rescuing units (TRU).

The TRU is a further generalisation of the concept of clonogenic survival after irradiation. Their existence is deduced:
(A) From the numerical equivalence of D_o values derived from the functional response of the tissue and values measured by stem cell assays.
(B) From the equivalence of clonogen survival at tissue-isoeffect doses after altered fractionation or dose-rate.
(C) From the limiting slopes of isoeffect graphs for tissue response to fractionated and continuous exposures as opposed to those deduced from target-cell models.

In many tissues the TRU model cannot be based on considerations of known pathogenic mechanisms or morphological features which can be directly and empirically tested, but on indirect comparisons between predictions from mathematical models for the analysis of dose-response relationships of the incidence of radiation injury. The biology of these hypothetical tissue-rescuing units is difficult to describe in complex organs such as lung, central nervous system or heart.

The various models described above attempt to link the pathogenesis of normal tissue radiation injury to cellular radiation responses. At present, they are unable to explain those functional side effects of radiotherapy which are not directly caused by a major decrease in the number of parenchymal cells. Thus, there is no cellular explanation for acute functional side effects of radiotherapy such as nausea, diarrhoea, or erythema. Moreover, the impairment of microcirculation in normal tissues for months after irradiation, which may lead to progressive atrophy (Section 8.2), cannot at present be related to any of the known cellular radiation effects.

5.5 Conclusions

The relation between cellular radiation effects and clinical tissue responses to radiotherapy is different with respect to three major endpoints, namely tumour control, acute side effects and chronic side effects.

Tumour control depends on the complete sterilisation of all tumour stem cells, local recurrences are equivalent to the progeny of surviving colony-forming cells in vitro. There is a close relation between clonogenic cell survival and local tumour control.

Most acute radiation injury is related to the decrease in number of functioning parenchymal cells as the steady state of cell production and cell loss is disturbed by radiation leading to a dose-dependent reduction of the amplification factor in the transit compartment. As the number of surviving stem cells decreases with increasing radiation dose, the duration and the severity of acute radiation injury increases. Most chronic radiation injury is not closely related to a decrease in the overall number of tissue-specific functional cells. Structural changes and atrophy may develop secondarily to impaired tissue microcirculation. In contrast to the early effects seen in intestinal epithelium and bone marrow, a close relation between clonogenic cell survival and radiation injury cannot be identified for late normal tissue damage.

References

Bond, V.P., Fliedner, T.M. and Archambeau, J.O. (1965) Mammalian radiation lethality, a disturbance in cellular kinetics. Academic Press, New York.
Elkind, M.M., Sutton, H. and Moses, W.E. (1961) Postirradiation survival kinetics of mammalian cells grown in culture. J. Cell. Comp. Physiol. 58 (Suppl. 1), 113–134.
Hewitt, H.B. (1958) Studies of the dissemination and quantitative transplantation of a lymphocytic leukaemia in CBA mice. Br. J. Cancer 12, 378–401.
Hurwitz, C. and Tolmach, L.J. (1969) Time-lapse cinemicrographic studies of X-irradiated HeLa S3 cells. I. Cell progression and cell disintegration. Biophys. J. 9, 607–633.
Michalowski, A. (1981) Effects of radiation on normal tissues: hypothetical mechanisms and limitations of in situ assays of clonogenicity. Radiat. Environm. Biophys. 19, 157–172.
Puck, T.T. and Marcus, P.I. (1956) Action of X-rays on mammalian cells. J. Exp. Med. 103, 653–666.
Suit, H.D. and Shalek, R.J. (1963) Response of spontaneous mammary carcinoma of the C3H mouse to X irradiation given under conditions of local tissue anoxia. J. Natl. Cancer Inst. 31, 479–509.
Suit, H.D., Shalek, R.J. and Wette, R. (1965) Radiation response of C3H mouse mammary carcinoma evaluated in terms of cellular radiation sensitivity in: Cellular Radiation Biology, Williams and Wilkins, Baltimore.
Thames, H.D. and Hendry, J.H. (1987) Fractionation in Radiotherapy. Taylor and Francis, London.
Thompson, L.H. and Suit, H.D. (1972) Proliferation kinetics of X-irradiated mouse L cells studied with time-lapse photography. Int. J. Radiat. Biol. 15, 347–362.
Trott, K.R., Maciejewski, B., Preuss-Bayer, G. and Skolyszewski, J. (1984) Dose-response curve and split-dose recovery in human skin cancer. Radiother. Oncol. 2, 123–129.
Van Peperzeel, H.A. (1972) Effects of single doses of radiation on lung metastases in man and experimental animals. Eur. J. Cancer 8, 665–675.

Wheldon, T.E., Michalowski, A.S. and Kirk, J. (1982) The effect of irradiation on function in self-renewing normal tissues with differing proliferative organisation. Br. J. Radiol. 55, 759–766.

Wilson, C.W. (1961) Possible implications of recent radiobiological observations for tumour – dose – fractionation schedules. Radiology 77, 940–945.

CHAPTER 6

Cell proliferation kinetics in tumours

G. GORDON STEEL

Radiotherapy Research Unit, The Institute of Cancer Research, Cotswold Road, Sutton, Surrey SM2 5NG, England

---

6.1   Descriptive and operational cell kinetics 77

6.2   The growth rate of tumours 78
     6.2.1   Shapes of tumour growth curves 79
     6.2.2   How fast do tumours grow? 80

6.3   Cell proliferation in tumours 80
     6.3.1   The cell cycle in tumours 81
     6.3.2   The growth fraction concept 82
     6.3.3   Cell loss from tumours: potential doubling time 83
     6.3.4   Repopulation during therapy 84

6.4   The kinetic status of clonogenic cells 86

6.5   Overview of cell proliferation and tumour response to treatment 87

6.1 Descriptive and operational cell kinetics

Studies of cell proliferation in normal and tumour tissues fall into two categories (Steel, 1974):

Descriptive. Studies based on the microscope or the flow-cytometer. Dividing and non-dividing cells can be identified and their proliferation can be related to cell morphology and to tissue architecture. With the aid of autoradiography (Rogers, 1973) it is possible to measure the time that cells take to migrate or to undergo various cellular processes. The flow cytometer documents the numbers of cells in defined proliferative or morphological categories.

Operational. The approach based on assays of tissue function. The operational measure of cell proliferation is colony-forming ability. The underlying notion is that

TABLE 6.1
Analogies between descriptive and operational concepts

Descriptive approach	Operational approach
Stem cells postulated as a source of continued proliferation	Stem cells registered by their ability to produce a discrete number of descendants under test conditions
Cycle phase specificity	Cell-survival curve falls to a plateau that depends on proliferation rate
Cells 'out of cycle'	Subpopulation that is resistant to protracted treatment with proliferation-dependent agents
Mobilisation or 'recruitment' of non-proliferating cells	Sensitivity to proliferation-dependent agents is increased by prior treatment

the regrowth of a tumour after treatment or the long-term integrity of an irradiated normal tissue depends upon the existence of stem cells that can give rise to a large family of descendents; the kinetic property that matters most in this situation is their ability to maintain this operational function. The Operational approach is thus based on cell-survival assays (Section 4.3).

The reason for setting out this distinction is because the information obtained by these two approaches is very different and often does not overlap. A drawback of the Descriptive approach for studies in cancer therapy is that, although cells can be classified as proliferating or non-proliferating, we cannot know whether they have colony-forming ability. The concept of 'stemness' in tissues is difficult to deal with by the Descriptive approach. On the other hand, a drawback of the Operational approach is that when we remove cells from a tissue and detect the formation of colonies in tissue culture it is often difficult to know which are the cells that gave rise to the colonies.

Phenomena detected by cell-survival studies are often interpreted in terms of ideas that are part of the Descriptive approach, but these connections are sometimes hard to draw. Some examples of such analogies are listed in Table 6.1.

6.2 The growth rate of tumours

The most basic Descriptive proliferative feature of tumours is their volume growth rate. It must be remembered that tumours do not consist only of neoplastic cells. A large part of the volume is taken up by stroma, by the differentiated (no longer malignant) products of neoplastic cells, and by necrosis and other acellular products.

6.2.1 Shapes of tumour growth curves

If every cell divides to produce two proliferative daughters, then the growth of the population is: 1, 2, 4, 8, 16 ..., an exponential series. If the generation time is constant, the population size will increase exponentially with time. Exponential growth is the simplest mode of population increase. The population doubling time is constant and when cell populations do not grow exponentially we have to invoke one or more processes to explain the retardation.

For this reason, exponential growth is the norm with which tumour growth must be compared. Many tumours do not grow exponentially, though over short periods of time they can be assumed to do so. The best way to specify the rate of tumour growth is by the *volume doubling time*.

An important property of exponential tumour growth is illustrated in Figure 6.1. The two panels show the same growth curve, plotted either on a linear scale of size (above) or on a logarithmic scale (below). On the logarithmic scale the growth curve is a straight line: the doubling time is constant. In equal time intervals the volume will increase from 1 mg to 1 g, or from 1 g to 1 kg (or any factor of 1000). On the linear scale it is impossible to represent a tumour volume below about 1 g and, more importantly, tumours below this approximate limit are usually clinically undetectable. There therefore appears to be a long 'silent interval' of undetected growth, and, when growth is detected, it gives the appearance of *accelerating*; yet the actual growth rate

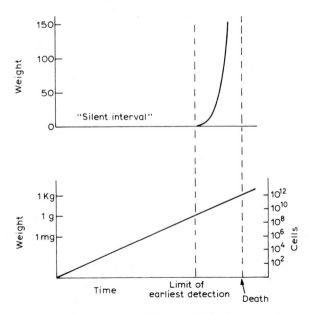

Figure 6.1. The implications of regular exponential growth. The same growth curve is displayed in both panels: above on a linear scale, below on a logarithmic scale. (From Steel, 1975.)

is constant. Since our perception of a tumour tends to be linear rather than logarithmic, it is easy to be misled about changes of growth rate with time. Moreover, since the minimally-detectable cancer may contain upwards of 10^9 cells and death may well occur when growth exceeds 10^{12}, regular exponential growth must always lead to a clinical phase of growth that is shorter than the silent period.

Many accurately determined growth curves for human tumours are close to exponential (Steel, 1977). Mostly, however, these data are on lung metastases whose environment may be ideal for unrestricted growth. But there are also many examples of human tumours that show irregular or decelerating growth. Careful studies of transplanted tumours in experimental animals usually show growth curves that are convex upwards on a semilogarithmic plot: the doubling time progressively increases. Such curves can be fitted with a variety of mathematical equations, but the popular form is the Gompertz equation (Steel, 1977). This can be regarded as a growth curve in which the doubling time increases exponentially with time as the tumour approaches a limiting maximum volume. It may be that this asymptotic maximum volume is related to total body size: tumours in small animals give more prominently Gompertzian growth curves than are found in man.

6.2.2 How fast do tumours grow?

A substantial amount of data accumulated up to the early 1970s on the growth rate of untreated human tumours. Since then the widespread use of chemotherapy has made such studies less feasible. The data consist mainly of measurements from serial chest X-rays of metastatic and primary lesions in the lung, some studies on involved lymph nodes, and a few on primary tumours in other sites (see Steel, 1977, for review). What they indicate is:

(i) Within any group of tumours there is usually a wide range of growth rates.
(ii) The average volume doubling time of lung metastases from common tumours is around 3 months.
(iii) More rapid growth is seen in lymphomas, teratomas, and some childhood tumours.

6.3 Cell proliferation in tumours

The rate of cellular proliferation in a tumour can be judged by a number of relatively simple methods: the mitotic index, thymidine labelling index, fraction of cells with S-phase DNA content (i.e., flow cytometry), incorporation of BUdR followed by staining for its presence in DNA by a monoclonal antibody, or from the rate of accumulation of blocked metaphases following the administration of a mitotic spindle poison. These methods give an indication of the rate of cell proliferation, although only the last one is a direct measure of mitotic rate (i.e., the rate at which cells enter mitosis).

6.3.1. The cell cycle in tumours

To obtain information on the duration of the cell cycle and its phases requires a more sophisticated type of experiment than those just referred to. The problem is how to determine this information when, as is invariably the case, non-proliferating cells are present. There are two principal methods: the technique of labelled mitoses, or by a kinetic study with flow cytometry.

The principle underlying the technique of labelled mitoses is to radioactively label the cells that at one time are undergoing DNA synthesis (and therefore are in the S-phase), then to observe their subsequent passage through the cell cycle (see Steel, 1977, for full review). Labelling is by a single administration of [^{3}H]thymidine. In autoradiographs of samples (biopsies in the case of human tumours) taken at various times afterwards, cells in mitosis are scored as labelled or unlabelled. The fraction of mitoses that are labelled shows a peak as the labelled cells move out of G$_2$ and through

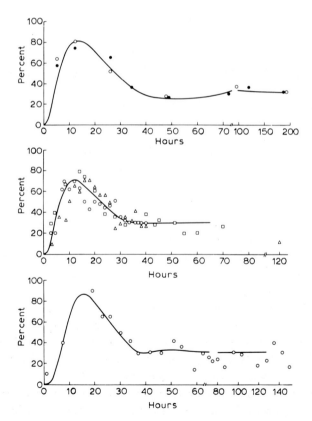

Figure 6.2. Labelled mitoses curves from three studies on human melanoma. These are taken from the review by Steel (1977).

into G_1; later it should peak again as the cells go through their second post-labelling division. The time from peak to peak is then a good indication of the duration of the intermitotic cycle. Furthermore, the width of the first peak is the duration of the S-phase, since this is the time taken for the labelled cohort to pass the fixed point of mitosis. The other cell-cycle phases can also be determined.

Figure 6.2 shows some examples of labelled mitoses curves obtained on human tumours. Two aspects stand out. First, duration of the S-phase, as indicated by the width of the first peaks at half-height, is approximately 20–25 h. Second, there is no evidence of a second peak in these data. This conclusion is also borne out by other data on human tumours (see Steel, 1977). The implication is that the cohort of labelled cells have completely lost synchrony in one passage through the cell cycle. The variability in cell-cycle duration must therefore be very wide. The overall picture is one of great heterogeneity in cell kinetics within an individual tumour: there is no regular 'cycle' and this is bad news for any attempt to achieve 'synchronisation therapy'.

The more recent use of flow-cytometry to determine the cell cycle is based on labelling S-phase cells with a fluorescent dye and in sequential FCM traces to follow the movement of cells through the cell cycle (Barlogie et al., 1983; also see Section 21.4). Although faster to perform, this method is not as precisely analysable as the thymidine method.

6.3.2 The growth-fraction concept

In most in vivo cell populations (tumour and normal tissues) proliferating and non-proliferating cells coexist. The growth fraction describes the proportion that are proliferating. Although this is often considered to be a simple concept, it is complicated by two factors. First, as has been indicated in the previous section, there is often a wide variation in cell-cycle duration within a tumour. Many cells are proliferating very slowly: should we include them in the growth fraction? The most reliable course of action is to use the shape of the labelled mitoses curve to describe the distribution of cell-cycle times, and tacitly therefore to use this as a definition of proliferating cells. But such a definition is not absolute.

The second factor is that cell populations of tumours are notoriously heterogeneous in terms of cell morphology. Which cells should be included in the assessment of growth fraction? Stromal cells should be excluded, as should cells that are clearly becoming necrotic, but there is still room to modify the growth fraction by adjusting the criteria for inclusion of other cell categories.

Growth fraction should be taken as a concept, rather than a precise quantity. It conveys the important therapeutic idea that some clonogenic cells may not be actively proliferating and may thus be resistant to proliferation-dependent cytotoxic drugs.

6.3.3 Cell loss from tumours: potential doubling time

Excessive cell production is the kinetic feature that is usually associated with cancer. There is a temptation to forget that carcinomas arise from epithelial tissues that are in balance between an often high rate of cell production and an equally high rate of cell loss. The loss occurs by differentiation leading, in the case of surface epithelia, to exfoliation. The histological appearance of a well-differentiated carcinoma derives from the fact that the normal process of cellular differentiation and cell loss is still taking place.

Necrosis is also a common feature of tumours, and this involves a further process of cell loss. Inadequacy of nutrient supply to a region of the tumour (coupled with the effects of cytotoxic tissue products) leads to progressive cell death.

Calculation of the rate of cell loss from tumours has been done by comparing the growth rate with the rate of cell production:

growth rate = cell-production rate − cell-loss rate

The growth rate is estimated by the doubling time of the cell population (often a volume doubling time is taken for this purpose, but this assumes that the number of viable cells per gram is constant over a short period of growth). By rate of cell production we mean the rate at which cells are being added to the tumour; every cell division adds one cell, thus the rate of cell production equals the mitotic rate (i.e., the rate at which cells are coming into mitosis). This can be found in a number of ways. A mitosis accumulation curve in the presence of a spindle poison such as colchicine or vincristine (Aherne, Camplejohn and Wright, 1977) is a direct measure of mitotic rate. Using [^{3}H]thymidine, the proportion of cells in the S-phase (LI, the labelling index after a single administration of thymidine) and the duration of the S-phase (T_s, from a labelled mitoses curve) can both be determined. Then:

$$\text{mitotic rate} \simeq \frac{LI}{T_s}$$

A fraction LI of the cells pass through the S-phase in T_s hours. The equation is not exact because the age distribution of cells in a growing population cannot be rectangular; there must always be more young cells than old. If we know the mitotic rate we can calculate the rate at which the cell population should grow in the absence of cell loss. We call this the

$$\text{potential doubling time } (T_{\text{pot}}) = \lambda \frac{T_s}{LI}$$

TABLE 6.2
Cell loss calculations for human tumours

	Thymidine labelling index (%)		Volume doubling time (days)		T_{pot}[b] (days)	Cell loss factor (%)
	cases	median (range[a])	cases	median (range[a])		
Colorectal carcinoma	12	15 (10–22)	56	90 (60–170)	3	96
Squamous cell carcinoma of head and neck	23	7 (5–17)	27	45 (33–150)	7	85
Undifferentiated bronchial carcinoma	23	19 (8–23)	55	90 (40–160)	3	97
Melanoma	25	3	8	52 (20–150)	14	73
Sarcoma	22	2 (0.3–6)	101	39 (16–78)	23	40
Lymphoma	28	3 (0.4–13)	11	22 (15–70)	16	29
Childhood tumours	14	13 (10–25)	4	20	4	82

[a] Range includes 68 % of the data ±1 SD).
[b] Calculated using $\lambda = 0.75$, $T_s = 15$ h.

where λ is a correction factor for the age distribution which lies between 0.7 and 1.0 (see Steel, 1977). Some examples of calculations of cell loss are given in Table 6.2. The cell-loss factor indicates the rate of cell loss as a fraction of the rate of cell production: 100% would indicate a steady-state situation in which loss just balances production. It can be seen that values for potential doubling time are often much less than the volume doubling time for human tumours and the derived cell-loss factors are therefore high.

The implication is that a tumour is a dynamic entity in which both cell production and cell loss are taking place; the actual growth rate is determined by the imbalance between these processes.

6.3.4 Repopulation during radiotherapy

The most interesting current application of tumour growth kinetics to radiotherapy is in the prediction of regrowth during treatment (Sections 13.2 and 21.4). To the extent that this occurs, there are more tumour cells to be killed and a higher radiation dose is required. The direct determination of repopulation rate is complicated by two factors:
  (i) Clonogenic cells are usually a small minority of tumour cells, and these are by definition the cells that we need to study. As indicated above, their properties cannot be determined using the microscope or flow cytometry because these techniques do not recognise them.
  (ii) After the start therapy, the fraction of surviving clonogenic cells becomes smaller still. A modest tumour response requires a surviving fraction of 1% or less (Section 4.5.1; Stephens and Steel, 1980). To identify such a small number of survivors among a large number of dead and dying cells is very difficult.

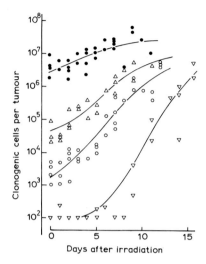

Figure 6.3. Repopulation in the Lewis lung tumour following irradiation. The tumours were implanted intramuscularly and irradiated at a size of about 0.15 g: (●) unirradiated controls, (△) 15 Gy, (o) 25 Gy, (▽) 35 Gy. The number of clonogenic cells per tumour recovers more rapidly as the radiation dose (and extent of depopulation) increases. (From Stephens and Steel, 1980.)

There is good evidence from sequential clonogenic assays on transplanted mouse tumours (Figure 6.3) that clonogenic cells can repopulate faster than the pretreatment growth rate of the tumour. It is unlikely that their doubling time for repopulation will be as short as the cell-cycle time, for non-proliferating cells may still be present. It has therefore been argued that the repopulation doubling time may be close to the potential doubling time. This implies that during repopulation cell loss from clonogenic cells is zero but that the growth fraction is the same as for the total cell population before treatment. Although this seems inherently unlikely, it may well be that T_{pot} is empirically correlated with repopulation rate. In support of this, Trott and Kummermehr (1985) found a positive correlation between time to local recurrence and T_{pot} among six types of human cancer (the correlation depended, however, on the values for prostate cancer whose T_{pot} and latency interval were twice as long as for other tumour types). The improvement in local control that comes from shortening treatment time (Section 13.2.4) also implies a doubling time that is in the region of T_{pot}.

In summary, although we have no reliable predictor of repopulation rate it seems a reasonable guess that the tumours that repopulate fast will be those that before treatment had a high S-phase fraction or short potential doubling time.

6.4 The kinetic status of clonogenic cells

The kinetic properties of clonogenic cells is a subject about which much is written but little is known. The concept of clonogenic cells derives from studies of cell proliferation in normal tissues (Section 7.4) where the maintenance of a hierarchy of differentiation requires the existence of a primitive stem cell. Tumours must arise from neoplastic transformation in stem cells. The detection of tumour stem cells requires making a single-cell suspension and testing for growth under artificial conditions (see Steel, 1977, for review). This may well distort the properties of stem cells, and it is therefore a useful convention to use the term 'clonogenic cells' for those stem cells whose properties are studied in this way. The often low in vitro cloning efficiencies of tumour cells and radiobiological arguments about curability lead to the view that the clonogenic fraction in human tumours may be very low, perhaps a fraction of 1% (see review by Steel and Stephens, 1983).

In normal tissues the most primitive stem cells often proliferate more slowly than the cells immediately derived from them (Lajtha, 1983; Lord, 1983; Potten and Hendry, 1983). This seems to be true of the pluripotent bone marrow stem cell under unstimulated conditions, also of the cells at the base of intestinal crypts. The same may not be true of tumours. Perhaps the neoplastic transformation switches on the proliferation of stem cells. We may well then have the situation described by Tannock (1968) in a transplanted mouse tumour: cells close to blood vessels proliferate rapidly but inevitably displace other cells further away from the source of nutrients. The proliferation of cells remote from blood vessels will therefore be impaired, perhaps to the point where cell death will occur, leading to necrosis. There will be a continual flow of cells away from blood vessels toward necrosis, this being one of the components of cell loss as described in Section 6.3.3. It is the cells close to blood vessels that proliferate the fastest and will be responsible for the long-term growth of the tumour. In so far as clonogenic tumour cells retain their capacity for unlimited proliferation within this worsening environment, there will be some that proliferate slowly and perhaps can be described as 'out of cycle'. This kinetic picture of tumours thus leads to the idea that, in contrast to the situation in normal tissues, clonogenic tumour cells may tend to proliferate rapidly, but that many may have a reduced growth rate because of their poor nutritive environment.

The killing effect of most cytotoxic agents depends on stage in the cell cycle. This is true of low LET radiation (Figure 3.1E) but more so of chemotherapeutic drugs. The classification by Bruce and Valeriote (1966) of cytotoxic agents in terms of their proliferation-dependence has been described in Section 4.4.1. The concepts of proliferation dependence and phase specificity are important. When combined with the ideas about slowly proliferating clonogenic cells described in the last section, they help to explain some of the causes of failure in clinical chemotherapy (see reviews by Steel, 1977; Tannock, 1978; Tubiana, 1982; van Putten, 1974).

6.5 Overview of cell proliferation and tumour response to treatment

During the 1960s and early 1970s there was considerable optimism that detailed information on the cell kinetics of tumours and critical normal tissues might allow rational and effective new treatment strategies to be developed. This has not proved to be the case. Some reasons may be listed as follows:
 (i) The kinetic heterogeneity of human tumours (Section 6.3.1)
 (ii) The difficulty of obtaining reliable kinetic data on surviving clonogenic cells (Section 6.4)
 (iii) The fact that the proliferative state of cells is usually only a minor determinant of sensitivity (except to highly proliferation-specific drugs, which therefore tend to be ineffective)

More realistic is the hope that cell kinetic data may be of empirical use in helping to predict disease progression or response to treatment. There are many published examples of correlations between proliferation rate and prognosis (for example, Silvestrini et al., 1985). The negative correlation between proliferation rate and time to recurrence is particularly clear. In recent years the detrimental effects of repopulation during fractionated radiotherapy have been recognised and a new role for kinetic studies is to select those patients that may benefit from accelerated treatment (see Sections 13.2 and 21.4).

References

Aherne, W.A., Camplejohn, R.S. and Wright, N.A. (1977) An Introduction to Cell Population Kinetics. Edward Arnold, London.
Barlogie, B., Raber, N.M., Schumann, J. et al. (1983) Flow cytometry in clinical cancer research. Cancer Res. 43, 3982–3997.
Bruce, W.R. and Valeriote, F.A. (1966) Comparison of the sensitivity of normal haemopoietic and transplanted lymphoma colony-forming cells to chemotherapeutic agents administered in vivo. J. Natl. Cancer Inst. 37, 233–245.
Lajtha, L.G. (1983) Stem-cell concepts, in: Stem Cells (Potten, C.S., ed.), Churchill Livingstone, Edinburgh.
Lord, B.I. (1983) Haemopoietic stem-cells, in: Stem Cells (Potten, C.S., ed.), Churchill Livingstone, Edinburgh.
Potten, C.S. and Hendry, J.H. (1983) Stem cells in murine small intestine, in: Stem Cells (Potten, C.S., ed.), Churchill Livingstone, Edinburgh.
Rogers, A.W. (1973) Techniques of Autoradiography, Elsevier, Amsterdam.
Silvestrini, R., Daidone, M.G., Valagussa, P. et al. (1987) Cell kinetics as a prognostic marker in locally advanced breast cancer. Cancer Treat. Rep. 71, 375–379.
Steel, G.G. (1975) Cell kinetics and cell survival, in: Medical Oncology (Bagshawe, K.D., ed.), Blackwells, Oxford.
Steel, G.G. (1977) Growth Kinetics of Tumours, Clarendon Press, Oxford.
Steel, G.G. and Stephens, T.C. (1983) Stem cells in tumours, in: Stem Cells (Potten, C.S., ed.), Churchill Livingstone, Edinburgh.

Stephens, T.C. and Steel, G.G. (1980) Regeneration of tumors after cytotoxic treatment, in: Radiation Biology in Cancer Research (Meyn, R.E. and Withers, H.R., eds.), pp. 385–395, Raven Press, New York.

Tannock, I.F. (1968) The relation between cell proliferation and the vascular system in a transplanted mouse mammary tumour. Br. J. Cancer 22, 258–273.

Tannock, I.F. (1978) Cell kinetics and chemotherapy: a critical review. Cancer Treat. Rep. 62, 1117–1133.

Trott, K.-R. and Kummermehr, J. (1985) What is known about tumour proliferation rates to choose between accelerated fractionation or hyperfractionation) Radiother. Oncol. 3, 1–9.

Tubiana, M. (1982) Cell kinetics and radiation oncology. Int. J. Radiat. Oncol. Biol. Phys. 8, 1471–1489.

Van Putten, L.M. (1974) Are cell kinetic data relevant for the design of tumour chemotherapy schedules? Cell Tissue Kinet. 7, 493–504.

CHAPTER 7

Radiation damage to early-reacting normal tissues

JOLYON H. HENDRY

Department of Radiobiology, Paterson Institute for Cancer Research, Christie Hospital and Holt Radium Institute, Manchester M20 9BX, England

7.1	Introduction	89
7.2	The acute response of the Central Nervous System (CNS)	90
	7.2.1 Prodromal responses	90
	7.2.2 The CNS syndrome	91
7.3	Modes of cell death in tissues	91
7.4	Hierarchical tissues	92
	7.4.1 Germinal tissue	94
	7.4.2 Haemopoietic tissues and the immune system	96
	7.4.3 Intestine	97
	7.4.4 Skin	98
7.5	Summary	99

7.1 Introduction

There are three types of early reacting normal tissue to irradiation. Firstly, those in which the functional ability of cells is affected by the energy deposition. Examples are the response of the central nervous system (CNS) after doses higher than 100 Gy, leading to incapacitation and death, and of the stomach after doses around 2 Gy, resulting in prodromal reactions, e.g., nausea. Secondly, those tissues in which the functional cells die quickly through apoptosis, a process previously called interphase death or shrinkage necrosis. Examples of this are thymic lymphocytes, germ cells and serous salivary-gland cells. Thirdly, those tissues which are rapidly renewed and where, although the mature functional cells may be radioresistant, their progenitor

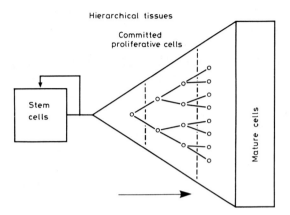

Figure 7.1. Diagrammatic representation of a cell population hierarchy where mature cells are produced from proliferative cells. The ancestors of the lineage are the stem cells which renew themselves (left arrow) and which also differentiate into various maturing cell lineages (right arrow).

cells are radiosensitive and die by mitotic failure. The cell populations in the latter tissues are 'hierarchical' in the sense that the mature functional cells are produced from divisions of precursor cells which in turn are produced from less-differentiated stem cells (Figure 7.1). Examples considered in detail here are spermatogenic epithelium, haemopoietic tissue, gastrointestinal mucosa, and epidermis. Others include oral mucosa, hair follicles and growing cartilage.

7.2 The acute response of the Central Nervous System (CNS)

7.2.1 Prodromal responses

Prodromal responses comprise the symptoms and signs appearing in individuals in the first 48 hours after irradiation of large regions of the body. After supralethal doses of several tens of grays in man, all individuals begin to experience characteristic symptoms within 15 minutes. The reactions are mediated through the response of the autonomic nervous system, and they are expressed as gastrointestinal and neuromuscular symptoms. The former are anorexia, nausea, vomiting, diarrhoea, intestinal cramps, salivation and dehydration. The neuromuscular symptoms are fatigue, apathy, listlessness, sweating, fever, headache and hypotension, followed by hypotensive shock. The reaction after high doses is maximal within 30 minutes, then it diminishes until it merges either closely with the neurological syndrome or later with the gastrointestinal syndrome (see below).

The prodromal reaction in leukaemia patients receiving 10 Gy whole-body irradiation (0.05 Gy/min) is characterised often by nausea and vomiting after the first 3–4

Gy, chills and then an acute fever in the first 24 hours. The effects are delayed, fewer and less severe following irradiation at lower dose rates or lower doses.

The doses required to produce effects in 50% of exposed subjects (i.e., ED_{50} values) for acute irradiation are about 1 Gy for anorexia and nausea, and 2–3 Gy for vomiting. The responses can be produced by separate irradiation of the head, thorax or abdomen, the last being the most sensitive region. Also, the region below the umbilicus is less responsive than the region above it.

The neural control mechanism for emesis is located in two distinct regions of the medulla oblongata in the brain: the area postrema containing the chemoreceptor trigger zone (CTZ) and the vomiting centre. The latter is the final pathway for emesis, whether the signal originates from the gastrointestinal tract or from the CTZ. Ablation of the CTZ eliminates prodromal vomiting in the dog, monkey and man. Small peptides are implicated as mediators of emesis. Inflammatory processes could be involved in post-irradiation vomiting, as suggested by the success of anti-inflammatory agents in controlling emesis in animals and in patients receiving large-field or whole-body irradiation.

7.2.2 The CNS syndrome

Doses higher than about 100 Gy to most mammalian species result in death from cerebrovascular injury within 2 days. Survival times are shorter for higher doses, and after 1000 Gy most species survive only a few hours or less. The CNS syndrome is characterised by severe prodromal symptoms and signs, followed by transient periods of depressed or enhanced motor activity before death. Histological studies in primates have shown perivascular infiltration, haemorrhages and oedema, followed by pycnosis of neurones.

7.3 Modes of cell death in tissues

The rapid death and lysis of cells (apoptosis) in a variety of tissues (Kerr et al., 1987) even after doses as low as a few centigray, is considered to be an increased incidence of the natural cell death which occurs in tissues such as the thymus and stem-cell zones in several epithelia. This mode of death is thought to be programmed so as to minimise genetic abnormalities in offspring (germ cells), minimise the risk of induced cancer (epithelia), and reduce the risk of developing auto-immune diseases (thymus). The primary event initiating the sequence is unknown, and both nuclear and cytoplasmic fragmentation are observed. The time-course extends over a period of several to many hours and is dose-dependent. The D_o can be as low as 10 cGy, and the response is independent of dose rate using such low doses. Apoptosis is important in radiotherapy regarding lymphocyte depletion, parotitis and germ-cell sterilisation.

Mitotic death is the major means of cell sterilisation and subsequent loss in most tissues (Hendry and Scott, 1987). Assays of colony-forming ability of cells in vivo or in vitro are now available for many tissues (Potten and Hendry, 1985). Stem cells in the bone marrow are more radiosensitive than stem cells in epithelia, e.g., in gut and skin. This relates in particular to the *initial slope* of the cell-survival curve, which is 3–5-times greater for bone marrow stem cells ($_1D_o \sim 1$ Gy) than for those in several epithelia (Table 7.1). This accounts in large part for the smaller dose rate and fractionation effect seen for cells in the marrow compared to epithelia after similar levels of depletion. Cells which are destined naturally to undergo only 1 or a few more divisions before maturation are usually more radioresistant then the colony-forming cells. For instance, in epidermis and in gastrointestinal mucosa there is evidence that the transit-cell divisions are very radioresistant (Potten, 1981).

7.4 Hierarchical tissues

The characteristic principal features of the radiation response of hierarchical tissues are shown in Figure 7.2, and they have been described in detail for various tissues (Potten and Hendry, 1983). If apoptosis does not occur in the mature cells, their numbers will be maintained for a short time if the last division or two of the precursor

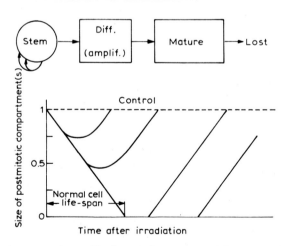

Figure 7.2. Theoretical response of a type H cell population to a range of single doses of irradiation. During the period of zero input to the mature cell compartment of new cells, the total number of these cells declines linearly at a rate equal to that which is characteristic of the steady-state conditions of the tissue concerned. The onset of complete depletion of the mature cells occurs at a time equal to the (postmitotic) lifetime of these cells. Recuperation sets in later the higher the dose (upward-pointing lines to the right of the figure), because of the lower number of surviving precursor cells. (Taken from Michalowski, 1981.)

cells is radioresistant. Then there will be a decline in the numbers of mature cells at their natural rate of senescence and loss from the tissue, with reduced or no replacement from the sterilised stem-cells.

After doses where a significant number of stem cells survive there will be a gradual regeneration of stem, committed precursor and mature cell populations. In many tissues the average cell-cycle time of the stem cells is considered to be normally around 10 days, and this reduces dramatically to round 6 hours during regeneration. However, in the latter case, the doubling time is much longer, around 24 hours, due to a concomitant differentiation of the stem cells at a rate of about 40% on average at each division (compared to 50% in the steady-state).

For those tissues where the mature cells are radioresistant and the progenitor cells are radiosensitive, the latter are the target cells for injury. If sufficient of these cells survive after a given dose, they will proliferate and differentiate to maintain the mature cell content above a critical level. As the number of surviving cells varies between samples (in mice or humans) according to a Poisson distribution there will be a dose for example where 50% of individuals survive and where 50% die (the LD_{50}). These percentages will be dose-dependent. If target theory (Section 4.2.1) is applied both to single cells and also to groups of cells required to rescue a tissue from failure (i.e., the tissue-rescuing units, TRU) or an animal from death, a combination of two exponential functions is required to relate dose and incidence of effect (Thames and Hendry, 1987).

In the simplest case of single-hit cell killing:

Fraction of cells with *no* lethal events $(S_c) = \exp(-D/D_o)$

For animal lethality:

fraction of K groups of cells (i.e., TRU) which all fail to survive $(L) = \exp(-KS_k)$

If the sensitivity $(1/D_o)$ of the TRU equates to that of the cells

$S_k = \exp(-D/D_o)$

Tissue survival is thus

$S_{tissue} = 1 - L$

and we have:

$-\ln[-\ln(1 - S_{tissue})] = D/D_o - \ln K$

94 J.H. Hendry

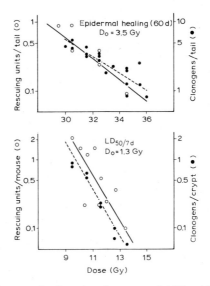

Figure 7.3. Correspondence between the D_o values for target-cell killing (right ordinates) and for the depletion of groups of cells (rescuing units, left ordinate), with respect to epidermal healing (top panel) and gut death ($LD_{50/7\,d}$ bottom panel). (Taken from Thames and Hendry, 1987.)

This has the common form $y = mx + c$. Thus the steepness of the dose-incidence curve for tissue failure, an important feature in radiotherapy (Chapter 5) depends in this way on the sensitivity of the target cells. The relationship holds only if the cells contribute independently to the regeneration of the tissue. This has been shown to be the case for the healing of small areas of the epidermis, and the survival of mice in the first week after whole-body irradiation, where comparisons are made with colony survival in vivo (Figure 7.3). However, there are other confounding features which will modify the correlation in other situations (Hendry and Moore, 1985). For example, heterogeneity among the patients or animals in the number or sensitivity of the target cells will flatten the dose-incidence curve for tissue failure, because the composite curve will be in effect a summation of a series of individually steeper curves.

The effects of fractionation and low dose rate on early-reacting hierarchical tissues mimic the corresponding effects on target cells in these tissues (Thames and Hendry, 1987). A summary of parameters is shown in Table 7.1.

7.4.1 Germinal tissue

The testis is very responsive to irradiation because the early differentiating forms of spermatogonia are extremely radiosensitive ($D_o \sim 0.2$ Gy). Spermatogonial cell necrosis can be detected in man at 4–6 hours after doses around 1 Gy. The more mature cells comprising the second and third phases of spermatogenesis are unaffected by

TABLE 7.1
Radiobiological parameters for early-reacting normal tissues

	$_1D_o$ [a] (Gy)	D_o [b] (Gy)	Exposure-time exponent (m) [c]	No. of fractions exponent [e] (n)	α/β (Gy)	Repair half-time (h)
Bone marrow	1	1.0–0.7	0.1	0.24–0.08	9–16	–
Epidermis	–	1.4–2.7[d]	0.3	0.3	10–20	1.3
Intestinal mucosa	3–4	1.3	0.3	0.3	7–12	0.5
Testis	5	1.8	–	0.3–0.07	11	–

[a] $_1D_o$ = initial inverse slope of survival curve (values quoted for target cells for long-term repopulation).
[b] D_o = final inverse slope of survival curve.
[c] $m = \dfrac{\log(D_2/D_1)}{\log(T_2/T_1)}$ and $n = \dfrac{\log(D_2/D_1)}{\log(N_2/N_1)}$ where D is total dose, T is the overall time, and N is the number of fractions in two regimens (subscripts 1 and 2).
[d] Site-dependent.
[e] Second figure applies for >4 fractions.

doses below 3 Gy. These cells mature normally after such doses, and they therefore maintain the normal sperm count in man for about 46 days, which is the time of development from preleptotene spermatocyte to spermatozoa. The sperm count begins to drop after 46 days, approaching azoospermia at about 10 weeks after doses higher than 1 Gy. The sperm count drops earlier after doses higher than 4 Gy, when the spermatids also become affected. Oligospermia in man is induced by lower doses down to 0.15 Gy.

Acute doses up to 4 Gy cause temporary or prolonged sterility in some men. The dose that induces permanent sterility in 100% of men is greater than 6 Gy. Concomitant with the histological changes, changes in testicular-hormone levels are also observed. Plasma and urinary levels of follicle-stimulating hormone increase after doses to the testis higher than 0.1 Gy, and after high doses the increase is up to four times. Plasma but not urinary levels of luteinising hormone are also elevated but not testosterone or urinary oestrogen. The target cells for long-term sterility are slowly cycling spermatogonial stem cells, which have survival characteristics similar to those for other epithelial stem cells (Table 7.1). Studies in mice have shown a good correlation between the level of stem-cell killing, the sperm count at a fixed time of recovery after irradiation, the final plateau level of recovery, and the length of the infertile period (Meistrich, 1986).

Acute doses of up to about 4 Gy cause temporary sterility in some women, and doses up to 10 Gy cause permanent sterility in an increasing proportion. Older women are more susceptible, probably because the number of follicles decreases with age. Germ cells killed by radiation become pycnotic and are removed by phagocytosis within a few days. Oocytes in different mammals show a wide variation in radiation response, the LD_{50} for primordial oocytes being of the order of 0.09 Gy in mice, higher in the rat and monkey, and reaching 4.5 Gy in women. This might reflect the different stages of arrest of the oocytes in the meiotic prophase among species.

7.4.2 Haemopoietic tissues and the immune system

Animals die from marrow failure within 30 days after whole-body acute doses between about 2 and 10 Gy, and the $LD_{50/30}$ is related to body weight (UNSCEAR, 1982). The values range from about 7 Gy for mice down to 2 Gy for sheep. In man, there are deaths up to 60 days, and the $LD_{50/60}$ is about 2.5–3.0 Gy for individuals receiving little or no medical treatment or for ill cancer patients receiving good medical care, and up to 5 Gy for healthy individuals receiving good medical care. The $LD_{50/60}$ can be further increased by successful marrow transplantation, probably to around 9 Gy. After these higher doses there may be some cases of pneumonitis occurring in the second month. After even higher doses (> 10 Gy) acute gastrointestinal injury becomes more prevalent.

Death from bone marrow failure is associated variously among species with granulocytopenia, thrombocytopenia and lymphopenia. In most species, anaemia is less severe than neutropenia or thrombopenia and does not correlate well with time of death. This is due partly to the radioresistance and long life span of red blood cells (120 days in man). Haemorrhage is not a major problem after doses in the LD_{50} range, but becomes increasingly important with higher doses. Similarly, thrombocytopenia, occurring because of the sensitivity of megakaryocytes and the relatively short life time of platelets in the blood (8 days in man) is not regarded as a major contributor to mortality in the LD_{50} range but becomes increasingly important after higher doses.

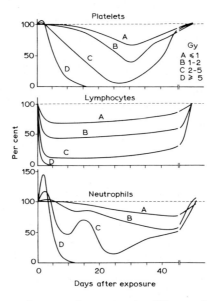

Figure 7.4. Schematic picture of average time-courses for different cells in the blood after various doses of radiation in man, derived from accident cases (Redrawn from Wald, 1971.)

A schematic picture of the average time-courses for the various blood cell types after different ranges of dose, deduced from accidental human exposures, is shown in Figure 7.4. The lymphocyte count is the most sensitive index of radiation injury in the blood in the sense that for the same dose, nadir levels are reached earlier than for the other cell types. Lymphocytes die in interphase, and doses of 1–2 Gy cause a decline to 50% of normal numbers by 48 hours. Neutrophil counts often show an initial abortive rise, probably due to a transient mobilisation of cells from marrow and/or extramedullary sites and to an accelerated maturation of precursor cells. This phase is followed by a dose-dependent decline, and then a second abortive rise starting at about day 10 after doses below 5 Gy. This is due to haemopoiesis recovering from the precursor cell populations, which is a good prognostic sign. Long-term recovery from surviving haemopoietic stem cells becomes apparent from day 25 in man, with sustained increases in neutrophils and platelets in the blood (Figure 7.4). The target cells at doses around the $LD_{50/60}$ are probably the granulocyte precursor cells, and survival and differentiation of these helps in counteracting infection long enough to allow haemopoietic repopulation from the stem cells. Attempts are currently being made to use growth factors (GM-CSF and G-CSF) to stimulate an earlier and greater recovery of granulocytes in cases of accidental whole-body irradiation or therapeutic cytotoxic treatments.

Marked alterations in the immune system are caused by doses of irradiation of the order of a few grays, leading in general to an increased susceptibility to infections. Immune responses involve both T and B lymphocytes, and suppressor T cells are more radiosensitive than helper T cells, with B cells having an intermediate sensitivity. There is also an impairment of the normal recirculation of lymphocytes. The overall effects are complex, and they may result in an augmented or suppressed response to the same antigen, depending on the dose and the time between irradiation and the introduction of the antigen (Anderson and Warner, 1976; Workshop, 1988).

Residual deficiencies in irradiated haemopoietic tissues include a persistently reduced complement of stem cells and a developing anaemia (Testa and Gale, 1988).

7.4.3 Intestine

Animals receiving doses of between about 10 and 50 Gy die between 3.5 and 9 days later with signs of intestinal damage. The symptoms in man follow those of the prodromal phase and include anorexia, increased lethargy, diarrhoea, infection and loss of fluids and electrolytes. Other signs include weight loss, diminishing food and water intake, gastric retention and decreased intestinal absorption. The leukocyte count falls dramatically, and there may be haemorrhages and bacteraemia which aggravate the injury. The incidence of intestinal death can be reduced by transfusions with balanced salt solutions and antibiotics. For example, the $LD_{50/5\ days}$ in rats can be increased by a factor 1.4.

Intestinal damage is due to sterilisation of the progenitor cells, with subsequent depletion of the intestinal mucosa (the villi) at a rate characteristic of the normal turnover time. This is about 3–4 days in man and in conventionally housed mice, and longer in germ-free animals. The $LD_{50/7\ days}$ is about 11 Gy in conventionally housed mice and other species, and higher following irradiation of the abdomen alone (with leukocyte influence largely preserved) or with whole-body irradiation of SPF animals. The $LD_{50/7\ days}$ in conventionally housed mice corresponds to the survival of about 40% of crypts. The correspondence of survival of animals and colony-forming cells is shown in Figure 7.3, and radiobiological parameters for the small intestine are quoted in Table 7.1. At present it is considered that there may be up to 30–40 colony-forming cells in each crypt, including a few (1–4) cells that operate as stem cells in the unirradiated crypt.

Residual injury in the intestinal mucosa is characterised by persistently fewer, larger and more radioresistant crypts, the latter being due to induced hypoxia.

7.4.4 Skin

The earliest effect in skin after high doses is a transient erythema which appears and disappears within hours (up to a day), followed by a second wave beginning at about a week after irradiation. A dose of about 6 Gy results in marked erythema in 50% of individuals using 10×10 cm^2 fields. Erythema has been quantified using spectrophotometry. Marked erythema is followed by desquamation in increasing proportions of individuals after doses above 12 Gy, and the severity of the reaction depends on many factors, e.g., anatomical location, vascularity and oxygenation of the skin, genetic background, age and hormonal status. Moist desquamation in 50% of individuals occurs after about 20 Gy, and the maximum reaction is at about 3 weeks.

Desquamation reactions are due primarily to the killing of cells in the basal layer of the epidermis and its associated hair follicles (Potten, 1985). This has been shown in pig skin by the use of radiations with different energies and hence different penetrations. The effects were the same for equal doses to the basal layer. The time to full depletion of the epidermis after high doses is independent of dose, and the time corresponds to the transit time from the least-differentiated but committed progenitor cell in the basal layer to the surface in unirradiated epidermis. After low doses the epidermis repopulates from surviving stem cells. These have radiobiological characteristics similar to those of other epithelial cells (Table 7.1). In mice, it has been shown that the colony-forming stem cells constitute 10% of the cells in the basal layer, with one stem cell at the origin of each epidermal proliferative unit (EPU).

Skin reactions have been used extensively in mice, pigs and man for assessing many radiobiological variables. Peak reactions, average reaction over a defined period, percentages of animals with reactions that heal, have all been used. In general, the parameters reflect those of the underlying target cells for the desquamatory reactions, namely the stem cells in the basal layer which colonise the depleted epidermis. There is a field-size effect for the skin, due largely to the lower tolerance of large desquamated areas of skin in healing satisfactorily.

Haemorrhages appear in the skin as small (petechiae) or large (purpura) lesions, within weeks after irradiation with doses of 4–6 Gy which also cause epilation. After high doses they are more severe and occur earlier. After very high doses to extremities, pain is often a feature which corresponds to the appearance of vascular lesions.

Residual effects in irradiated skin include a thin and dry epidermis, a lower density of colony-forming cells in the basal layer, and the appearance of dermal injury, e.g., induration, dermal necrosis and fibrosis (Jammet et al., 1986).

7.5 Summary

Radiation damage to early-reacting tissues is due to injury to cell function in a few specific tissues or to cell loss in the majority. The characteristics of cell loss can be described adequately in terms of a target-cell framework of responses of hierarchical-type tissues. Current studies are aimed in particular at elucidating the regulatory mechanisms for these cell populations, normally and during recovery from injury, which involves the stroma.

References

Anderson, R.E. and Warner, N.L. (1976) Ionising radiation and the immune response. Adv. Immunol. 24, 215–335.

Hendry, J.H. and Moore, J.V. (1985) Is the steepness of the dose incidence curves for tumour control or complications due to variation before, or as a result of irradiation? Br. J. Radiol. 57, 1045–1046.

Hendry, J.H. and Scott, D. (1987) Loss of reproductive integrity of irradiated cells, and its importance in tissues, in: Perspectives on Cell Death. (Potten, C.S. ed.), pp. 160–183, Oxford University Press, Oxford.

Jammet, H., Dabuson, F., Gerber, G.B. et al. (eds.) (1986) Radiation damage to skin; fundamental and practical aspects. Br. J. Radiol. (Suppl. 19), 1–159.

Kerr, J.F.R., Searle, J., Harmon, B.V. and Bishop, C.J. (1987) Apoptosis. in: Perspectives on Cell Death. (Potten, C.S., ed.), pp. 93–128, Oxford University Press, Oxford.

Michalowski, A.S. (1981) Effects of radiation in normal tissues: hypothetical mechanisms and limitations of in situ assays of clonogenicity. Radiat. Environ. Biophys. 19, 157–172.

Meistrich, M.L. (1986) Relationship between spermatogonial cell survival and testis function after cytotoxic therapy. Br. J. Cancer 53, (Suppl. VII), 89–101.

Potten, C.S. (1981) The cell kinetic mechanism for radiation-induced cellular depletion of epithelial tissues based on hierarchical differences in radiosensitivity. Int. J. Radiat. Biol. 40, 217–225.

Potten, C.S. and Hendry, J.H. (eds.) (1983) Cytotoxic Insult to Tissue: Effects on Cell Lineages. Churchill Livingstone, Edinburgh.

Potten, C.S. (1985) Radiation and Skin. Taylor and Francis, London.

Potten, C.S. and Hendry, J.H. (1985) Cell Clones: Manual of Mammalian Cell Techniques. Churchill

Livingstone, Edinburgh.
Testa, N.G. and Gale, R.P. (eds.) (1988) Hematopoiesis; Long-Term Effects of Chemotherapy and Radiation. Hematology, Vol. 8, Marcel Dekker, New York.
Thames, H.D. and Hendry, J.H. (1987) Fractionation in Radiotherapy, Taylor and Francis, London.
UNSCEAR (1982) Non-stochastic effects of irradiation. Annex J, United Nations Committee on the Effects of Atomic Radiation. Report to the General Assembly, New York, pp. 571–654.
Wald, N. (1971) Hematological parameters after acute radiation injury, *in*: Manual on Radiation Haematology. pp. 253–264, I.A.E.A., Vienna.
Workshop on low-dose radiation and the immune system (1988) Int. J. Radiat. Biol. 53, No. 1.

CHAPTER 8

Radiation effects on blood vessels: role in late normal tissue damage

JOHN W. HOPEWELL[1], W. CALVO[2] and HUIBERT S. REINHOLD[3]

[1]*CRC Normal Tissue Radiobiology Research Group, Research, Institute (University of Oxford), The Churchill Hospital, Headington, Oxford OX3 7LJ, England,* [2]*Department of Clinical Physiology and Occupational Medicine, University of Ulm, Ulm, F.R.G. and* [3]*Department of Experimental Radiotherapy, Erasmus University, Rotterdam and Radiobiological Institute TNO, Rijswijk, The Netherlands*

8.1 Introduction 101

8.2 Radiation effects on potential target cells 102
     8.2.1 Endothelial cells 102
     8.2.2 Smooth muscle cells 106

8.3 Blood vessels at risk after irradiation 107

8.4 Vascular changes and normal tissue damage 109
     8.4.1 Pig skin 109
     8.4.2 Rat brain 110

8.5 Conclusion 112

8.1 Introduction

Irradiation with therapeutic doses of ionising radiation may result in damage to the normal tissues included within the treatment volume. In the so-called early reacting normal tissues, damage may appear shortly after irradiation with single doses or during the course of therapy with fractionated doses. In late-reacting normal tissues, damage may develop several months or even years after therapy. This chapter deals predominantly with the likely pathogenesis of lesions appearing in the late-responding normal tissues.

Since the very early observations by Gassman (1899) and Wolbach (1909) that blood vessels in irradiated tissues showed changes, a general consensus appears to have developed amongst pathologists that blood vessels are sensitive to radiation. This view was later developed into a general hypothesis (Rubin and Casarett, 1968) which proposed that radiation-induced damage to blood vessels was the dose-limiting component in the development of lesions in late-responding normal tissues. Although this hypothesis has been rightly challenged (Withers et al., 1980) there is still a wealth of information linking late-radiation effects with damage to the vasculature. However, the exact role of the vasculature in the development of late effects still remains uncertain.

In order to identify direct evidence for the role of vascular damage, two key questions need to be answered: (a) what are the time and dose-related changes in the number of potential target cells within the blood vessel wall? and (b) what are the vessel types predominantly at risk after irradiation?

These basic questions can be answered by examining the results of experiments obtained using simple tissue systems such as the hamster cheek pouch and the gut mesentery of the mouse. The observations can then be used to help interpret the changes seen in more complex tissues. In complex tissues the question of whether effects seen in the parenchyma, after therapeutic doses of radiation, are a primary or secondary lesion still has to be answered. Recent studies in the skin and the central nervous system point to a primary role for the vasculature in the development of late effects in these tissues. Parenchymal cell loss may be secondary to vascular damage in these tissues.

8.2 Radiation effects on potential target cells

8.2.1 Endothelial cells

There have been relatively few quantitative studies showing the time-scale of changes in the endothelium after irradiation. However, in the two most detailed investigations on the vasculature of the mouse mesentery (Hirst et al., 1980) and on the choroid plexus in the rat brain (Calvo et al., 1987), there was general agreement that a relatively early loss of endothelial cells occurred after irradiation with single doses of 17.5–30 Gy of X-rays. A significant reduction in the number of endothelial cells was seen after 6 weeks in the arteries and arterioles of the mesentery (Figure 8.1). In the choroid plexus, endothelial cells in vessels of differing morphology were counted. The results suggested a small reduction in the number of endothelial cells after 1 week, and the reduction reached a plateau beyond 12–26 weeks after irradiation (Figure 8.2).

The curves showing the time-course of the radiation-induced loss of endothelial cells from the choroid plexus could be well fitted by an equation which included a single-exponential function plus a constant. The constant represents the plateau level,

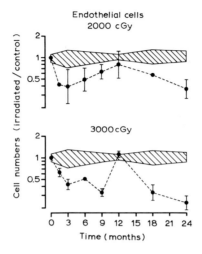

Figure 8.1. Time-related changes in the relative number of endothelial cells in the walls of arterioles in the irradiated mesentery of the mouse. Hatched areas show controls; error bars indicate ±SE. (Redrawn from Hirst et al., 1980.)

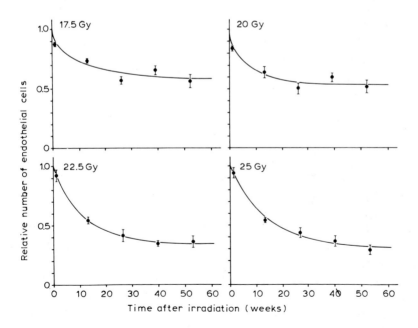

Figure 8.2. Time-related changes in the relative number of endothelial cells in the walls of vessels of the choroid plexus in the irradiated rat brain (from Calvo et al., 1987). The dose-effect curves were redrawn using the equation $Y = a\,e^{bX} + c$. Error bars indicate ±SE. (Courtesy of A. v.d. Berg.)

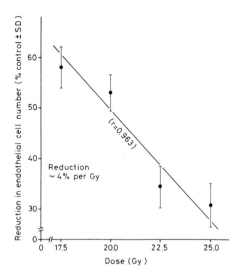

Figure 8.3. Dose-related changes in the maximum reduction (c in the legend to Fig. 8.2) in the relative number of endothelial cells in the vessels of the choroid plexus of the irradiated rat brain. Error bars indicate ±SE.

or the maximum reduction in endothelial cell number, and this level was slightly lower at the higher radiation doses. The slopes of the initial exponential part of the curves were consistent with a mean half-time of 8.4 ±0.6 weeks (range 6.7–9.6 weeks). The rate of endothelial cell loss was independent of the radiation dose. The results obtained for the mesenteric vessels are consistent with these findings. This strongly indicates that the endothelium is not an homogeneous population of cells with a uniformly long cell-cycle time, but that it contains a small subpopulation of cells with a relatively rapid turnover. The average turnover time of endothelial cells in normal tissues, based on the low labelling index, has been estimated to be in excess of 100 days (Hobson and Denekamp, 1984). Clearly, more information is needed on the cell-population kinetics of the endothelium if its response to radiation is to be fully understood.

The maximum reduction in endothelial cell number in both the above systems was dose-related, but not markedly so. In the case of the choroid plexus, when the residual plateau levels were plotted against dose, a linear dose-effect curve could be fitted to the data with a slope suggesting only a small (4%) reduction in the number of endothelial cells per gray (Figure 8.3). This value is similar to that reported by Ward et al. (1985) for the dose-related reduction in angiotensin-converting enzyme (ACE) in the lung of rats at 2 and 6 months after irradiation. ACE may simply be acting as a marker of endothelial cells and hence this decline in ACE actively represents the dose-related reduction in endothelial cell number in the lung at these late times. Alternatively, it could simply reflect a radiation-induced change in endothelial cell function.

In marked contrast to these findings, dose-effect curves obtained from assays which have attempted to assess clonogenic survival in endothelial cells were much steeper (for review see Reinhold et al., 1985). The curves showed approximately two decades of 'cell kill' for a 10 Gy increment in dose. The D_o values obtained from such curves were in the range 1.7–2.6 Gy, comparable to those for endothelial cells and other cell types in culture (Hopewell, 1983). It is of interest to note that in assay systems which have involved the counting of capillary sprouts, where it is possible that only subclonogenic endothelial cell proliferation was assessed, the D_o values were significantly higher. The slopes of such curves were more akin to those for the loss of endothelial cells in intact tissues. This adds weight to the suggestion (Reinhold et al., 1985) that the radiobiological concept of unlimited cell proliferation may be inappropriate in such slowly dividing tissues as the endothelium where tissue integrity may, to some extent, be preserved by only a few cell divisions.

Evidence for an attempt at endothelial cell repopulation was reported in the choroid plexus and the gut mesentery after the initial loss of endothelial cells. In the case of the mesenteric arteries there was a temporary recovery in the density of endothelial cells (Figure 8.1). In the choroid plexus, evidence for an attempt at repopulation was shown by the appearance of mitotic figures, endothelial cell nuclear enlargement and the presence of pairs or groups of endothelial cell nuclei randomly distributed along the walls of blood vessels that were otherwise devoid of endothelial cell nuclei. These groups of cells sometimes occluded the lumen of the blood vessels. Similar changes have been reported in the vasculature of many tissues after irradiation (Hopewell et al., 1986) but have been quantified for the first time in the vessels of the choroid plexus (Figure 8.4). This phenomenon occurred frequently: pairs or groups of endothelial

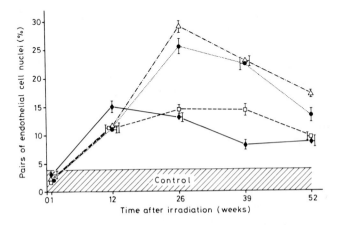

Figure 8.4. Time-related changes in the proportion of endothelial nuclear pairs or groups in the vasculature of the choroid plexus after single doses of X-rays. Error bars indicate ±SE, the shaded area represents the error for unirradiated control animals. (Redrawn from Calvo et al., 1987.) ♦ —— ♦, 17.5 Gy; □ – –□, 20 Gy; ●····●, 22.5 Gy; △ · – · △, 25 Gy.

cell nuclei occupied around 30% of all endothelial nuclear sites 26 weeks after 22.5 and 25 Gy.

The differences in the time-course of the change in the number of endothelial cells between 12 weeks and 52 weeks after irradiation in the mesentery (Figure 8.1), as compared with the choroid plexus (Figure 8.2), might in part be explained by the differences in the types of vessel examined in the two studies. It might also reflect a difference in the time-course of responses of other components in the blood vessel walls in the two vascular networks.

8.2.2 Smooth muscle cells

Smooth muscle cells are a major component of the walls of arteries and arterioles, forming the tunica media. Degeneration of this layer and its replacement by hyaline material, fibrinoid or fibrotic tissue is a common finding in human radiation pathology. However, experimental studies involving smooth muscle cells are fewer in number than those involving endothelial cells. The time-scale for the loss of smooth muscle cells may depend on the radiation dose and the type of tissue irradiated. This can be illustrated by a comparison of effects seen in the mesenteric vessels and those of the choroid plexus (Table 8.1). The degeneration of smooth muscle cells occurred earlier in the choroid plexus. The median latency time for the appearance of this effect in this tissue was also dose-related.

In the studies by Hirst et al. (1980), the second wave of depletion of endothelial cells (Figure 8.1) was attributed to the later degeneration of the tunica media. The failure of the endothelium of the choroid plexus to show any increase in the number of cells after 26–52 weeks, in the presence of some evidence for an attempt at repopulation, might be explained by the earlier degeneration of the tunica media in this tissue.

TABLE 8.1
Time of onset of degenerative changes in the smooth muscle cells of arteries and arterioles in the vasculature of the choroid plexus of the rat brain and of the mouse mesentery after irradiation

X-ray dose (Gy)	Estimated *minimum* latency time (weeks)	
	choroid plexus[a]	mesentery[b]
20	>26 (>52)[c]	>52
22.5	>20 (46.4+4.0)[c]	–
25	>13 (29.8+3.8)[c]	–
30	–	>39

[a] Estimated from Hopewell et al. (1989).
[b] Estimated from Hirst et al. (1980).
[c] Values in parentheses indicate the *median* latency $\pm$SE.

Clearly, interaction between endothelial and smooth muscle cells is possible but is little understood.

8.3 Blood vessels at risk after irradiation

The radiation pathology and radiobiological literature is inundated with reports outlining the types of lesion that may be seen in vessels after irradiation (for recent review see Reinhold et al., 1989). Of the vessels at risk, the capillaries are frequently reported to be the most sensitive: a reduction in the capillary density is one of the most important mechanisms leading to delayed normal-tissue injury. However, the frequently proposed link between the radiosensitivity of endothelial cells and the loss of capillaries may be over simplistic. The loss of a single endothelial cell does not necessarily lead to the loss of a capillary. The cytoplasm of endothelial cells has a large capacity for expansion, even in vitro, and so the death of a single cell is very unlikely to result in the loss of a segment of the capillary bed.

Time-related changes in the vasculature of the hamster cheek pouch were investigated systematically (Hopewell et al., 1989) after irradiation with a single dose of 25 Gy (Figure 8.5). The first significant changes were seen as early as 1 month after

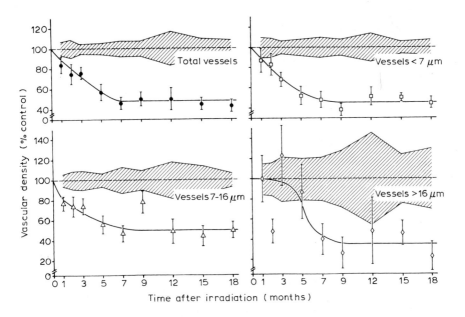

Figure 8.5. Time-related changes in the relative number of blood vessels of different sizes in the vasculature of the hamster cheek pouch after irradiation with 25 Gy. Error bars indicate ±SE; the shaded areas represent the errors on age-matched unirradiated control values. (Redrawn from Hopewell et al., 1989.)

irradiation, a reduction in the number of vessels 7–16 μm in diameter; this possibly represents the smaller arterioles. These changes corresponded with the time of appearance of macroscopic focal occlusive changes in the arterioles. At these early times after irradiation there was no evidence for a significant reduction in the number of vessels below 7 μm in diameter. However, the number of capillaries was significantly reduced after 3 months. The number of vessels of less than 7 μm and 7–16 μm in diameter then declined further, reaching a plateau level approximately half that in unirradiated cheek pouches beyond 5 months after irradiation. Although there was much scatter in the data, a consistent reduction in the number of vessels of less than 16 μm in diameter was seen only beyond 7 months after irradiation.

At 7 months after irradiation, reduction in the number of vessels of less than 7 μm and 7–16 μm in diameter were dose-related (Figure 8.6). The dose-effect curves were shallow and suggested a reduction in the vessel density of approximately 4% per gray for doses in the range 15–25 Gy. These results show remarkable similarity to those previously reported for the loss of endothelial cells from the choroid plexus after irradiation (Figure 8.3). At 7 months, only the cheek pouches irradiated with 25 Gy showed a significant reduction in the number of vessels of greater than 16 μm in diameter.

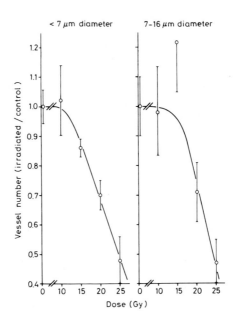

Figure 8.6. Dose-related changes in the relative number of vessels of less than 7 μm and 7–16 μm in diameter in the vasculature of the hamster cheek pouch 30 weeks after irradiation. Error bars indicate ±SE.

8.4 Vascular changes and normal tissue damage

8.4.1 Pig skin

A number of the changes in blood vessels that have been documented in simple tissue systems can also be found in the vasculature of the dermis after irradiation. These vessel changes precede and contribute to the development of late injury in this tissue. Late tissue injury in the dermis is characterised by atrophy and, after higher doses, necrosis. A schematic representation of the time-related changes in the dermal tissue of the pig after irradiation is given in Figure 8.7.

A reduction in the number of endothelial cells and an associated decline in the vascular density was seen at relatively early times after irradiation (Archambeau et al., 1984). There was also an increased separation between the remaining endothelial cell nuclei. This greater cell separation may result in an increased vascular permeability with the appearance of oedema, manifest by 6 weeks after a single dose of approximately 18 Gy of X-rays.

The reduction in the number of endothelial cells was also associated with an abortive attempt at regeneration, and groups of endothelial cells were found to occlude the lumen of many arterioles (Hopewell, 1983). The presence of occluded vessels and of oedema would be expected to produce a further reduction in the vascular density and in the dermal blood flow. At 12 weeks, after irradiation with single doses of

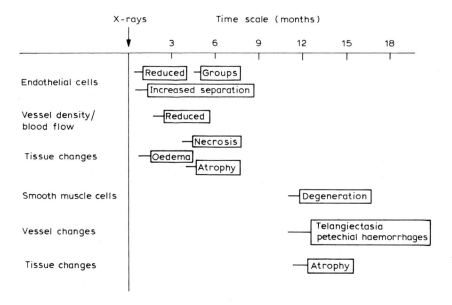

Figure 8.7. Time-scale of radiation-induced changes in pig skin.

18–23.4 Gy, the reduction in blood flow was dose-related (Moustafa and Hopewell, 1979). The additional reduction in blood flow over this dose-range, when assessed by isotope clearance, was again of the order of 4% per gray.

Reduction in vascularity was associated with the development of ischaemic dermal necrosis after high doses (>20 Gy, equivalent single dose) and dermal atrophy after lower doses. Dermal atrophy developed rapidly, between 14 weeks and 22 weeks after irradiation (Hopewell et al., 1989) with no additional changes occurring between 22 weeks and 52 weeks. Resting blood flow and vascular density were apparently normal in atrophic dermal tissue. There was no reduction in the number of parenchymal fibroblast nuclei prior to the development of dermal atrophy. A loss of fibroblast nuclei only seemed to occur in association with the development of general tissue atrophy, after longer than 14 weeks (Hamlet and Hopewell, 1988).

Measurements of dermal thickness (Hopewell et al., 1989) also indicated a further phase of dermal thinning between 52 weeks and 65 weeks after irradiation. Although the underlying mechanisms responsible for these later effects are uncertain, this gross change was associated with histological evidence for the degeneration of the tunica media of arterioles, the presence of petechial haemorrhages and of foci of necrosis. Telangiectatic vessels were also seen in histological sections at these late times. The time-scale for the appearance of telangiectatic vessels in pig skin parallelled the development of these changes in human skin after radiotherapy (Turesson and Notter, 1986).

8.4.2 Rat brain

The patterns of changes in the vasculature are more complex in an heterogeneous structure such as the brain than in dermal tissue. In the brain there again are two phases of development of late radiation-induced damage. However, these are not so clearly separated in time as in dermal tissue. The two phases of damage have been characterised by a selective necrosis of white matter with a latency of less than 12 months and a more generalised telangiectasia with a latency of greater than 12 months. The suggested relationships of these two phases of damage to vascular effects are illustrated in Figure 8.8. Not illustrated is the fact that the latency for the appearance of these effects and many of the changes that preceded them are dose-related.

The role of vascular damage in the development of selective white matter necrosis has been evaluated recently in the fimbria of the hippocampus (Calvo et al., 1988). The first detectable change, already present 3 months after irradiation, was a reduction in the density of endothelial cells and in the vascular density. The vessels present in the fimbria were predominantly capillaries and venules. Reactive changes were seen in the remaining blood vessels. These were characterised by a dilation of the blood vessels, an enlargement of endothelial cell nuclei, a thickening of the blood vessel wall, and the hypertrophy of perivascular astrocytes. The incidence of these

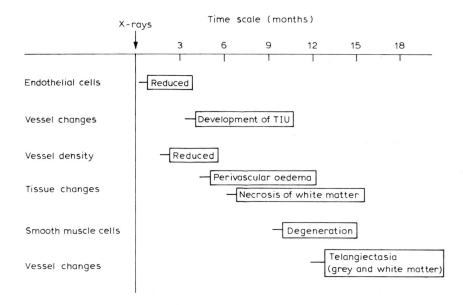

Figure 8.8. Time-scale of radiation-induced changes in the rat brain. TIU = tissue-injury unit (see text).

four factors was highly correlated and collectively they were referred to as a 'tissue-injury unit' (TIU). These phenomena appeared to increase in severity and incidence until necrosis ensued. Perivascular oedema and the appearance of groups or pairs of endothelial cell nuclei in the walls of the blood vessels were associated features and both could have contributed to an additional reduction in the vascular density, ischaemia eventually resulting in the development of necrosis.

At no time prior to the onset of white matter necrosis, after single doses of 22.5 and 25 Gy of X-rays, was there evidence for a reduction in the number of parenchymal glial cells, indeed just prior to the development of necrosis the number of astrocytes was increased. This suggested that the astrocyte component of the TIU was represented both by hypertrophy and a limited hyperplasia. There was also histological evidence of possible oligodendrocyte hyperplasia in areas adjacent to the necrosis. It thus would seem that glial cells proliferate, at least to a limited extent, after single doses of 20–25 Gy.

The underlying mechanism responsible for the development of late telangiectasia in both grey and white-matter regions of the brain, after doses which did not produce necrosis, is less certain. However, the degeneration of the smooth muscle cells of the tunica media of arterioles and its replacement by hyaline material is an associated feature. This may lead to a failure in the control of capillary pressure. Alternatively, telangiectatic vessels may represent a gross expression of the TIU; histological evidence for changes consistent with TIU were found at earlier times after doses which did not lead to the development of necrosis.

8.5 Conclusion

In any review of this type only a simplified view of the pattern of change observed can be presented. This is particularly true in the study of radiation-induced late effects. There is a complex relationship between cells in the vessel wall and the vasculature, and between the vasculature and the parenchyma of the tissue it supplies. These may produce tissue-specific changes which are of interest but this does not influence the general pattern of reaction.

There is general agreement, in both simple and more complex tissues, for an early loss of endothelial cells. The magnitude of that loss is not strongly dose-related for doses close to what might conventionally be termed 'late normal-tissue tolerance'. It amounts to a 4% reduction in cell number per gray. The dose-effect relationships for the loss of blood vessels and for reduction in tissue blood flow are of the same order of magnitude.

An attempt by endothelial cells to repopulate depleted areas of the vessel wall can lead to the presence of groups of cells that may themselves occlude the lumen of a vessel. This change and the presence of tissue oedema may be a further contributing cause to the reduction in the size of the capillary bed. It is the reduction in the size of the capillary network that leads to the development of late tissue injury within 12 months of irradiation.

The mechanisms responsible for tissue changes developing at later times, including telangiectasia, are less well understood. However, evidence for a delayed degeneration of the smooth muscle cells of the tunica media of arterioles may represent a possible mechanism responsible for their development and for other changes developing at very late times after irradiation. This is an important avenue for future research.

References

Archambeau, J.O., Ines, A. and Fajardo, L.F. (1984) Response of the swine skin microcirculation to acute single exposures of X-rays: quantification of endothelial cell changes. Radiat. Res. 98, 37–51.

Calvo, W., Hopewell, J.W., Reinhold, H.S., Van den Berg, A.P. and Yeung, T.K. (1987) Dose-dependent and time-dependent changes in the choroid plexus of the irradiated rat brain. Br. J. Radiol. 60, 1109–1117.

Calvo, W., Hopewell, J.W., Reinhold, H.S. and Yeung, T.K. (1988) Time and dose-related changes in the white matter of the rat brain after single doses of X-rays. Br. J. Radiol. 61, 1043–1052.

Gassman, A. (1899) Zur Histologica der Röntgenulara. Fortschr. Roentgenstr. 2, 199–207.

Hamlet, R. and Hopewell, J.W. (1988) A quantitative assessment of changes in the dermal fibroblast population of pig skin after single doses of X-rays. Int. J. Radiat. Biol. 54, 675–682.

Hirst, D.G., Denekamp, J. and Hobson, B. (1980) Proliferative studies of the endothelia and smooth muscle cells of the mouse mesentery after irradiation. Cell Tissue Kinet. 13, 91–104.

Hobson, B. and Denekamp, J. (1984) Endothelial proliferation in tumours and normal tissues: continuous labelling studies. Brit. J. Cancer 49, 405–413.

Hopewell, J.W. (1983) Radiation effects on vascular tissue, in: Cytotoxic Insult to Tissue: Effects on Cell

Lineages. (Potten, C.S. and Hendry, J.H., eds.), pp. 228–257, Churchill Livingstone, Edinburgh.

Hopewell, J.W., Calvo, W., Campling, D., Reinhold, H.S., Rezvani, M. and Yeung, T.K. (1989) Effects of radiation on the microvasculature: implications for normal tissue damage. Front. Radiat. Ther. 23, in press.

Hopewell, J.W., Campling, D., Calvo, W., Reinhold, H.S., Wilkinson, J.H. and Yeung, T.K. (1986) Vascular irradiation damage: its cellular basis and likely consequences. Br. J. Cancer 53 (Suppl. VII), 181–191.

Moustafa, H.F. and Hopewell, J.W. (1979) Blood flow clearance changes in pig skin after single doses of X-rays. Br. J. Radiol. 52, 138–144.

Reinhold, H.S., Fajardo, L.F. and Hopewell, J.W. (1989) The vascular system, in: Relative Radiosensitivity of Human Organ Systems, Vol. II, (Lett, J.T. and Altman, K.I., eds.), Academic Press, New York.

Reinhold, H.S., Hopewell, J.W. and Busman, G.H. (1985) Colony regeneration technique in vascular endothelium, in: Cell Clones; Manual of Mammalian Cell Techniques. (Potten, C.S. and Hendry, J.H., eds.), pp. 160–169, Churchill Livingstone, Edinburgh.

Rubin, P. and Casarett, G.W. (1968) Clinical Radiation Pathology, Vols. I and II, W.B. Saunders, Philadelphia.

Turesson, I. and Notter, G. (1986) The predictive value of skin telangiectasia for late effects in different normal tissues. Int. J. Radiat. Oncol. Biol. Phys. 12, 603–609.

Ward, W.F., Moltoni, A., Solliday, N.H. and Jones, G.F. (1985) The relationship between endothelial dysfunction and collagen accumulation in irradiated rat lung. Int. J. Radiat. Oncol. Biol. Phys. 11, 1985–1990.

Withers, H.R., Peters, L.J. and Kogelnik, H.D. (1980) The pathobiology of late effects of irradiation, in: Radiation Biology in Cancer Research (Meyn, R.E. and Withers, H.R., eds.), pp. 439–448, Raven Press, New York.

Wolbach, S.B. (1909) The pathological histology of chronic X-ray dermatitis and early X-ray carcinoma. J. Med. Res. 21, 415–449.

CHAPTER 9

Physiological hypoxia and its influence on radiotherapy

JULIANA DENEKAMP

CRC Gray Laboratory, Mount Vernon Hospital, Northwood, Middlesex HA6 2RN, England

---

9.1 Hypoxic radioresistance results from vascular insufficiency 115

9.2 Reoxygenation 118
    9.2.1   Detection of hypoxic cells 121

9.3 Chemical radiosensitizers 123
    9.3.1   Enhancing sensitizer efficiency by thiol depletion 124

9.4 Sensitization by increased oxygen delivery 125

9.5 Utilising hypoxic radioresistance 127
    9.5.1   Induction of normal-tissue hypoxia 127
    9.5.2   Chemical radioprotection 128

9.6 Combined tumour radiosensitizers and normal-tissue radioprotectors 130

9.7 Conclusions 131

9.1 Hypoxic radioresistance results from vascular insufficiency

The vascular network that has evolved in all higher animals is an efficient method of delivering oxygen and other nutrients to each cell in the body. The erythrocytes contain haemoglobin which has a very high affinity for oxygen and can carry approximately 10-times as much oxygen as would be dissolved in a simple liquid. Because high concentrations of haemoglobin are toxic to cells, it is contained within the cell membrane of the highly deformable erythrocyte which can pass through very small capillaries. Oxygen is taken up across the thin membrane between the alveolar gas space in the lungs and the blood in the adjacent capillary space. The average oxygen tension in venous blood is 40 mmHg, and this increases to 100 mmHg as it passes through the lungs towards the arterial circuit.

In early development, the capillary bed in each tissue is developed with a characteristic architecture, so that the metabolic requirements of all cells in that tissue will be met. Most tissues have an excess of vessels, many of which are intermittently closed, but can open to meet additional demands. The capillary flow is controlled by precapillary sphincters, the arterial and venous flow and the cardiac output by the sympathetic nervous system and by various hormones (e.g., angiotensin, adrenalin). The rate at which oxygen is supplied to the blood is controlled by the depth and rate of respiration, which is itself dependent upon the level of carbon dioxide in the blood.

This elaborate system has evolved to keep all cells supplied with enough oxygen for their metabolic needs, whilst protecting them from the toxic effects of excessive oxygen. Many years ago Krogh (1919) described the geometry of cylinders around each vessel with an oxygen gradient away from the vessel, occasionally leading to a 'hypoxic corner' where cells will be unable to survive if the vessels are too far apart or the oxygen supply in the blood falls to a critical level. Such necrotic foci are rarely seen in normal tissues, but it is well recognised that a variation in the oxygen tension exists, with cells adjacent to the vessels having the highest levels (Figure 9.1).

In solid tumours, angiogenic factors are produced which induce new vessel formation to supply the metabolic needs. However, there is often an imbalance between the rate of tumour cell proliferation, and the proliferation and branching of the blood vessels. It is quite common to see necrotic areas, often developing towards the centre of the tumour where the quality of the blood in long vessel loops will be poorest. These necrotic foci eventually merge to form a large accumulation of dead tissue within which cords of tumour cells around the patent blood vessels can be detected. As tumours enlarge, the fraction that is necrotic usually increases. Several workers

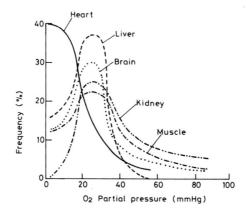

Figure 9.1. The distribution of oxygen tensions in a variety of normal tissues, as measured with microelectrodes. In each tissue values well below 40 mmHg are seen (Redrawn from Schuchhardt, 1973.)

Physiological hypoxia 117

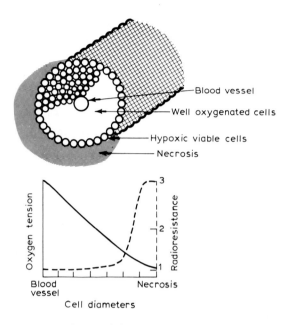

Figure 9.2. Schematic illustration of the corded structure that develops in tumours as oxygen becomes depleted by metabolism. At 5–6 cell diameters from the vessel, the cells may be transiently viable but radioresistant.

have calculated which nutrient is first likely to fall to a critically low level and lead to cell death (Thomlinson and Gray, 1955). Oxygen seems to be the most likely candidate. It therefore follows that a layer of cells which is alive but desperately short of oxygen will lie at the boundary between the cord and the necrotic region (Figure 9.2). The radius of the cords is approximately 90–150 μm. Within untreated tumours the process of cell death will be continuous, with some cells constantly passing these boundary regions. The existence of such hypoxic tumour cells is of great concern to radiotherapists and radiobiologists because hypoxia confers a 3-fold greater radio-resistance than if the same cells are irradiated in air. This is true across a broad spectrum from bacteria to mammalian cells.

It has long been recognised that hypoxia influences the response of cells and tissues to radiation. Considerable efforts were made in the 1950s to quantify the oxygen effect. Eventually, a curve relating radiosensitivity to oxygen tension was published for bacteria (Alper and Howard Flanders, 1956) and for mammalian cells (Deschner and Gray, 1959). The radiosensitivity of cells increases rapidly at first as the oxygen concentration increases from zero, with half the maximum effect being achieved in vitro with about 0.5% oxygen bubbled over the cells (Figure 9.3). The oxygen concentration that gives half the full enhancement is referred to as the 'K value'. It was shown that this represents an oxygen partial pressure of about 5 mmHg (Gray et al., 1953). It has subsequently been found that this form of curve is a reasonable

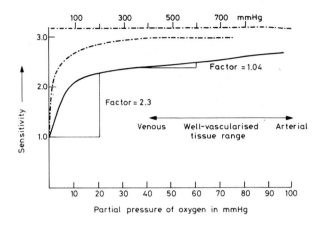

Figure 9.3. The variation in radiosensitivity with oxygenation (the 'K curve'). Most of the variation occurs over the first 20 mmHg partial pressure of oxygen, with an asymptote at higher levels. The range of values in arterial and venous blood are shown, but many cells exist below the venous tension. The broken line shows the same curve plotted on the upper scale, 10 times contracted.

representation for most cell systems. However, a fine structure of the K curve giving two separate components of the oxygen effect (of about equal magnitude) has been detected by very small alterations of oxygen concentration (Millar et al., 1979), and by rapid mix experiments (Michael and Harrop, 1980).

Gray (1957) showed that the oxygen tension in arterial and in venous blood were both well above the steep part of the curve and deduced that radiobiological hypoxia was of little importance in normal tissues, but might be a cause of radioresistance in tumours. This confirmed studies on several normal and malignant systems which were published in the classical papers of Gray et al. (1953) and Thomlinson and Gray (1955). However, it is now recognised that moderate hypoxia is a feature of some normal tissues (e.g. cartilage and skin in mice). The sensitivity of these tissues can be increased if the mice breathe higher concentrations of oxygen. Cells most distant from capillaries will exist well below the venous oxygen tension since they are at the low end of an oxygen gradient radially from the vessel.

9.2 Reoxygenation

It was recognised in the 1960s that an improvement in the oxygen supply to the hypoxic cells could occur after an initial dose of radiation (Thomlinson, 1967). This was termed re-oxygenation.

Tumours exposed to single doses of radiation become increasingly resistant at higher and higher doses, as the hypoxic subpopulation dominates the response (Figure 9.4). The dose-response curve breaks towards that for tumours made totally hypoxic

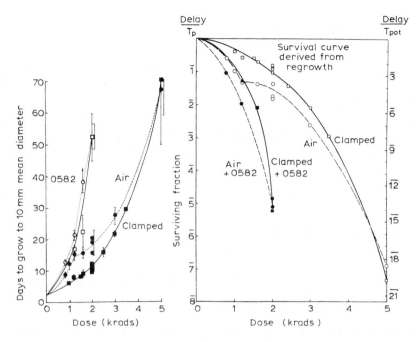

Figure 9.4. Growth delay as a function of X-ray dose for tumours treated in air or after applying an occlusive clamp. The addition of 0582 (i.e., misonidazole) sensitized both aerobic and clamped tumours. Pseudo-survival curves can be derived from these data (right panel) by converting to specific growth delay and assuming one doubling in cell number compensates for a factor of two in cell killing. From Denekamp and Harris (1975).

and radioresistant by the application of an occlusive clamp. The use of hyperbaric oxygen or an oxygen-mimetic agent such as misonidazole can shift the curve greatly to the left, i.e., cause radiosensitization. It is the relative positions of the clamped, air and sensitized lines that are used to calculate the hypoxic fraction.

If radiation is administered as a series of fractions it is less effective on clamped or sensitized tumours but it is as effective as a single dose in aerobic tumours. The sparing effect of fractionation, resulting from repair of sublethal lesions in DNA, is counterbalanced in the aerobic tumours by an increased sensitivity of hypoxic cells as their oxygen supply improves (i.e., reoxygenation). If reoxygenation is complete, there is no further sensitization when misonidazole or hyperbaric oxygen is added. It is the reoxygenation of the hypoxic cells that rescues them from an anoxic death and hence makes them a threat to the patient (Figure 9.5).

It was also recognised that, at the time of maximum reoxygenation, the tumour cell population would become more sensitive to a subsequent dose of radiation. For this reason a knowledge of the reoxygenation kinetics is important and could perhaps be used to tailor radiotherapy more effectively to different tumour types. Carcinomas exhibit extensive reoxygenation (after a large single dose of 10–15 Gy), whereas

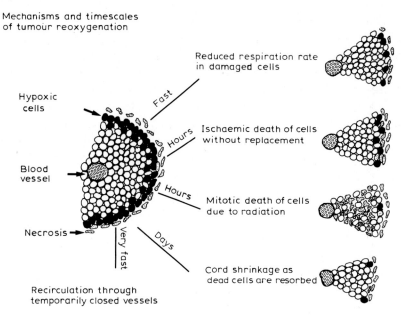

Figure 9.5. Illustration of the different methods by which the hypoxic fraction may change between sequential treatments.

sarcomas show less effective and more complex patterns of reoxygenation (Figure 9.6). The different patterns have been attributed to the rates of shrinkage of the tumours, which in turn have been related to the natural cell loss factor for different

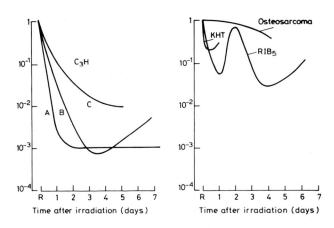

Figure 9.6. Schema to show the extensive reoxygenation seen within 1–2 days after large single doses in three studies of C3H mammary carcinomas (left panel), in contrast to the poor reoxygenation in three types of sarcoma (right panel). The ordinate is a logarithmic scale of hypoxic fraction. (From Denekamp and Fowler, 1977.)

Physiological hypoxia 121

tumour types (Denekamp, 1982). Untreated carcinomas are characterised by rapid cell proliferation with extensive cell loss. When radiation halts cell production, the natural cell loss leads to rapid shrinkage and hence to an improvement of the oxygen supply to the distant tumour cells. Untreated sarcomas, by contrast, have lower cell loss factors and exhibit delayed or a smaller amount of shrinkage after irradiation. Since rapid removal of dead cells will permit oxygen to diffuse to the more distant hypoxic cells, it is easy to envisage that shrinkage and reoxygenation will be causally related. Indeed, shrinkage during fractionation has also been shown to influence the curability of individual tumours within one tumour type, both in mice and in the clinic (Denekamp, 1977; Dische and Saunders, 1980). However, it is not sufficiently predictable to be used as a prognostic indicator in order to modify the treatment of each patient (Suit and Walker, 1980).

Extensive reoxygenation could obviously eliminate the problem of hypoxic radioresistance within a fractionated course of therapy. We have calculated the amount of reoxygenation that would be necessary to render a perfect radiosensitizer totally ineffective (Denekamp and Joiner, 1982). This is illustrated in Figure 9.7. These curves are based on calculations of cell kill in a mixed population, initially containing 90% oxic and 10% hypoxic cells. The redistribution of survivors into these two compartments has been calculated over the range 0–100% and the effect of reoxygenation has been estimated in terms of the reduction in the sensitizer enhancement ratio for the fractionated treatment. It can be seen that even a small amount (25%) of reoxygenation may be adequate with 30 small fractions of 2 Gy, but more extensive reoxygenation is needed to overcome the influence of hypoxic cells with six large fractions of 6 Gy. These calculations have direct relevance for trials of hyperbaric oxygen, chemical radiosensitizers and high linear-energy transfer radiations such as neutrons which also have as their main advantage a reduction in the oxygen enhancement ratio (Chapter 17).

Since, as shown in Fig. 9.7, the effect of a perfect sensitizer ($SER = 2.7$ and no toxicity) could be reduced in a clinical schedule to only 1.1 or less as a result of reoxygenation, hyperbaric or even normobaric oxygen may in fact be the perfect sensitizer. Its modest results in the clinic may be due to limited reoxygenation in the tumours. The clinical results (Henk, 1981; Dische, 1979) may represent the maximum gain that will ever be achieved from overcoming hypoxic radioresistance. The much larger factors expected on the basis of OER 2.5–3.0 were grossly over-optimistic estimates, based on single-dose studies and the assumption of no reoxygenation, which we now know to be unrealistic.

9.2.1 Detection of hypoxic cells

Figure 9.4 shows the way in which radioresistance due to the presence of hypoxic cells can be demonstrated. From such studies it has been found that hypoxic cells

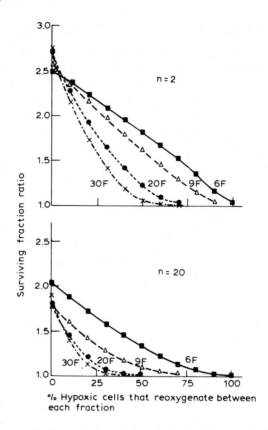

Figure 9.7. Enhancement ratios for a mixed population of cells in a fractionated schedule associated with differing degrees of reoxygenation. The calculations were made for survival curve characteristics with extrapolation numbers of 2 or 20, (see text.) (Denekamp and Joiner, 1982.)

exist before treatment in at least 38 of 40 types of animal tumours. The hypoxic fraction is usually estimated at 5–40%. The two exceptions are a very slow-growing fibrosarcoma and a mouse glioma (Denekamp and Fowler, 1978). Similar studies of patients with multiple subcutaneous or pulmonary nodules have yielded very similar values (1–80%) in patients. However, all these values relate to untreated tumours. If reoxygenation is a common phenomenon in rodent tumours it is important to ask:

If hypoxic cells *exist* in a particular tumour will they *persist* to influence the response throughout a course of radiotherapy?

This question is clearly of crucial importance, since if the answer is 'no' there is no need for hyperbaric oxygen, fast neutrons or radiosensitizers to overcome the problem of hypoxic tumour radioresistance. Unfortunately, no direct methods exist for identifying hypoxic viable cells, and the radiobiological techniques used to obtain hypoxic fractions in animal tumours cannot be applied to most human tumours.

A great effort has been invested in developing chemicals that specifically bind to hypoxic cells and hence allow their identification. Chapman et al. (1981) have shown that the product of [^{14}C]misonidazole produced by hypoxic metabolism is bound in hypoxic regions of spheroids and human tumours and can be identified in autoradiographs. To date, 16 patients have been studied and only 10 of them have shown clear evidence of hypoxic cells (Urtasun et al., 1989). Seven out of seven small-cell lung carcinomas, however, have shown significant evidence of hypoxia.

Fluorescent derivatives could also be useful, since cell sorters would allow the accurate quantification of small subpopulations of fluorescent cells. This principle has been demonstrated using a nitro-acridine which becomes a fluorophor on reduction, and appears to be stably bound in hypoxic cells (Begg et al., 1983). Such a compound must be administered in vivo and problems of delivery and toxicity have proved to be a major stumbling block. The ideal approach would be if an immunoassay could be developed to detect small quantities of a reduced metabolite of a clinically known compound such as misonidazole, so that toxic or radioactive doses would not need to be administered in vivo; detection could be done on biopsies or on histological sections.

Such an approach has yielded a useful antibody to another bound nitroimidazole (Raleigh et al., 1988). Unfortunately, the original agent cannot be freely administered to man, but it shows that this approach is likely to be a successful one. An intriguing and exciting result was recently described by Hlatky et al. (1989) who showed what they believe to be direct chemodevelopment of a photographic film laid over a 'sandwich preparation' consisting of cells in an oxygen gradient. The material released by the hypoxic cells which produced latent images in the film in the absence of any radioisotopes has yet to be identified.

It is necessary to develop a technique which will identify viable hypoxic cells in untreated and partially treated tumours (i.e., against a background of many dead cells) in order to predict which patients should be allocated to trials of sensitizers, oxygen or fast neutrons. At present, such trials are likely to show no significant effect if many of the tumours undergo efficient reoxygenation with conventional therapy. The non-reoxygenating subset needs to be identified, since these are the only patients likely to benefit.

9.3 Chemical radiosensitizers

The effect of oxygen as a potent radiosensitizer is believed to relate to its ability to interact with radiation-induced radicals, acting as an electron acceptor. This mechanism of damage fixation is in competition with chemical restitution of the damage in which thiols play an important role, presumably by proton donation or electron transfer. There is still considerable debate about the precise mechanism by which oxygen and thiols influence radiosensitivity, since they may influence direct damage inflicted by ionisation events in the DNA, or indirect damage caused by the products of water radiolysis, particularly hydroxyl radicals and the hydrated electron (Section 1.1.2).

Basic studies of the 'oxygen effect' led to the development of drugs which would mimic oxygen in its sensitizing action (Adams et al., 1978). It was quickly recognised that such compounds might be useful clinically if they were non-toxic and not metabolised and hence could diffuse to tissue regions that oxygen could not reach. The first of these, a 5-nitroimidazole in routine clinical use (metronidazole, trade name Flagyl, May and Baker) was shown to be effective in several systems in vitro and in vivo (Foster and Willson, 1973; Willson et al., 1974). As predicted, it had a sensitizing effect only in the *absence* of oxygen. The search for analogues led to the more active 2-nitroimidazoles, especially misonidazole (Roche 07-0582). This was extremely effective when used with a single dose of radiation on hypoxic skin or on tumours in mice breathing normal air (Figure 9.8). No effect was seen on the skin of mice breathing oxygen (Fowler and Denekamp, 1979). The uniform response in a wide variety of experimental studies led to clinical trials throughout the world (Section 10.3). The search for more effective analogues of misonidazole is dealt with in Section 11.4.

9.3.1 Enhancing sensitizer efficiency by thiol depletion

Prolonged thiol depletion prior to irradiation has been found to lead to increased efficiency of misonidazole (Wong et al., 1978). This resulted in loss of the shoulder on the cell survival curve and hence to increased effectiveness at low, clinically-relevant X-ray doses. This finding led to an interest in alternative means of decreasing the thiol content in order to enhance sensitizer efficiency. Glutathione (GSH)-binding agents, such as diethyl maleate and dimethyl fumarate, increased the efficiency of misonidazole (Bump et al., 1982). The development of a specific biochemical inhibitor of glutathione synthesis, buthionine sulphoximine (BSO), which interferes with γ-glutamyl synthetase was an important development (Griffith and Meister, 1979; Hodgkiss and Middleton, 1982; Shrieve et al., 1985). Subsequent studies, using prolonged exposure of animals to repeated doses of BSO have shown that it is relatively easy to deplete glutathione, the main intracellular non-protein thiol, in several normal tissues, but it is extremely hard to deplete *tumour* GSH levels below 10% (Minchinton et al., 1984). Since the object is to increase the effectiveness of sensitizers in the poorly perfused regions of tumours, this is a distinct disadvantage. Furthermore, hypoxia itself may lead to glutathione depletion, since its production is an energy-requiring process. It is possible to deplete tumour GSH more effectively by combining BSO with a binding agent (e.g., DEM) but the combination of this drastic pretreatment with misonidazole administration is extremely toxic and therefore does not effectively lead to a therapeutic advantage.

9.4 Sensitization by increased oxygen delivery

In the 1960s it was considered obvious that oxygen would be the best radiosensitizer if some way could be devised of carrying extra oxygen to the distant tumour cells. Normobaric oxygen, carbogen (i.e., 95% O_2/5% CO_2) and hyperbaric oxygen were all tested in clinical trials, with a limited success (Henk, 1981; Dische, 1979). The advent of misonidazole diverted attention from the gaseous sensitizers but recently they have been re-evaluated. The most obvious approach to improve tumour oxygenation is to increase the content of oxygen in the inspired gas. Initial experimental studies with oxygen and carbogen were promising (Suit et al., 1972; Siemann et al., 1977) and even led to some clinical trials. However, the potential advantages seemed to be greater if the patient could be enclosed in a pressurized chamber and given oxygen or carbogen at elevated pressures. This would force more oxygen into the plasma, thereby

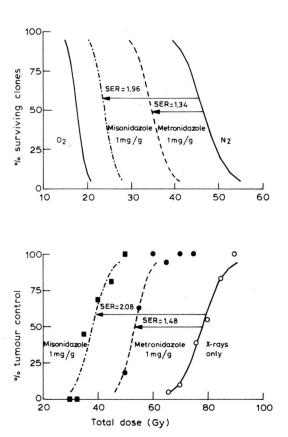

Figure 9.8. Sensitization of anoxic mouse skin (upper panel) or aerobic tumours (lower panel) with metronidazole and misonidazole.

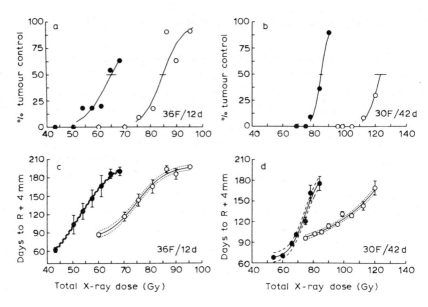

Figure 9.9. Enhancement by inhaled normobaric oxygen of local tumour control (a and b) or growth delay (c and d) in schedules using 30 daily fractions in 6 weeks or 36 fractions in 12 days. Significant sensitization of this mouse tumour is seen with these clinically relevant schedules. (Rojas et al., 1989.)

supplementing the reservoir carried in the haemoglobin. Again, many clinical trials were undertaken which superseded the normobaric studies (Dische, 1979). A distinct improvement was seen in certain patient subgroups, especially those presenting with anaemia, but the rewards did not seem to justify the continuance of this difficult and time-consuming addition to routine radiotherapy.

Recently, interest in normobaric oxygen and carbogen has been revived, because of the possibility that tumour oxygenation was compromised in the early studies by peripheral vasoconstriction under hyperbaric conditions resulting from the *prolonged* exposure to oxygen during the pressurisation and 'soaking' time. Animal studies have shown that even with normal-pressure oxygen or carbogen, the sensitizing effect is greatest if a short time elapses between inhaling the gas and irradiation. Fig 9.9 shows recent results from studies with inhaled oxygen in mice treated with up to 36 fractions of radiation. This is a tumour previously thought to show extensive reoxygenation, because of the limited sensitization seen with fractionated X-rays and misonidazole (Denekamp and Harris, 1976). Rojas (1989) and Rojas et al. (1989) have shown extensive sensitization, by a factor of 1.3 to 1.5, when using 12, 30 or 36 fractions in schedules that exactly mimic those used in the clinic. These results have led to a revived interest at Mount Vernon Hospital in using oxygen at normal pressures (or carbogen), given through a simple face mask for a *short* time before and during treatment.

Recent developments in blood-transfusion technology have added another element to this approach. Chemical substitutes have been developed as alternatives to fresh or frozen blood for transfusion (Rockwell, 1985). These consist of fine organic micelles containing a mixture of perfluorochemicals which can dissolve large amounts of oxygen. Water and plasma dissolve about 2% oxygen by volume, whole blood 20%, and perfluorochemicals can dissolve 40% or more. However, they have a limited oxygen-transport capacity at normal pressure. The volume of dissolved oxygen changes linearly with oxygen partial pressure and therefore to fully exploit their use in vivo, high partial pressures of oxygen are being used. Several animal studies have shown an increased tumour response using perfluorochemicals and high oxygen concentration (Teicher and Rose, 1984; Martin et al., 1987).

Interest has also developed in chemicals which influence the affinity of haemoglobin for oxygen, thus altering its ability to give up the oxygen in the tumour microvasculature. Groups of agents are under study which shift the oxygen-haemoglobin dissociation curve to the left, increasing its affinity for oxygen or to the right, making oxygen more readily available to cells (Section 11.2).

Alterations in blood viscosity, e.g., by reducing the haematocrit, could also anomalously increase the tumour oxygenation if it encouraged plasma flow through small vessels that are poorly perfused due to partial blocking by erythrocytes. Pharmacological agents which influence cardiac output, vascular tone and differential blood flow to different regions of the body are receiving increasing attention. Most of the vasodilators are not capable of causing tumour blood flow to *increase* because of the passive nature of the non-innervated tumour blood supply. Indeed most vasodilators and antihypertensive agents cause a *reduction* in tumour blood flow as the 'steal' effect of increased flow to other regions diminishes the blood available to the tumour.

9.5 Utilising hypoxic radioresistance

An alternative approach to dealing with the differential sensitivity of hypoxic tumour cells and well oxygenated normal cells is to attempt to get uniform radioresistance. This can be attempted by excluding oxygen from the normal tissues, or by using a chemical radioprotector. In this way larger radiation doses could perhaps be administered which should have a greater probability of curing the tumour.

9.5.1 Induction of normal tissue hypoxia

Several clinical studies have been undertaken in which normal tissue radioprotection was attempted by inducing local or systemic hypoxia (Section 10.4.1). Trials of systemic hypoxia induced by breathing reduced oxygen tensions have been initiated in the Soviet Union and East Germany (Neumeister et al., 1977; Yarmonenko, 1980).

Whilst reduced oxygen tensions in the inspired gas can have a very marked effect on some normal tissues (e.g., 5% oxygen protects mouse skin by a factor of 2 or more), the same inspired gas may have little effect on other dose-limiting normal tissues, such as kidney or lung. Furthermore, it increases the radioresistance of tumours, particularly in response to low doses (Stevens et al., 1989). Thus hypoxy-radiotherapy may be useful in certain limited circumstances, but is unlikely to produce a general therapeutic advantage.

9.5.2 Chemical radioprotection

The ability to protect cells against radiation injury by addition of thiols has been recognised for some 30 years. However, addition of non-protein thiols is not easy to achieve. Cysteine and cysteamine are relatively toxic, whilst glutathione itself is not readily transported into cells. Because of the potential value of radioprotection of military personnel when under nuclear attack, an enormous research programme at the Walter Read Hospital has been undertaken to develop various thiol radioprotectors. One of these is the aminothiol WR-2721, which is less toxic in its phosphorylated administered form and needs dephosphorylating in vivo before entering cells. It has been shown to be an effective radioprotector, especially against bone marrow death. Yuhas and Storer (1969) tested this compound in normal tissues and tumours and deduced that it might be useful in cancer radiotherapy because it showed little protection of the tumour. In subsequent work, Yuhas (1981) claimed that the drug was excluded from tumour cells in 16/17 tumour types. This led to widespread interest in the clinical application of radioprotectors both alone and in combination with tumour radiosensitizers.

Radioprotectors have been reviewed in detail in several publications (Denekamp et al., 1983; Denekamp and Rojas, 1988). Briefly, the level of radioprotection varies from tissue to tissue, being much lower in many other normal tissues than that seen in bone marrow. It does not correlate well with the measured drug concentrations in the tissues, mainly because of the variable levels of oxygen in the critical target cells and, perhaps also due to differences in the endogenous levels of thiols. The addition of thiols effectively competes with the oxygen, thereby shifting the oxygen concentration needed to achieve half-maximal sensitization to higher values. This is the obvious corollary of the attempts to increase sensitizer efficiency by depleting thiol levels. Figure 9.10 shows examples of oxygen 'K curves' derived from clonogenic assays of bacterial and mammalian cells in culture and rodent skin cells in vivo. All three systems show that when thiols are added the 'K curves' are shifted to higher oxygen concentrations. The protective effect of the thiol therefore varies depending on the oxygen level that is present (Denekamp and Rojas, 1988). In anoxic cells and in very well oxygenated cells, adding thiols has little or no effect. In marginally oxygenated cells, adding thiols makes a very large difference to the radiosensitivity, because the balance between reducing and oxidising species can be easily tipped. The protection factors (PF) have been plotted in the right hand panels and they show very convincingly that PF is critically dependent on oxygen.

Since tumours and normal tissues have cells at a range of oxygen tensions, different subpopulations become dominant as the dose increases and therefore the effect of thiol radioprotectors can vary with radiation dose level (and the level of effect). Careful analysis of both tumour and normal-tissue data indicates a complex dependence of the protection factor on the size of each X-ray dose. At equivalent low X-ray doses, the advantage of WR-2721 in giving normal tissue protection but no tumour protection disappears. At clinically relevant doses of a few grays it is quite unpredictable whether

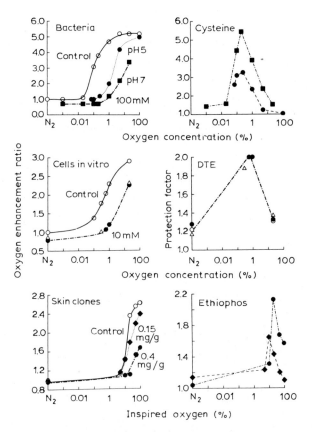

Figure 9.10. Radiosensitivity as a function of oxygen concentration can be altered by adding exogenous thiols. Results are shown for three experimental systems: bacteria protected by cysteine (top panels), mammalian cells in vitro protected by dithioerithritol (middle panels), and mouse skin protected by Ethiophos (i.e., WR2721, bottom panels). In each case the left-hand panels show the *OER* as a function of oxygen concentration, with or without the protector. The right-hand panels show corresponding calculated values of the protection factor relative to same gas without added thiols. (From Denekamp and Rojas, 1988.)

130 J. Denekamp

the protective effect is more marked in any tumour than in any normal tissue. These findings have led to less clinical interest, though WR-2721 may still be useful for local or intracavitary administration. It is currently being tested with a few large fractions in palliative radiotherapy and in chemotherapy (Kligerman et al., 1981).

9.6 Combined tumour radiosensitizers and normal tissue radioprotectors

Since the toxicities of WR-2721 and of misonidazole are quite different it has been postulated that benefit could be obtained by combined administration. This would be true if there were no additive toxicity, and no reason for an interference in the mode of action of the two drugs; early studies indicated that these two requirements might be met. Unfortunately, more detailed studies showed that the toxicity of misonidazole was greatly modified by the addition of WR-2721 (Figure 9.11). Likewise the toxicity of WR-2721 was directly influenced by the addition of misonidazole. The radioprotective effect of WR-2721 on skin could be reduced by adding the sensitizer. Furthermore, the enhancement of tumour sensitivity by misonidazole could be reduced by thiol addition. Indeed as might be predicted from a simple redox competition model, the degree of sensitization of anoxic cells by misonidazole can be titrated against

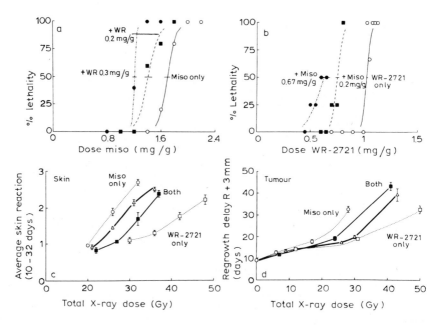

Figure 9.11. Illustration of the interaction of a thiol radioprotector and an electron-affinic radiosensitizer. The two drugs interact for their effect in toxicity (top panels) in tumour sensitization and skin protection (lower panels). (Rojas et al., 1983).

protection induced by the thiol. Likewise, the protective effect of the thiol can be titrated against sensitization either from added misonidazole or from added oxygen (Rojas et al., 1983).

9.7 Conclusions

Physiological hypoxia is extremely important as a concept in radiotherapy, because it can confer a high degree of radioresistance. Hypoxic cells occur in most tumours prior to treatment as a result of the imbalance between tumour cell production and the expansion of the vascular network. These cells create a great problem if tumours are treated with large single doses of radiation. However, if small doses are given in a series of repeated fractions the influence diminishes because of the natural process of reoxygenation. Methods of recognising and quantifying hypoxic cells are still difficult to use and it is not yet possible to select those tumours with a long-term hypoxic population for specific forms of treatment. Among the possible methods of overcoming the hypoxic resistance are: increasing the oxygen in the inspired gas, providing chemical substitutes for oxygen, or using high LET radiations such as neutrons. The option of increasing normal tissue resistance, either alone or combined with the sensitizers has also been considered.

References

Adams, G.E., Barnes, W.H., Du Boulay, C., Loutit, J.F., Cole, S., Sheldon, P.W., Stratford, I.J., Van den Aardweg, G.J.M.J., Hopewell, J., White, R.D., Kneen, G., Nethersell, A.B.W. and Edwards, J.C. (1986) Induction of hypoxia in normal and malignant tissues by changing the oxygen affinity of haemoglobin – implications for therapy. Int. J. Radiat. Oncol. Phys. 12, 1299–1302.

Adams, G.E., Fowler, J.F. and Wardman, P. (eds.) (1978) Hypoxic cell sensitizers in radiobiology and radiotherapy, Proceedings 8th L.H. Gray Conference. Br. J. Cancer 37, Suppl. III, 1–321.

Alper, T. and Howard Flanders, P. (1956) The role of oxygen in modifying the radiosensitivity of *E. coli* B. Nature 178, 978–979.

Begg, A.C., Engelhardt, Hodgkiss, R.J., McNally, N.J., Terry, N.H.A. and Wardman, P. (1983) Nitroacridine: a fluorescent stain for hypoxic cells. Br. J. Radiol 56, 970–973.

Brown, J.M. (Ed.) (1986) Proceedings 5th Conference on Chemical Modifiers of Cancer Treatment. Int. J. Radiat. Oncol. Biol. Phys. 12, pp. 1021–1545.

Bump, E.A., Yu, N.Y. and Brown, M.J. (1982) Radiosensitization of hypoxic tumour cells by depletion of intracellular glutathione. Science 217, 544–545.

Chapman, J.D., Franko, A.J. and Sharplin, J. (1981) A marker for hypoxic cells in tumours with potential clinical applicability. Br. J. Cancer 43, 546–550.

Denekamp, J. (1982) Cell Kinetics and Cancer Therapy (Dewey, W.C., ed.), pp. 1–162, C.C. Thomas, Springfield, IL.

Denekamp, J. (1977) Tumour regression as a guide to prognosis: a study with experimental animals. Br. J. Radiol. 50, 217–279.

Denekamp, J. (1983) Prediction and Quantitation of Tumour Response, *in*: Biological Bases and Clinical Implications of Tumour Radioresistance (Fletcher, G.H., Nervi, C. and Withers, H.R., eds.), pp. 91–102, Masson, New York.

Denekamp, J. and Fowler, J.F. (1977) Cell proliferation Kinetics and Radiation Therapy, *in*: Cancer: A Comprehensive Treatise (Becker, F.F., ed.), Vol. 6, pp. 101–137, Plenum Press, New York.

Denekamp, J. and Fowler, J.F. (1978) Radiosensitization of solid tumours by nitroimidazoles. Int. J. Radiat. Oncol. Biol. Phys. 4, 143–151.

Denekamp, J. and Harris, S.R. (1975) Tests of two electron- affinic radiosensitizers in vivo using regrowth of an experimental tumour. Radiat. Res. 61, 191–203.

Denekamp, J. and Harris, S.R. (1976) The response of a transplantable tumor to fractionated irradiation. 1. X-rays and the hypoxic cell radiosensitizer Ro 07-0582. Rad. Res. 66, 66–75.

Denekamp, J., Rojas, A. and Stevens, G. (1988) Redox competition and radiosensitivity: implications for testing radioprotective compounds in pharmacology. Therapy 39, 59–66.

Denekamp, J., Stewart, F.A. and Rojas, A. (1983) Is the outlook grey for WR-2721 as a clinical radioprotector? Int. J. Radiat. Oncol. Biol. Phys. 9, 1247–1249.

Denekamp, J. and Joiner, M.C. (1982) The potential benefit from a perfect radiosensitizer and its dependence on reoxygenation, Br. J. Radiol. 55, 657–663.

Denekamp, J. and Rojas, A. (1988) Radioprotection in vivo: cellular heterogeneity and fractionation, *in*: Anticarcinogenesis and Radiation Protection (Cerutti, P.A., Nygaard, O.F. and Simic, M.G., eds.), pp. 421–430, Plenum Press, New York.

Deschner, E. and Gray, L.H. (1959) Influence of oxygen tension on X-ray-induced chromosomal damage in Ehrlich ascites tumour cells irradiated in vitro and in vivo. Radiat. Res. 11, 115–146.

Dische, S. (1979) Hyperbaric oxygen: the Medical Research Council trials and their clinical significance, Br. J. Radiol. 51, 888–894.

Dische, S. and Saunders, M.I. (1980) Tumour regression and prognosis: a clinical study. Br. J. Cancer 41, Suppl. IV, 11–13.

Dische, S. (1985) Chemical sensitizers for hypoxic cells: a decade of experience in clinical radiotherapy. Radiother. Oncol. 3, 97–115.

Dische, S., Saunders, M.I., Anderson, P., Stratford, M.R.L. and Minchinton, A. (1982) Clinical experience with nitroimidazoles as radiosensitizers. Int. J. Radiat. Oncol. Biol. Phys. 8, 335–338.

Foster, J.L. and Willson, R.L. (1973) Radiosensitization of anoxic cells by metronidazole. Br. J. Radiol. 46, 234–235. (correspondence).

Fowler, J.F. and Denekamp, J. (1979) A review of hypoxic cell radiosensitization in experimental tumors. Pharmacol. Ther. 7, 413–444.

Gray, L.H. (1957) Oxygenation in radiotherapy. I. Radiobiological consideration. Br. J. Radiol. 30, 403–406.

Gray, L.H., Conger, A.D., Ebert, M., Hornsey, S. and Scott, O.C.A. (1953) The concentration of oxygen dissolved in tissues at the time of irradiation as a factor in radiotherapy. Br. J. Radiol. 26, 638–648.

Griffith, O.W. and Meister, A. (1979) Potent and specific inhibition of glutathione synthesis by buthionine sulfoxime (S-n-butylhomocysteine sulfoximine). J. Biol. Chem. 254, 7558–7560.

Hendry, J.H. (1979) Quantitation of the radiotherapeutic importance of naturally hypoxic normal tissues from collated experiments with rodents using single doses. Int. J. Radiat. Oncol. Biol. Phys. 5, 971–976.

Henk, J.M. (1981) Editorial: Does hyperbaric oxygen have a future in radiation therapy? Int. J. Radiat. Oncol. Biol. Phys. 7, 1125–1128.

Hirst, D.G. (1986) Oxygen delivery to tumors. Int. J. Radiat. Oncol. Biol. Phys. 12, 1271–1277.

Hlatky, L., Hong, C. and Sachs, R. (1989) An intrinsic marker for hypoxia. Int. J. Radiat. Oncol. Biol. Phys., in press.

Hodgkiss, R.J. and Middleton, R.W. (1982) Enhancement of misonidazole radiosensitization by an inhibitor of glutathione biosynthesis. Int. J. Radiat. Biol. 43, 179–183.

Kligerman, M.M., Blumberg, A.L., Glick, J.H., Nelson, D.F., Glover, D., Yuhas, J.M., Amols, H.I. and

Goodman, R.L. (1981) Phase I trials of WR-2721 in combination with radiation and with the alkylating agents cyclophosphamide and *cis*-platinum. Cancer Clin. Trials 4, 469–474.
Krogh, A.I. (1919) I. The rate of diffusion of gases through animal tissue, with some remarks on the coefficient of invasion. II. The number and distribution of capillaries in muscles with calculations of the oxygen pressure held necessary for supplying the tissue. III. The supply of oxygen to the tissues and the regulation of the capillary circulation. J. Physiol. 52, 391–474.
Malaise, E.P., Adams, G.E., Dische, S. and Guichard, M. (1989) Chemical modifiers of cancer treatment. Int. J. Radiat. Oncol. Biol. Phys., in press.
Martin, D.F., Porter, E.A., Rockwell, S. and Fischer, J.J. (1987) Enhancement of tumor radiation response by the combination of a perfluorochemical emulsion and hyperbaric oxygen. Int. J. Radiat. Oncol. Biol. Phys. 13, 747–51.
Michael, B.D. and Harrop, H.A. (1980) Time-scale and mechanism of radiosensitization and radioprotection at the cellular level, *in*: Radiation Sensitizers; Their Use in the Clinical Management of Cancer (Brady, L.W., ed.), pp. 14–21, Masson, New York.
Millar, B.C., Fielden, E.M. and Steele, J.J. (1979) A biphasic radiation survival response of mammalian cells to molecular oxygen, Int. J. Radiat. Biol. 36, 177–180.
Minchinton, A.I., Rojas, A., Smith, K.A., Soranson, J.A., Shrieve, D.C., Jones, N.R. and Bremner, J.C. (1984) Glutathione depletion in tissues after administration of buthionine sulphoximine. Int. J. Radiat. Oncol. Biol. Phys. 10, 1261–1264.
Neumeister, K., Kamprad, F., Arnold, P., Jahns, J., Mehlhorn, G., Johannsen, U., Koch, F. and Bolck, M. (1977) A basis for applying hypoxic hypoxia for optimising radiotherapy: information based on animal tests. IAEA-SM-212/7, pp. 197–207, Proceedings of International Symposium on the Radiobiological Research needed for the Improvement of Radiotherapy held by the IAEA in Vienna 22–26 November 1976.
Raleigh, J.A., Miller, G.G., Franko, A.J., Koch, C.J., Fuciarelli, A.F. and Kelly, D.A. (1987) Fluorescence immunohistochemical detection of hypoxic cells in spheroids and tumours. Br. J. Cancer 50, 395–400.
Rockwell, S. (1985) Use of perfluorochemical emulsion to improve oxygenation in a solid tumour. Int. J. Radiat. Oncol. Biol. Phys. 11, 97–103.
Rojas, A. (1989) Oxygen: a clinical reality or a mirage? *in*: The Scientific Basis for Modern Radiotherapy (BIR report 19). Br. J. Radiol., 86–90.
Rojas, A., Carl, U., Tanton, J.K. and Reghebi, K. (1989) Effect of normobaric oxygen on tumour radiosensitivity: fractionated studies. Int. J. Radiat. Oncol. Biol. Phys., submitted for publication.
Rojas, A., Stewart, F.A. and Denekamp, J. (1983) Interaction of misonidazole and WR-2721-II. Modification of tumour radiosensitization. Br. J. Cancer 47, 65–72.
Schuchhardt, S. (1973) Comparative Physiology of the Oxygen Supply, *in*: Oxygen Supply, Theoretical and Practical Microcirculation of Tissue, (Kessler, M., Bruley, D.F., Clark, L.C., Lübbers, D.W., Silver, I.A. and Strauss, J., eds.), pp. 223–229, Urban Schwarzenberg, Munich.
Shrieve, D.C., Denekamp, J. and Minchinton, A.I. (1985) Effects of glutathione depletion by buthionine sulphoximine on radiosensitization by oxygen and misonidazole in vitro. Radiat. Res. 102, 283–296.
Siemann, D.W. and Macler, L.M. (1986) Tumor radiosensitization through reductions in hemoglobin affinity. Int. J. Radiat. Oncol. Biol. Phys. 12, 1295–1297.
Siemann, D.W., Hill, R.P. and Bush, R.S. (1977) The importance of the pre-irradiation breathing times of oxygen and carbogen (5% CO_2/95% O_2) on the in vivo radiation response of a murine sarcoma. Int. J. Radiat. Oncol. Biol. Phys. 2, 903–911.
Stevens, G., Joiner, B. and Denekamp, J. (1989) Radioprotection by hypoxic breathing. Proceedings 6th Conference on Chemical Modifiers of Cancer Treatment, Paris, March 1988. Int. J. Radiat. Oncol. Biol. Phys., in press.
Suit, H.D. and Lindberg, R. (1968) Radiation therapy administered under conditions of tourniquet-induced local tissue hypoxia. Am. J. Roentgenol. 102, 27–37.

Suit, H.D. and Walker, A.M. (1980) Assessment of the response of tumours to radiation: clinical and experimental studies, Br. J. Cancer 41, Suppl. IV, 1–10.

Suit, H.D., Marshall, N. and Woerner, D. (1972) Oxygen, oxygen plus carbon dioxide, and radiation therapy of a mouse mammary carcinoma. Cancer 30, 1154–1158.

Teicher, B.A. and Rose, C.M. (1984) Perfluorochemical emulsions can increase tumor radiosensitivity. Science 223, 934–936.

Thomlinson, R.H. (1967) Oxygen Therapy: Biological Considerations. Modern Trends in Radiotherapy (Deeley, T. and Wood, C.P., eds.), pp. 52–72, Butterworths, London.

Thomlinson, R.H. and Gray, L.H. (1955) The histological structure of some human lung cancers and the possible implications for radiotherapy. Br. J. Cancer 9, 539–549.

Urtasun, R.C., Chapman, J.D., Raleigh, J.A., Franko, A.J., Koch, C.J. and McKinnon, S. (1989) Proceedings 6th Conference on Chemical Modifiers of Cancer Treatment. Int. J. Radiat. Oncol. Biol. Phys., in press.

Willson, R.L., Cramp, W.A. and Ings, R.M.J. (1974) Metronidazole ('Flagyl'): Mechanisms of Radiosensitization. Int. J. Radiat. Biol. 26, 557–569.

Wong, T.W., Whitman, G.F. and Gulyas, S. (1978) Studies on the toxicity and radiosensitizing ability of misonidazole under conditions of prolonged incubation. Rad. Res. 75, 541–55.

Yarmonenko, S.P. (1980) Hypoxyradiotherapy of tumours, *in*: progress in Radio Oncology (Karchev, K.H., Kogelnik, H.D. and Meyer, H.J., eds.), pp. 144–150, Georg Thieme Verlag, New York.

Yuhas, J.M. (1981) On the potential application of radioprotective drugs in solid tumor radiotherapy, *in*: Radiation – Drug-Interaction in the Treatment of Cancer, Chapter 6 (Sokol, G.H. and Maickel, R.P., eds.), pp. 113–135. John Wiley Sons, New York.

Yuhas, J.M. and Storer, J.B. (1969) Chemoprotection against three modes of radiation death in the mouse. Int. J. Radiat. Biol. 15, 233–237.

CHAPTER 10

The clinical consequences of the oxygen effect

STANLEY DISCHE

Marie Curie Research Wing, Regional Centre for Radiotherapy and Oncology, Mount Vernon Hospital, Northwood, Middlesex HA6 2RN, England

10.1   Introduction 135

10.2   Anaemia and impaired pulmonary function 136

10.3   Evidence that oxygen is important in modifying radiation response in humans 137

10.4   Current clinical efforts to sensitize hypoxic cells 138
       10.4.1   Anaemia 138
       10.4.2   New hypoxic cell radiosensitizers 138
       10.4.3   The combination of chemical sensitizing agents 139
       10.4.4   Intra-tumoural introduction of hypoxic cell sensitizers 140
       10.4.5   Use of carbogen breathing 140
       10.4.6   Fluorinated hydrocarbons 140
       10.4.7   Effect of blood pressure on tumour perfusion 140

10.5   Manipulation of the oxygen effect 141

10.6   Reoxygenation and accelerated radiotherapy 142

10.1 Introduction

The earliest demonstration of the oxygen effect has been traced to the demonstration by Schwarz in 1910 that the radiation reaction of his own skin was reduced when it was compressed at the time of treatment (Schwarz, 1910). It was Mottram who in 1935 first suggested that oxygen was important in determining sensitivity and that human tumour cells may be resistant to radiation because they lie distant from a capillary, but Gray and his co-workers (Gray et al., 1953) brought all the evidence together and gained the attention of clinicians.

The laboratory basis for the clinical application of the oxygen effect is one of the strongest in oncology (Chapter 9). However, despite 30 years of endeavour, we have yet to show in man that any method of hypoxic cell radiosensitization can give therapeutic benefit and have an accepted place in management.

10.2 Anaemia and impaired pulmonary function

In animal tumour studies, anaemia has been shown to be important in reducing radio-responsiveness and there is now considerable evidence to show that this is so in humans. There are nine publications concerned with anaemia and the response of tumours of the uterine cervix; in seven a direct relationship was found between haemoglobin level and response (Dische, 1988). There is also evidence of the effect of anaemia in carcinoma of the bladder and in tumours of the head and neck region. We have shown in a group of patients with carcinoma of the bronchus a significantly greater survival in those with a high level of haemoglobin and in these same patients the incidence of radiation myelitis was also greater. This showed that the haemoglobin concentration can influence the radiation response of normal tissues (Dische et al., 1986a). With all these data one must be careful in interpretation, for anaemia is associated with advancing disease and, therefore, a poor prognosis. There also is evidence, however, that restoration of anaemia leads to improved local control, and in many studies it has an effect upon local tumour control rather than distant disease. It is of special interest that in patients with head and neck tumours, and also lung cancer, none showed more than a minor depression in haemoglobin level: differences in haemoglobin level which are within the range of normality were associated with differences in response (Dische et al., 1986a; Overgaard et al., 1989). No explanation other than the oxygen effect has been proposed to account for the results observed.

The demonstration in hyperbaric oxygen trials that there was a sub-group of patients with carcinoma of the cervix where conventional therapy gave very poor local tumour control, but where treatment in hyperbaric oxygen led to a high level of control, suggested that hypoxia could be an important cause for failure under certain conditions (Dische et al., 1983). The sub-group in this case comprised those who were severely anaemic prior to treatment so as to require blood transfusion. It is of interest that in the DAHANCA trial the striking effect of anaemia on prognosis affected patients with pharyngeal tumours and not laryngeal, and it was with the same pharyngeal group that a further benefit was achieved with misonidazole (Overgaard et al., 1989). Once again this suggests that there are sub-groups where hypoxia is a severe problem and where a method of sensitization can give benefit. Sealy has made patients anaemic and then, after restoration of haemoglobin, treated them in hyperbaric oxygen. There was some initial promise, but with accumulation of more cases the method did not seem to be giving results superior to those obtained with conventional radiotherapy (Sealy et al., 1988a). It might be that the response pattern seen in the sub-groups of cervix and head and neck cancer was not due to anaemia followed by transfusion but that both anaemia and the response pattern were related to a defect in the vascular structure of the tumour.

As anaemia appears to influence the radio-responsiveness of tumours, it might be expected that a similar relationship would exist between lung function and radiation effect, for with impaired respiratory function a similar deprivation of oxygen may occur. The majority of patients receiving treatment for head and neck tumours and lung cancer do show impairment of pulmonary function but nearly all appear to be able to saturate their haemoglobin under the resting conditions which apply during treatment. Unless lung function is grossly impaired it is likely to have no significant influence on tumour oxygenation at rest (Hong, 1988).

10.3 Evidence that oxygen is important in modifying radiation response in humans

Thomlinson and Gray (1955) studied material from patients with carcinoma of the bronchus and described a model based on this human evidence. Hypoxic cells existing at the edge of the viable cells in a tumour cord could be resistant to radiation, survive, and cause regrowth after treatment. In many human tumours other than carcinoma of the bronchus such cords can be demonstrated. It should be added, however, that it was not suggested that this pattern was universal in all parts of all human tumours. Certainly in some areas of tumour the oxygen supply to cells may depend on several, rather than one capillary. Nevertheless, there may be a more general, though modest, local reduction in oxygen tension, leading to a slight impairment of response rather than the high resistance associated with the very low levels of oxygen tension at the edge of the tumour cord of the Thomlinson and Gray model.

In the early clinical studies direct comparisons were made in the same patient of the response of areas of tumour treated under normal conditions with those treated using a sensitizer – hyperbaric oxygen or one of the chemical agents. In seven of eight cases where hyperbaric oxygen was tested, Churchill-Davidson et al. (1955) found histological evidence for an increased response. With the chemical sensitizing agent, misonidazole, tumours in 13 of 22 patients were found to show an enhanced response by measuring regression and regrowth of tumour deposits (Thomlinson et al., 1976; Dawes et al., 1978; Ash et al., 1979). Nearly all these experiments, however, were performed under conditions which in the laboratory showed the oxygen effect to be at its greatest, i.e., the use of a single large radiation dose. Although one cannot extrapolate to the conditions of multi-fraction radiotherapy used in clinical practice, these studies gave firm evidence that hypoxia is present in human tumours and that a sensitizing agent can overcome the associated radioresistance.

Using radio-labelled misonidazole, Urtasun and his colleagues (1989) have shown that in a series of 16 human tumours 10 contained over 5% of hypoxic cells. All seven oat-cell carcinomas and both melanomas studied showed hypoxic cells, but these were not found in three of four sarcomas. These variations may relate to different vascular patterns associated with different types of tumour.

The measurement of reaction in skin made artificially hypoxic has clearly demonstrated the oxygen effect in humans; furthermore, resistance due to hypoxia was considerably overcome using a chemical sensitizing method (Dische, 1988).

Although there has been a general disappointment in the clinical trials which have taken place, there are three with hyperbaric oxygen and two with chemical sensitizing agents where significant benefit would seem to have been achieved. These trials do suggest that hypoxia may be a cause of radiation failure and that in some circumstances improved tumour control can be achieved with a method to sensitize hypoxic tumour cells (Dische, 1988).

10.4 Current clinical efforts to sensitize hypoxic cells

10.4.1 Anaemia

Blood transfusion is clearly indicated for patients who are anaemic, before attempts at curative radiotherapy. The results of the DAHANCA study (Overgaard et al., 1989) would suggest that a haemoglobin concentration well within the normal range is desirable and so in men this should be raised above 14 g% and in women above 13 g%. The availability of blood for transfusion may require, for practical reasons, a modest reduction in both these levels. In clinical trials, particularly those of any radiosensitizing method, it is important to standardise the conditions of requirement for blood transfusion.

10.4.2 New hypoxic cell radiosensitizers

Two chemical sensitizers of hypoxic tumour cells which give promise for improvement over misonidazole have now reached Phase III study. With SR-2508 (etanidazole), the dose-limiting effect is again peripheral neuropathy, but considerably higher doses may be given than with misonidazole before there is a significant incidence of this dose-limiting effect (Coleman et al., 1984). With Ro 03-8799 (pimonidazole) peripheral neuropathy does not occur, but there is an immediate disturbance of the central nervous system giving rise to a feeling of heat and malaise which limits the amount which can be given on any one occasion (Saunders et al., 1984). The drug, however, shows a several-fold concentration in tumours.

We have performed tumour concentration studies after both new drugs were given together with misonidazole. These allowed an estimate of the radiosensitizing concentrations likely to be achieved, and a direct comparison was made with misonidazole in the same human tumour. Our conclusions were that in multi-fraction radiotherapy both are likely to give a sensitization of hypoxic cells equal to a 5-fold increase in misonidazole dose. Therefore, sensitization will be achieved equal to that given by a total of 60 g instead of 12 g of misonidazole per square metre of surface area which was the maximum allowable due to the incidence of peripheral neuropathy (Dische et al., 1986b).

Particularly high tumour concentrations of pimonidazole (Ro 03-8799) have been detected in some cases of malignant melanoma where these may be 10-fold greater than in the plasma at the time of tumour sampling. A small series of patients with malignant melanoma who have been treated with the objective of local cure have shown a high incidence of complete and lasting local clearance (Dische, 1987).

Randomised controlled clinical trials have commenced on an international basis with etanidazole in head and neck cancer and with pimonidazole in advanced carcinoma of cervix. It is in these studies that the combination of a second generation chemical sensitizing agent with conventional fractionated courses of radiotherapy will be assessed.

Use of a low activity but well-tolerated nitroimidazole has been advocated and nimorazole has been incorporated into the current Danish head and neck study. Laboratory studies suggest that only a modest radiosensitization will be achieved – no greater than with misonidazole, but tolerance has been, as expected, good and the results of the study are awaited (Overgaard, personal communication).

10.4.3 The combination of chemical sensitizing agents

The use of a combination of chemical sensitizing agents follows logically from the differing toxicities of the two new chemical sensitizing agents etanidazole and pimonidazole. A Phase I dose-escalation study using single agents was followed by a multi-dose study. It was found that there was a small cross-over of toxicities with a slightly greater incidence of peripheral neuropathy due to etanidazole when pimonidazole was given. Nevertheless, it was shown that the two agents could be combined so as to achieve a considerably greater degree of radiosensitization than with each alone (Bleehen et al., 1989). Unfortunately, problems of drug availability and anticipated problems with Drug Regulation Authorities have considerably hampered this development. The manipulation of thiol concentrations in conjunction with chemical radiosensitizers is described in Section 9.3.1.

10.4.4 Intra-tumoural introduction of hypoxic cell sensitizers

In order to achieve the very highest concentrations in tumour, with the minimum systemic toxicity, attempts have been made to introduce hypoxic cell sensitizers directly into tumour (Hong et al., 1984; Sealy et al., 1988b). With the high concentrations achieved in this way the direct cytotoxic effect of these drugs, independent of radiation, is likely to contribute to cell kill. The use of a powdered form of misonidazole introduced through special needles did result in particularly striking local tumour regression. However, recurrence in the areas immediately around the primary tumour site led to less satisfactory longer-term results (Sealy et al., 1988b). It was obviously difficult to produce a good distribution of drug throughout the tumour.

More recently, dramatic regression in carcinoma of the cervix after direct injection into the tumour and parametrial tissues of a solution of metronidazole have been shown (Balmukhanov et al., 1989; Garcia 1989). The follow-up of patients treated in this manner will be of much interest.

10.4.5 Use of carbogen breathing

Breathing of pure oxygen or carbogen at normal atmospheric pressure was tested clinically, but there was no evidence for improved response and the method was discarded (Rubin et al., 1979). Recently, in a laboratory tumour model, it was shown that normobaric oxygen or carbogen was more effective than any other method of hypoxic cell radiosensitization in a variety of fractionation regimes (Rojas, 1989) (Section 9.4). This has stimulated a further interest in its clinical application. The timing of oxygen or carbogen breathing with the radiotherapy is important. The method has been developed and preliminary studies are underway.

10.4.6 Fluorinated hydrocarbons

The development of fluorinated hydrocarbons as substitutes for blood transfusion has led to their testing as hypoxic cell radiosensitizers (Section 11.3.2). Laboratory studies were followed by a pilot study in head and neck cancer when promising increases in tumour control were observed (Rose et al., 1986). The fluorinated hydrocarbon is given once weekly during therapy and oxygen breathing applied during each treatment. A randomised controlled trial in head and neck cancer is now underway.

10.4.7 Effect of blood pressure on tumour perfusion

In general, tumours have a less adequate vascular supply than normal tissues and thus can respond less effectively to alterations in blood pressure. With a fall in blood pressure tumours are likely to be deprived selectively of an effective blood supply, and therefore of oxygen, but with an increase in blood pressure there is likely to be an increase in perfusion and oxygen availability. In a review of our cases of carcinoma of the bronchus treated by radiotherapy, patients with a higher systolic or pulse pressure appeared to survive longer than those with a lower (Dische et al., 1986a). The use of drugs to raise systolic pressure has not been explored.

10.5 Manipulation of the oxygen effect

The importance of the oxygen concentration in determining radiation response has led to attempts to manipulate rather than simply achieve a greater concentration of oxygen in tumour at the time of treatment.

In the management of limb tumours the circulation has been arrested and radiotherapy given under hypoxic conditions (Suit and Lindberg, 1968). Total radiation doses at least twice those normally used were required. Although there were some striking responses, there were complications when the interruption of vascular supply was not as complete as was expected and, furthermore, since the fractionation regimes incorporated few treatments in order to make the regime tolerable, late effects were seen in some cases and the technique was discontinued.

In Russia and East Germany radiotherapy has been given while breathing 10% oxygen. It is believed that under such conditions there is protection of normal tissues, but not of tumour. Randomised clinical trials are now underway (Neumeister and Révész, 1987).

The use of vaso-dilators can lead to a fall in systolic blood pressure and severe deprivation of blood supply to tumours: extensive necrosis can thus be induced. Under such conditions a nitroimidazole can be expected to exert an additional cytotoxic effect, as well as giving hypoxic cell sensitization when radiation is applied (Adams et al., 1989; Chaplin et al., 1989). Vaso-active drugs are now being given to patients in order to explore this effect.

Drugs have been developed which modify the function of haemoglobin, moving the oxygen dissociation curve to the right (Section 11.2.1). Such drugs give the effect of anaemia and so may, like the vaso-active drugs, be used to induce tumour hypoxia and increase the effect of a nitroimidazole drug (Siemann et al., 1989). This technique is yet to be applied to man.

By the use of hypothermia the oxygen requirement of tissues may be decreased and therefore, effectively, the oxygen tension be increased. Sealy has experimented with the use of hypothermia and irradiation using hyperbaric oxygen. Unfortunately the technique is a complex one and difficult to apply, and can only be used on one or two radiation treatments (Sealy et al., 1986).

10.6 Reoxygenation and accelerated radiotherapy

In recent years it has become evident that many human tumours have a potential for rapid cellular growth. Cell kinetic studies suggest that a considerable number will repopulate at a rapid rate once tumour cell kill occurs during a course of radiotherapy (Wilson et al., 1988). Applying this knowledge we have employed a scheme of continuous, hyperfractionated, accelerated radiotherapy (CHART) in which 36 fractions are given on 12 consecutive days with a minimum interval of 6 hours (see Chapter 14). Results in head and neck, and in advanced primary carcinoma of the bronchus, have been striking (Saunders et al., 1989). Using such short durations for radiotherapy, the time for re-oxygenation is reduced and there may be, at least in some cases, a problem of resistance due to hypoxic tumour cells. It is of note that a preliminary analysis of tumour regression in a series of 52 patients with carcinoma of the bronchus has shown a relationship between completeness of tumour regression and haemoglobin concentration.

It is probable that tumours with an ability to rapidly repopulate are also those with radioresistant hypoxic cells and so the best tumour control will be achieved by combining continuous, hyperfractionated, accelerated radiotherapy with hypoxic cell radiosensitization.

In the reports of the effect of anaemia upon response to radiotherapy and also of those methods of hypoxic cell radiosensitization where positive results have been achieved, there is a trend for the greatest effect to be seen where there was a short overall duration of treatment. The apparent similarity in result between the use of short and long overall treatment times in the radiotherapy of tumours at any one site may be related to a balance of greater effect upon repopulation with shorter treatment times against the overcoming hypoxia with more time for reoxygenation during the longer treatment periods.

The oxygen effect remains important as a determinant of radioresponsiveness but can only be exploited in clinical radiotherapy in the context of all factors determining the responsiveness of a tumour. Cell kinetics, inherent sensitivity, time of shrinkage and reoxygenation must all be considered together with hypoxic cell sensitizers in order to optimise radiotherapy.

References

Adams, G.E., Stratford, I.J., Godden, J. and Howells, N. (1989) Effect of vasoactive agents on the efficiencies of electron affinic radiation sensitizers in vivo. Int. J. Radiat. Oncol. Biol. Phys., in press.

Ash, D., Peckham, M. and Steel, G.G. (1979) The quantitative response of human tumours to radiation and misonidazole. Br. J. Cancer 40, 883–889.

Balmukhanov, S.B., Beisebaev, A.A., Aitkoolava, Z.I., Mustaphin, J.S., Philippenko, V.I., Rismuhamedova, R.S., Aisarova, A.M., Abdrahmanov, J.N. and Révész, L. (1989) Intratumoral and parametrial infusion

of metronidazole in the radiotherapy of uterine cervix cancer. Int. J. Radiat. Oncol. Biol. Phys. 16, 1061–1063.
Bleehen, N.M., Newman, H.F.V., Maughan, T.S. and Workman, P. (1989) A multiple dose study of the combined radiosensitizers Ro 03-8799 (pimonidazole) and SR 2508 (etanidazole). Int. J. Radiat. Oncol. Biol. Phys. 16, 1093–1096.
Chaplin, D.J., Acker, B. and Olive, P.L. (1989) Potentiation of the tumour cytotoxicity of melphalan by vasodilating drugs. Int. J. Radiat. Oncol. Biol. Phys. 16, 1131–1135
Churchill-Davidson, I., Sanger, D. and Thomlinson, R.H. (1955) High pressure oxygen and radiotherapy. Lancet i, 1091–1095.
Coleman, C.N., Urtasun, R.C., Wasserman, T.H., Hancock, S., Harris, J.W., Halsey, J. and Hirst, V.K. (1984) Initial report of the phase I trial of the hypoxic cell radiosensitizer SR 2508. Int. J. Radiat. Oncol. Biol. Phys. 10, 1749–1753.
Dawes, P.J.D.K., Peckham, M.J. and Steel, G.G. (1978) The response of human tumour metastases to radiation and misonidazole. Br. J. Cancer 37 (Suppl. III), 290–296.
Dische, S., Anderson, P.J., Sealy, R. and Watson, E.R. (1983) Carcinoma of the cervix – anaemia, radiotherapy and hyperbaric oxygen. Br. J. Radiol. 56, 251–256.
Dische, S., Saunders, M.I. and Warburton, M.F. (1986a) Hemoglobin, radiation morbidity and survival. Int. J. Radiat. Oncol. Biol. Phys. 12, 1335–1337.
Dische, S., Saunders, M.I., Dunphy, E.P., Bennett, M.H., Des Rochers, C., Stratford, M.R.L., Minchinton, A.I. and Orchard, R.A. (1986b) Concentrations achieved in human tumours after administration of misonidazole, SR-2508 and Ro 03-8799. Int. J. Radiat. Oncol. Biol. Phys. 12, 1109–1111.
Dische, S. (1987) Radiotherapy using the hypoxic cell sensitizer Ro 03-8799 in malignant melanoma. Radiother. Oncol. 10, 111–116.
Dische, S. (1988) Radiation sensitizers in clinical radiotherapy, in: Radiobiology in Radiotherapy (Bleehen, N.M., ed.), pp. 165–176, Springer Verlag, London.
Garcia, A.H. (1989) Radiosensitizer metronidazole plus standard radiation therapy for advanced cervical carcinoma: preliminary results. Int. J. Radiat. Oncol. Biol. Phys., in press.
Gray, L.H., Conger, A.O., Ebert, M., Flockhart, I.R. and Foster, J.L. (1953) The concentration of oxygen dissolved in tissue at the time of irradiation as a factor of radiotherapy. Br. J. Radiol. 26, 638–648.
Hong, A. (1988) Lung function and radiation response. Proceedings Annual Meeting Royal College of Radiologists, Exeter, 7–9 September 1988.
Hong, S.S., Abe, Y., Kaneta, K. and Matsuzawa. T. (1984) Combined treatment of radiation and local injections of misonidazole. Int. J. Radiat. Oncol. Biol. Phys. 10, 2369–2373.
Mottram, J.C. (1935) Mount Vernon Hospital and Radium Institute, Northwood, England, Annual Report.
Neumeister, K. and Révész, L. (1987) Advances in hyporadiotherapy. Int. J. Radiat. Oncol. Biol. Phys. 13, 427–431.
Overgaard, J., Sand Hansen, H., Andersen, A.P., Hjelm-Hansen, M., Jørgensen, K., Sandberg, E., Rygård, J., Hammer, R. and Pedersen, M. (1989) Misonidazole combined with split-course radiotherapy in the treatment of invasive carcinoma of larynx and pharynx, Final Report of the DAHANCA Study. Int. J. Radiat. Oncol. Biol. Phys. 16, 1065–1068.
Rojas, A. (1989) Oxygen – a clinical reality or a mirage? Br. J. Radiol., BIR Report 19, 86–90.
Rose, C., Lustig, R., McIntosh, M. and Teicher, B. (1986) A clinical trial of fluosol DA 20% in advanced squamous cell carcinoma of the head and neck. Int. J. Radiat. Oncol. Biol. Phys. 12, 1325–1328.
Rubin, P., Hanley, J., Keys, H.M., Marcial, V. and Brady, L. (1979) Carbogen breathing during radiation therapy. The Radiation Therapy Oncology Group Study. Int. J. Radiat. Oncol. Biol. Phys. 5, 1963–1970.
Saunders, M.I., Dische, S., Anderson, P.J., Tothill, M., Stratford, M.R.L. and Minchinton, A.I. (1984) The clinical testing of Ro 03-8999 – pharmacokinetics, toxicology, tissue and tumor concentrations. Int. J. Radiat. Oncol. Biol. Phys. 10, 1759–1763.
Saunders, M.I. and Dische, S. (1989) Continuous hyperfractionated accelerated radiotherapy in non-small-

cell carcinoma of the lung. Br. J. Radiol., BIR Report 19, 47–51.

Schwartz, W. (1910) Wien. Klin. Wochenschr. No. 11 S, 397.

Sealy, R., Harrison, G.G. and Morrell, D. (1986) A feasibility study of a new approach to clinical radiosensitisation: hypothermia and hyperbaric oxygen in combination with pharmacological vasodilation. Br. J. Radiol. 59, 1093–1098.

Sealy, R., Harrison, G. and Morrell, D. (1988a) Hypothermic, hyperbaric irradiation. Br. J. Cancer, 61, 269.

Sealy, R., Cridland, S., Blekkenhorst, G., Barry, L. and Rombouts, T. (1988b) Interstitial misonidazole: clinical experience in advanced mouth cancer. Clin. Radiol. 39, 182–185.

Siemann, D.W., Alliet, K.L. and Macler, L.M. (1989) Manipulations in the oxygen transport capacity of blood as means of sensitizing tumors to radiation therapy. Int. J. Radiat. Oncol. Biol. Phys. 16, 1169–1172.

Suit, H. and Lindberg, R. (1968) Radiation therapy administered under conditions of tourniquet-induced local tissue hypoxia. Am. J. Roentgen. 102, 27–37.

Thomlinson, R.H. and Gray, L.H. (1955) The histological structure of some human lung cancers and the possible implications for radiotherapy. Br. J. Cancer 9, 539–549.

Thomlinson, R.H., Dische, S., Gray, A.J. and Errington, L.M. (1976) Clinical testing of the radiosensitizer Ro 03-0582. III. Response of tumours. Clin. Radiol. 27, 167–174.

Urtasun, R.C., Chapman, J.D., Raleigh, J.A., Franko, A.J., Koch, C.J., McKinnon, S. (1989) Measurement of the hypoxic fraction in solid human tumors utilizing the [^{14}C]misonidazole binding in vivo technique. Int. J. Radiat. Oncol. Biol. Phys., in press.

Wilson, G.D., McNally, N.J., Dische, S., Saunders, M.I., Des Rochers, C., Lewis, A.A. and Bennett, M.H. (1988) Measurement of cell kinetics in human tumours in vivo using bromodeoxyuridine incorporation and flow cytometry. Br. J. Cancer 58, 423–431.

CHAPTER 11

Radiation sensitizers and bioreductive drugs

IAN J. STRATFORD and GERALD E. ADAMS

MRC Radiobiology Unit, Chilton, Didcot, Oxfordshire OX11 0RD, England

11.1	Introduction	145
11.2	Effect of haemoglobin status on tumour response to radiotherapy	146
	11.2.1 Modification of haemoglobin/oxygen association	147
11.3	Modification of oxygen transport	148
	11.3.1 Alterations in tumour blood flow	148
	11.3.2 Perfluorocarbons	150
11.4	Electron-affinic radiosensitizers	150
	11.4.1 Etanidazole	151
	11.4.2 Pimonidazole	152
	11.4.3 Dual-function radiosensitizers	153
11.5	Bioreductive cytotoxicity	155
11.6	Chemosensitization	157
11.7	Exploitation of tissue hypoxia for diagnosis	158

11.1 Introduction

The development of methods that lead to an increase in the radiosensitivity of hypoxic cells in tumours remains an important area of research aimed at reducing local failure in radiotherapy. A major focus of attention has been the use of electron affinic radiosensitizers and one of these, misonidazole, has undergone extensive clinical trial. Some benefit is indicated in some situations (Overgaard et al., 1986; 1987) but it is clear that the usefulness of this compound is severely limited by neurotoxic side effects. A variety of compounds potentially superior to misonidazole have been synthesized and some are undergoing clinical investigation, e.g., pimonidazole, Ro

03-8799 (Saunders et al., 1984; Roberts et al., 1984); etanidazole, SR 2508 (Coleman et al., 1984); and RSU1069 (Horwich et al., 1986). Radiation sensitizers of this type are also considerably more toxic to hypoxic than oxic cells. This differential hypoxic cytotoxicity is due to bioreductive activation of the drug under anaerobic conditions and is potentially exploitable in cancer therapy. Alternative strategies against hypoxia in tumours have been aimed at modulating O_2 delivery by: controlling anaemia, modifying the association kinetics of O_2 with haemoglobin, changing tumour blood flow, or using perfluorocarbons as O_2 carriers. These topics are reviewed together with a discussion of the possibility for exploiting the presence of hypoxia in tumours for various diagnostic purposes.

11.2 Effect of haemoglobin status on tumour response to radiotherapy

Clinical experience in relation to the oxygen effect is considered in the previous chapter.

A particularly surprising finding in regard to the importance of haemoglobin status comes from a re-examination, by Dische et al. (1983), of data from a multi-centre trial of radiotherapy in hyperbaric oxygen for a large group of patients with advanced carcinoma of the cervix. The trial showed a significant improvement in local control rate for patients treated in oxygen. However, the analysis of the outcome of patients who presented with anaemia and therefore required transfusion before treatment with radiotherapy produced the data shown in Figure 11.1. A total of 39 patients received transfusion, of which, by chance, 23 were treated in air and 16 in oxygen.

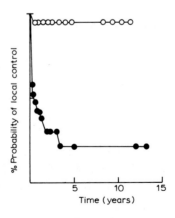

Figure 11.1. Sub-group analysis of patients entered into the MRC trial of hyperbaric oxygen with radiotherapy. Local tumour control in patients with stage III cancer of the cervix requiring blood transfusion, i.e., Hb < 10 g%. Patients were divided according to treatment in air (●) 23 cases, and hyperbaric oxygen (o) 16 cases. The difference between the two groups is significant at $P = 0.0003$ (from Dische et al., 1983).

Despite receiving transfusion, the former group showed a relatively poor response compared with the non-transfused patients who were treated in air. However, the group of transfused patients treated in oxygen showed a very good response, even better than the response rate in the total group of patients treated in oxygen. The explanation of this behaviour is still not clear but it is suggested that prior anaemia could have a *beneficial* effect on the outcome of treatment with radiotherapy and oxygen provided the *anaemia is corrected before treatment*. This encourages continued laboratory research on the various effects of chronic and acute anaemia, with and without transfusion, on the radiation response of experimental tumours (Hirst, 1986).

11.2.1 Modification of haemoglobin/oxygen association

Oxygen delivery to tissues is mediated in part by the equilibrium:

$$HbO_2 \rightleftharpoons Hb + O_2$$

The equilibrium is shown diagrammatically in Figure 11.2A. Most normal tissues are adequately supplied with oxygen by the pool of Hb, which in arterial blood is almost completely saturated under normal conditions. This equilibrium can be displaced in a variety of ways which will be expressed by a change in the value of P_{50} (the partial pressure of oxygen at which half the Hb exists in the oxy conformation). For example, small decreases in pH or temperature result in a decrease in P_{50} i.e., a displacement of the equilibrium to the left.

Similarly, decreases in erythrocyte concentrations of 2,3-diphosphoglycerate (2,3-DPG), an allosteric effector for the binding of O_2 to Hb, can also decrease the value of P_{50}. The effect of left-shifting will be to reduce the level of free oxygen in tissues and thus should induce radioprotection: in contrast, a right-shift could induce some radiosensitization.

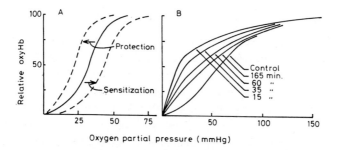

Figure 11.2. (A) Diagrammatic representation of the relationship between oxygen association with Hb and the oxygen partial pressure. (b) Oxygen association curves for haemoglobin taken from CBA/He mice at various times after i.v. administration of 70 mg/kg BW12C (Adams et al., 1987).

Alterations in P_{50} can be achieved by holding mice for 48 hours in an atmosphere of 10% O_2 (raises P_{50}) or 100% O_2 (lowers P_{50}), and these changes are thought to reflect alterations in erythrocyte concentrations of 2,3-DPG (Siemann et al., 1979). Subsequent exchange transfusion of blood from mice exposed to the two different O_2 concentrations into tumour-bearing animals results in tumour radiosensitization in the former group and radiation resistance in the latter (Hirst and Wood, 1987).

There are a number of drugs that right-shift the oxygen/haemoglobin association curve in vitro and the most potent of these is bezafibrate. This drug and a closely related analogue, clofibrate, are able to radiosensitize the murine RIF-1 tumour (Hirst et al., 1987). However, the drug doses used were very high and there was an indication that other drug-induced phenomena contributed to the overall effect. Nevertheless, the study demonstrates the potential usefulness of this approach.

The compound BW12C, under development as an anti-sickling agent, is a potent left-shifter. Figure 11.2 B reproduces data on the left-shifting activity in CBA mice treated with BW12C (Adams et al., 1987). The left-shift is considerable and is still evident for at least 2-3 hours in this strain of mice. A recent study has shown that the reduction of free oxygen levels in tissue caused by the left-shift produces significant radioprotection in experimental systems (Adams et al., 1986; 1987). BW12C protects against the whole-body acute radiation syndrome in CBA mice and radiation-induced skin damage in both experimental mice and pigs. It also induces hypoxia in lymph nodes infiltrated by an experimental mouse T-cell lymphoma. Treatment of mice with multiple doses of BW12C induces necrosis of tumour tissue in the infiltrated nodes. There is no evidence of necrosis induction in normal tissue, suggesting a differential deprivation of available oxygen in or around the tumour tissue.

11.3 Modification of oxygen transport

11.3.1 Alterations in tumour blood flow

There is much experimental evidence that even small tumours are considerably restricted in their oxygen supply compared with most normal tissues. The possibility, therefore, that further deprivation of oxygen could induce tumour necrosis and render tumours *more* susceptible to subsequent therapy, has prompted much investigation into ways of artificially increasing tumour hypoxia. This may be achieved with vaso-active agents that reduce blood flow to tumours. Recent data for 5-hydroxytryptamine (5-HT) is given in Figure 11.3A, which shows survival of RIF-1 tumour cells irradiated in vivo at various times following treatment of mice with a single i.p. dose of 5 mg/kg 5-HT. The dashed line indicates the level of survival obtained when irradiated tumours are taken from mice not receiving drug. Animals given 5-HT and irradiated a few minutes later show a marked radiation resistance which is maximal when the drug

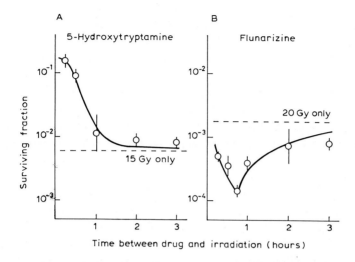

Figure 11.3. Time-course for the effect of vasoactive agents on the radiosensitivity of murine tumours. (A) Response of the RIF-1 tumour in mice injected i.p. with 5 mg/kg 5-hydroxytryptamine and irradiated with 15 Gy. (B) Response of the SCCVII tumour in mice injected i.p. with 50 mg/kg flunarizine and irradiated with 20 Gy (Wood and Hirst, 1988). The dashed lines give the survival for tumour cells from mice treated with radiation only. Points are mean values ± SE from at least three tumours.

is administered 15 minutes prior to irradiation. Further, this high level of survival is similar to that obtained when the blood supply to the tumour is physically occluded by clamping, i.e., the tumour is rendered 100% radiobiologically hypoxic. However, the effect of 5-HT is transient, such that when the drug is given more than 1 hour before X-rays, tumour cell survival is identical to that for cells from tumours in mice not treated with the vaso-active agent.

Alteration in blood flow caused by 5-HT, with the consequent induction of tumour hypoxia, has been used to exploit the properties of certain therapeutic regimes. For example, Chaplin (1986) found that 5-HT enhanced the effectiveness of the hypoxic cytotoxin RSU 1069 (see also Section 11.5). Similarly, tumour response to hyperthermia was found to be enhanced by 5-HT (Knapp et al., 1985). Such an approach will also allow the manipulation of the tumour pharmacokinetics of cytotoxic drugs, since lack of tumour perfusion can result in prolonged exposure to cytotoxic drug, particularly if the vaso-active agent is given *after* the chemotherapeutic agent. This has been demonstrated by using melphalan in combination with 5-HT or hydralazine (Stratford et al., 1988; Adams et al., 1989a).

Hydralazine, a drug used in the treatment of acute hypertension, also induces 100% hypoxia in a range of different tumours (Stratford et al., 1987). It acts mainly on the vascular smooth muscle causing peripheral vaso-dilation and decreased arterial blood pressure, which leads to a reduction in blood flow in a variety of experimental tumours. In contrast, other vaso-active agents such as the calcium antagonists verapamil and flunarizine have been shown to *increase* tumour blood flow in experimental animals. In principle, this property could therefore be exploited in radiation therapy, where enhanced tumour oxygenation brought about by the increase in blood flow could be beneficial. This is illustrated by the data of Wood and Hirst (1988) in Figure 11.3B which shows the time-course for the effect of 50 mg/kg flunarizine injected i.p. on the response of the SCCVII tumour to 20 Gy X-rays in vivo. Clearly, this vaso-active agent caused radiosensitization such that a 10-fold increase in cell killing was obtained when the drug was given 45 minutes before irradiation. In the same study, little effect of flunarizine was observed on the response of the RIF-1 tumour. This variation between tumour types was attributed to the presence of a much higher proportion of 'acutely' hypoxic cells (see Chaplin et al., 1986) in the SCCVII compared to the RIF-1 tumour and it was thought these acutely hypoxic cells were those whose oxygen supply is limited by perfusion. If the oxygenation status of chronically hypoxic cells in tumours is not affected by treatment with agents such as flunarizine, then this approach may have limitations; this is currently being investigated.

11.3.2 Perfluorocarbons

Emulsions of perfluorocarbons (PFC) are artificial blood substitutes that can efficiently act as oxygen carriers to tissue, particularly when combined with breathing oxygen at high concentrations. PFCs have been used as oxygen transport agents to minimise ischaemic damage after myocardial infarction or in place of blood transfusion (Nunn et al., 1983). Particles of PFCs are small (<0.2 μm diameter). O_2 solubility is linearly related to O_2 tension and thus uptake and release of O_2 can be extremely rapid. Hence, these oxygen-rich particles would be expected to diffuse through the vascular network of tumours and sensitize hypoxic cells to radiation therapy.

In experimental systems, administration of Fluosol-DA (20%) while breathing carbogen or 100% O_2 shortly before irradiation, can reduce the fraction of radiobiologically hypoxic cells in a range of animal tumours. Further, it has been shown that PFCs can also increase the effectiveness of certain chemotherapeutic agents, presumably by enhancing drug delivery (Teicher and Holden, 1987). These pre-clinical findings have stimulated Phase I/II trials of Fluosol-DA as an adjuvant in radiation therapy (Rose et al., 1986).

11.4 Electron-affinic radiosensitizers

Structure-activity relationships have identified one-electron reduction potential as the important physicochemical parameter for determining sensitizing efficiency in vitro. Such a relationship is wholly consistent with O_2 and the electron-affinic agents increasing the radiation sensitivity of hypoxic cells by a fast free-radical mechanism.

Radiation sensitizers 151

All oxygen-mimetic sensitizers so far examined clinically, operate, at least in part, in this manner.

11.4.1 Etanidazole (SR-2508)

Neurotoxicity is dose-limiting for misonidazole but analogues with reduced lipophilicity (lower octanol/water partition coefficients) show reduced uptake in neural tissue and appear to be less neurotoxic. Studies with a series of nitroimidazoles related to misonidazole have led to the clinical development of SR-2508, etanidazole (Figure 11.4). This compound has a sensitizing efficiency similar to that of misonidazole, is substantially less neurotoxic and may possibly show an improved tumour uptake (Brown et al., 1981). Phase I and II clinical studies have confirmed the much reduced neurotoxicity and total doses over 30 g/m^2 have been successfully administered to patients over a 6 week course of radiotherapy without undue neurological complications (Coleman et al., 1984). Randomised trials with this drug are now being initiated in the U.S.A. It has been calculated that sensitizer enhancement ratios (dose modification

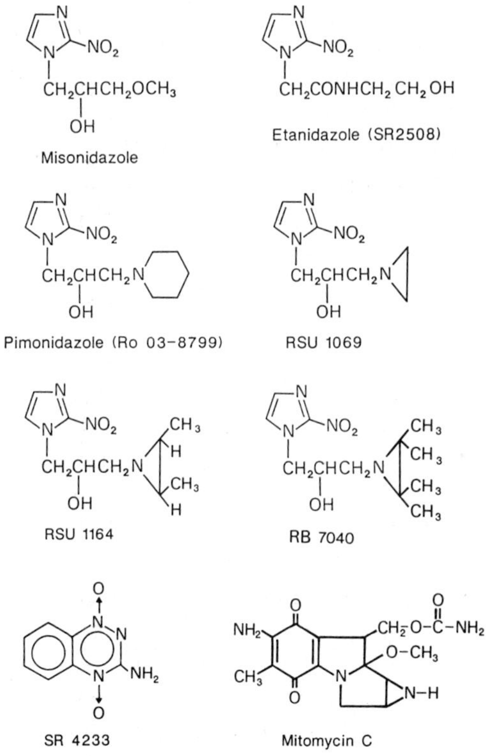

Figure 11.4. Chemical structures of some radiation sensitizers and bioreductive drugs.

factors) up to about 1.7 may be obtainable with this sensitizer. If this is realised, substantial improvements over misonidazole should be demonstrable.

11.4.2 Pimonidazole (Ro 03-8799)

Experimental and clinical studies have shown that misonidazole penetrates well into the tumour regions where hypoxic cells are likely to be present. However, in no instance have gross tumour levels in excess of those in plasma been reported. This is not the case for pimonidazole which is a misonidazole analogue with a side-chain containing a weakly basic piperidine group (Figure 11.4). Clinical studies involving drug uptake measurements in tumour biopsy specimens have shown generally that peak tumour levels of the drug can substantially exceed peak serum levels (Roberts et al., 1984; Dische et al., 1986). Studies in vitro (Dennis et al., 1985; Watts and Jones, 1985) demonstrated that the intracellular uptake of the drug and, consequently, its sensitizing efficiency are highly dependent on the pH of the extracellular medium. This is illustrated in Figure 11.5 where it can be seen that, at low pH, intracellular uptake of pimonidazole is only modest (intra:extracellular concentration of drug = 0.8 at pH 6.2). In contrast, at high values of pH, drug accumulation is increased and this is reflected by an increase in sensitizing efficiency. This effect is not seen with misonidazole. It is proposed that access of pimonidazole into the cell is via the neutral (unprotonated) form of the molecule. In the extracellular fluid in hypoxic regions of tumours, the relatively lower pH allows the drug to be concentrated in its water-soluble protonated form. According to this hypothesis, intracellular levels build up as the drug is transported into the tumour cells in the non-protonated form (Wardman, 1982).

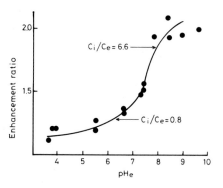

Figure 11.5. Enhancement ratio for sensitization of hypoxic V79 cells by 0.1 mmol/dm^3 pimonidazole as a function of extracellular pH (pH$_e$). The measured values of intra:extra-cellular concentrations of pimonidazole at pH$_e$ = 6.2 and pH$_e$ = 7.9 are indicated (redrawn from Dennis et al., 1985).

Pimonidazole has a slight advantage in sensitizing efficiency over misonidazole on the basis of its increased electron affinity. Further, it is undoubtably less toxic in patients (Saunders et al., 1984). These facts, taken together with the observation that substantially higher tumour levels can be obtained with pimonidàzole have led to the proposal that the therapeutic efficiency of this drug should be 5–7-times greater than that of misonidazole. Phase III trials of pimonidazole with radiation in the treatment of advanced carcinoma of the cervix have commenced.

11.4.3 Dual-function radiosensitizers

These are nitro-containing compounds that also possess alkylating properties. The lead compound is the 2-nitroimidazole, RSU 1069 (Figure 11.4), which contains an aziridine group in the side-chain (Adams, 1984a; b). This drug is a more active radiation sensitizer in vivo than any other nitroheterocyclic compound so far investigated, and it also displays a particularly high cytotoxic activity towards hypoxic cells (Section 11.5). The radiosensitizing efficiencies of RSU 1069 and misonidazole in vivo are shown in Figure 11.6.

KHT tumours implanted subcutaneously in C3H mice were irradiated with 10 Gy 1 hour after administration of sensitizer. Tumour response was measured by clonogenic assay in vitro. This tumour has a hypoxic fraction of about 10% and with this dose of radiation, the surviving cells are derived predominantly from the radiation resistant hypoxic fraction. Thus the data points show changes in the surviving fraction of the hypoxic cells in the tumour. Clearly, RSU 1069 is more efficient than misonidazole by at least a factor of 10, which is consistent with previous studies in vitro (Adams, 1984a). It is of interest that, at the highest dose of RSU 1069 (0.38 mmol/kg), the surviving fraction is reduced to $1.4 \cdot 10^{-3}$. In comparison, the surviving

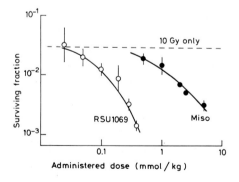

Figure 11.6. Surviving fraction of cells from KHT tumours in mice irradiated with 10 Gy X-rays 60 min after i.p. injection of various doses of misonidazole (●) or RSU 1069 (o). The horizontal dashed line gives the survival for tumour cells from mice treated with radiation only (Stratford et al., 1989).

fraction of aerobic KHT cells in vitro given 10 Gy is about $2 \cdot 10^{-3}$, which suggests that RSU 1069 achieves a level of sensitization in this tumour close to the value of the oxygen enhancement ratio.

The enhancement efficiency of radiation sensitization by RSU 1069 relative to that of misonidazole is not in line with the finding that the one-electron reduction potentials of the two compounds are similar. However, the sensitizing efficiency of the former compound over the range 4–37°C is very temperature-dependent whereas that of misonidazole is much less so. Further, rapid-mix studies have shown that misonidazole and RSU 1069 show similar radiosensitizing efficiencies at room temperature for pre-irradiation contact times up to about 1 second. Thus, both drugs act in part, over a sub-second time-scale in mechanisms involving intracellular free-radical processes. However, the enhanced sensitizing efficiency of RSU 1069 compared to that of misonidazole is likely to be due to 'slow' processes associated with metabolic activation of RSU 1069.

A preliminary clinical study of RSU 1069 showed that the drug induced severe gastro-intestinal toxicity depending on the dose level administered (Horwich et al., 1986). This has stimulated the search for equally effective, but less toxic analogues of RSU 1069. One series includes a group of compounds in which the aziridinyl group of RSU 1069 is progressively substituted with methyl groups (Figure 11.4).

Studies of radiation sensitization in mammalian cells in vitro show very little change in sensitization efficiency with increasing methylation of the aziridine. However, in vivo there is a slight decrease in efficiency, but for one compound (RSU 1164) this is accompanied by a substantial decrease in toxicity and, overall, provides the possibility for therapeutic gain when compared to RSU 1069. A potentially important factor in the development of this series of agents is that the methylation increases the efficiency of cellular drug uptake. This effect is associated with the influence of methyl substitution on the acid-base properties of the side-chain and is in line with the results of previous investigations of the rôle of such properties on the uptake of pimonidazole in vitro and in vivo (Section 11.4.2).

The property of differential uptake may be a general characteristic of weakly basic nitroimidazole sensitizers. If so, this may be exploitable, particularly in melanoma. It has already been established clinically that pimonidazole appears to concentrate in melanoma even more so than in other tumour types (Dische, 1987). This is also observed with RSU 1069, RSU 1164 and RB 7040 in experimental tumours (Walling et al., 1989). These authors found that the AUC (area under the curve in the plot of tissue level against time after administration) for RSU 1069 and RSU 1164 was 7.6- and 3.6-times higher in B16 melanoma compared to either the KHT or Lewis lung tumours. However, the therapeutic implications of these observations remain to be determined.

11.5 Bioreductive cytotoxicity

Bioreductive drugs are chemical agents that are activated by metabolic biochemical reduction. Such processes have long been known to be involved in the mechanisms of action of various anaerobic antibiotics. Preferential hypoxic toxicity against mammalian cells has also been observed for various nitroimidazoles such as metronidazole, misonidazole and RSU 1069, as well as mitomycin C and the benzotriazine-di-N-oxide, SR 4233. There is little doubt that the enhanced cytotoxicity under hypoxic conditions is caused by highly toxic substances formed by enzyme-mediated reduction of the drugs. In aerobic cells, the formation of such cytotoxic metabolites is inhibited by oxygen and this results in 'futile reductive cycling'; illustrated for nitroimidazoles below:

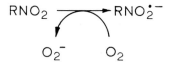

The position of this equilibrium will depend primarily on the one-electron reduction potential of the nitroheterocycle and on the oxygen tension. Should the equilibrium lie to the right, then disproportionation of $RNO_2^{\cdot -}$ will occur to yield cytotoxic metabolites. It would be expected that compounds of higher (i.e. less negative) reduction potential would show less dependence on O_2, i.e., be active at relatively high O_2 tensions. This has been demonstrated by Mohindra and Rauth (1976) who compared metronidazole with nitrofurazone. Further, it would be predicted that, under hypoxic conditions, toxicity would increase as the reduction potential increases. This is illustrated in Figure 11.7 for a range of nitroheterocycles (Adams et al., 1980). The concentration of compound required to achieve a given level of toxicity is plotted as a function of reduction potential and there is a significant correlation ($r = 0.94$). The full square shows data for RSU 1069 and the hypoxic activity of this agent is far in excess (10^3-fold) of that expected from its redox potential.

The differential toxicity of RSU 1069 (i.e., the ratio of concentrations required to give similar levels of toxicity in air and N_2) is approximately 100, whereas the ratio for many other compounds in Figure 11.7 is between 2 and 10 (Stratford and Stephens, 1989). The reason for the high differential toxicity of RSU 1069 is as follows. Under oxic conditions, the drug acts merely as a *mono*-functional alkylating agent, involving interaction of the aziridine group with intra-cellular DNA. In hypoxia, bioreduction of the nitro group leads to the formation of metabolites that are much more cytotoxic due to their ability to act bifunctionally in their reactivity with DNA. Such processes are also likely to contribute to the high radiation sensitizing efficiency of RSU 1069 (Section 11.4.3).

Bioreductive agents should be useful for therapy in combination with other modal-

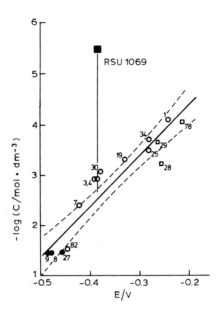

Figure 11.7. Dependence of hypoxic toxicity (the concentration required to reduce survival to 10^{-2} in 5 hours) on one-electron reduction potential: o, 2-nitroimidazoles; •, 5-nitroimidazoles; □, 5-nitrofurans. The solid line is the regression represented by $-\log C = B_0 + b_1 E_7^1$. The curved broken lines are the 95% confidence limits (Adams et al., 1980).

ities, including drugs or radiation that would otherwise be limited by the presence of tumour hypoxia. However, it is only recently that compounds, other than mitomycin C, have been developed which have substantial activity against solid tumours. This is because, as single agents, the bioreductive drugs will be much less active against the oxic tumour cells. Activity in vivo can be demonstrated in two ways: firstly, by giving the bioreductive agent after irradiation when the surviving cell population will be predominantly hypoxic, and secondly, by the use of bioreductive drugs in combination with agents that selectively induce 100% tumour hypoxia. This can be achieved with hydralazine (Section 11.3). Treatment of mice with this vaso-active agent can increase the efficacy of RSU 1069, SR 4233 and mitomycin C. The data in Figure 11.8 show this effect in three experimental murine tumours, KHT, RIF-1 and the Lewis lung tumour, which normally have hypoxic fractions of 10, 1–3 and 10–20%, respectively. The plots show the surviving fractions of tumour cells treated in vivo with increasing single doses of RSU 1069. The closed circles show that, as expected, the drug has only a small effect on tumour response. The drug is primarily active only against hypoxic cells and therefore the oxic clonogenic cells in the tumour will be relatively unresponsive. In contrast, the tumours treated with hydralazine 5–15 minutes after

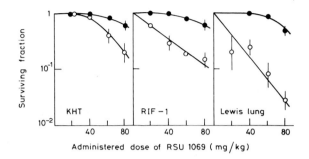

Figure 11.8. Cell-survival data for various tumour types in mice given RSU 1069 alone (●) or RSU 1069 followed 5–15 minutes later by hydralazine 5 mg/kg i.v. (o). Data points are means (± SE) of survival determinations of up to six individual tumours (Adams et al., 1989).

administration of RSU 1069 (open circles) show a greater response, indicative of the greater degree of hypoxia induced by hydralazine. It is of interest that the extent of the increased effect of RSU 1069 appears to be greatest in the Lewis lung tumour. This variation does *not* reflect differences in the hypoxic status normally present in these tumours; but may indicate differences in the enzymology of each tumour type, which will also influence the amount of bioreductive activation that will occur.

11.6 Chemosensitization

The phenomenon of bioreductive toxicity led to speculation that drugs that are more effective against hypoxic cells could be added to existing chemotherapy schedules in order to increase therapeutic effectiveness. Independently, Rose et al., (1980) and Clement et al. (1980) investigated the effect of misonidazole on the anti-tumour activity of various alkylating agents. Enhancement of efficacy was observed in various tumour systems, although the effect was variable depending on the nature of the tumour and the type of alkylating agent used. In particular, both groups observed enhancement factors of up to about 2, which in terms of numbers of cells killed represents a considerable increase in effectiveness. Since that time, numerous reports have been published confirming the phenomenon in a variety of different experimental tumour systems with various nitroheterocyclic compounds including misonidazole. Further, a significant effect using the combination of melphalan and misonidazole has recently been demonstrated in the clinical treatment of non-small-cell lung cancer (Coleman et al., 1988).

Chemosensitization by nitroimidazoles can still be demonstrated using doses of the drug that, alone, cause little or no cell kill. Experiments of this type have shown unequivocally that the phenomenon is a true potentiation of the cytotoxic effect of the alkylating agent and not simply an expression of the additivity of the independent

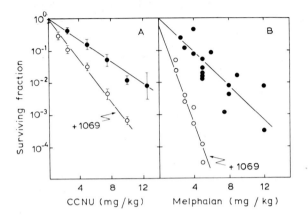

Figure 11.9. Chemosensitisation by RSU 1069. ●, chemotherapeutic drug alone; ○, chemotherapeutic drug plus 0.38 mmol/kg RSU 1069. (A) mice with the KHT tumour given RSU 1069 30 minutes before various doses of CCNU (Siemann et al., 1985). (B) mice with the MT tumour given RSU 1069 60 minutes before various doses of melphalan (Adams et al., 1984b).

cytotoxic actions of each agent. Experimental data on the chemosensitizing effects of the nitroimidazole RSU 1069 on the anti-tumour activities of CCNU (Siemann et al., 1985) and melphalan (Adams et al., 1984b) are shown in Figure 11.9. Tumour-bearing mice were treated with single doses of the appropriate drugs and tumour responses were measured quantitatively by the clonogenic cell assay method. The compound RSU 1069 sensitizes the anti-tumour effect of both CCNU and melphalan in the respective tumours. The dose modification factors calculated from the slopes of the survival curves are 2.0 for sensitization of CCNU and about 3.0 for melphalan. In terms of increase in cell killing efficacy, the sensitization is very large in both cases. At the doses of RSU 1069 used in the two sets of experiments, the cell kill induced by the sensitizer alone was negligible, indicating that the enhancing effects are true potentiations.

Overall, the mechanism of chemosensitization in tumours is undoubtedly complex and can be influenced by various factors: the nature of the nitroheterocyclic compound, the type of alkylating agent, tumour size and histological type, and the drug sequence and timing. However, the evidence supporting the role of hypoxia-mediated bioreductive processes in chemosensitization provides a sound rationale for the development of new strategies in cancer chemotherapy.

11.7 Exploitation of tissue hypoxia for diagnosis

Bioreductive drugs of the nitroheterocycle type (e.g. misonidazole) selectively bind in oxygen-deficient mammalian cells of various types both in vitro and in vivo

(Garrecht and Chapman, 1983). The binding is known to involve DNA but other intercellular binding sites are not excluded. The binding occurs through metabolites that arise directly from enzyme-mediated reduction of the ring-substituted nitro group and appears to be irreversible. Some binding *can* occur in some normal tissues (e.g., liver) where reductive enzyme levels may be high or where some degree of hypoxia exists. Nevertheless, it is now clear that differential binding in regions of solid tumours is high. Further, this differential can be increased by techniques which enhance tumour hypoxia: for example, blood flow modification by hydralazine (Stratford et al., 1988). Binding of isotopically labelled misonidazole has been used clinically in attempts to identify those human tumours where hypoxic cell resistance may be particularly important in treatment by radiotherapy (Urtasun et al., 1986).

This approach can be extended in a variety of ways.

Firstly, bioreductive drugs labelled with energetic γ-ray emitters will have application in the detection of pre-ischaemic and ischaemic lesions in cardiac and cerebral dysfunction (Hoffman et al., 1987) as well as in applications in oncology. Studies with a nitroimidazole labelled with ^{131}I have already suggested that this may be feasible (Jette et al., 1986).

Secondly, using ^{19}F-NMR spectroscopy, Raleigh et al., (1986) demonstrated that a fluorinated analogue of misonidazole localises well in the EMT6 tumour. Subsequent studies by Maxwell et al. (1989) have shown that this localisation can be followed spectroscopically in situ with doses of the compound that are tolerated by tumour-bearing mice. A recent report has indicated that the equivalent ^{18}F positron emitter has potential for application in PET scanning (Rasey et al., 1987).

Acknowledgement

This work was supported in part by NCI grant No. RO1 CA44126.

References

Adams, G.E., Ahmed, I., Sheldon, P.W. and Stratford, I.J. (1984a) Radiation sensitization and chemopotentiation: RSU 1069, a compound more efficient than misonidazole in vitro and in vivo. Br. J. Cancer. 49, 571–578.
Adams, G.E., Ahmed, I., Sheldon, P.W. and Stratford, I.J. (1984b) RSU 1069, a 2-nitroimidazole containing an alkylating group: high efficiency as a radio- and chemosensitizer in vitro and in vivo. Int. J. Radiat. Oncol. Biol. Phys. 10, 1653–1656.
Adams, G.E., Barnes, D., Loutit, J., Cole, S., Sheldon, P., Stratford, I.J., Van den Aardweg, G.J.M.J., Hopewell, J., White, R., Kneen, G., Nethersell, A. and Edwards, C. (1986) Induction of hypoxia in normal and malignant tissues by changing the oxygen affinity of haemoglobin: implications for therapy. Int. J. Radiat. Oncol. Biol. Phys. 12, 1299–1302.
Adams, G.E., Stratford, I.J., Ahmed, I. and Sheldon, P.W. (1987) Some new developments in tumour

radiosensitization. in: Progress in Radio-Oncology III, (Kärcher, K.H., Kogelnik, H.D. and Szapasi, S., eds.), pp. 81–88, ICRO, Vienna.

Adams, G.E., Stratford, I.J., Godden, J. and Howells, N. (1989a) Enhancement of the anti-tumour effect of melphalan by some vaso-active agents in experimental mice. Int. J. Radiat. Oncol. Biol. Phys. 16, 1137–1140.

Adams, G.E., Stratford, I.J. and Nethersell, A.B.W. (1989b) Manipulation of the oxygenation status of tumours: activation of bioreductive drugs. Br. J. Radiol. BIR Report 19, 71–75.

Adams, G.E., Stratford, I.J., Wallace, R.G., Wardman, P. and Watts, M.E. (1980) Toxicity of nitro compounds toward hypoxic mammalian cells: dependence upon reduction potential. J. Natl. Cancer Inst. 64, 555–560.

Brown, J.M., Yu, N.Y., Brown, D.M. and Lee, W. (1981) SR 2508: a 2-nitroimidazoleamide which should be superior to misonidazole as a radiosensitizer for clinical use. Int. J. Radiat. Oncol. Biol. Phys. 7, 695–703.

Chaplin, D.J. (1986) Potentiation of RSU 1069 tumour cytotoxicity by 5-hydroxytryptamine. Br. J. Cancer 54, 727–731.

Chaplin, D.T., Durand, R.E. and Olive, P.L. (1986) Acute hypoxia in tumours: implications for modifiers of radiation effects. Int. J. Radiat. Oncol. Biol. Phys. 12, 1279–1282.

Clement, J.J., Gorman, M.S., Wodinsky, I., Catane, R. and Johnson, R.K. (1980) Enhancement of anti-tumour activity of alkylating agents by the radiation sensitizer misonidazole. Cancer Res. 40, 4165–4172.

Coleman, C.N., Carlson, R.W., Halsey, J., Kohler, M., Gribble, B.I. and Jacobs, C. (1988) Enhancement of the clinical activity of melphalan by the hypoxic cell sensitizer misonidazole. Cancer Res. 48, 3528–3532.

Coleman, C.N., Urtasun, R.C., Wasserman, T.H., Hancock, S., Harris, J.W., Halsey, J. and Hirst, V.K. (1984) Initial report of the phase I trial of the hypoxic cell radiosensitizer SR 5208. Int. J. Radiat. Oncol. Biol. Phys. 10, 1749–1753.

Dennis, M.F., Stratford, M.R.L., Wardman, P. and Watts, M.E. (1985) Cellular uptake of misonidazole and analogues with acidic or basic functions. Int. J. Radiat. Biol. 47, 629–643.

Dische, S. (1987) Radiotherapy using the hypoxic cell sensitizer Ro 03-8799 in malignant melanoma. Radiother. Oncol. 10, 111–116.

Dische, S., Anderson, P.J., Sealy, R. and Watson, E.R. (1983) Carcinoma of the cervix: anaemia, radiotherapy and hyperbaric oxygen. Br. J. Radiol. 56, 251–255.

Dische, S., Saunders, M.I., Bennett, M.H., Dunphy, E.P., Des Rochers, C., Stratford, M.R.L., Minchington, A.I. and Wardman, P. (1986) A comparison of the tumour concentrations obtainable with misonidazole and Ro 03-8799. Br. J. Radiol. 59, 911–917.

Garrecht, B.M. and Chapman, J.D. (1983) The labelling of EMT-6 tumours with [^{14}C]misonidazole. Br. J. Radiol. 56, 745–754.

Hirst, D.G. (1986) Anaemia: a problem or opportunity in radiotherapy? Int. J. Radiat. Oncol. Biol. Phys. 12, 2009–2017.

Hirst, D.G. and Wood, P.J. (1987) The influence of haemoglobin affinity for oxygen on tumour radiosensitivity. Br. J. Cancer 55, 487–491.

Hirst, D.G., Wood, P.J. and Schwarz, H.C. (1987) The modification of haemoglobin affinity for oxygen and tumour radiosensitivity by antilipidemic drugs. Radiat. Res. 112, 164–172.

Hoffmann, J.M., Rasey, J.S., Spence, A.M., Shaw, D.W. and Krohn, K.A. (1987) Binding of the hypoxic tracer [^{3}H]misonidazole in cerebral ischaemia. Stroke 18, 168–176.

Horwich, A., Holliday, S.B., Deacon, J.M. and Peckham, M.J. (1986) A toxicity and pharmacokinetic study in man of the hypoxic cell radiosensitizer RSU 1069. Br. J. Radiol. 59, 1238–1240.

Jette, D.C., Wiebe, L.I., Flanagan, R.J., Lee, J. and Chapman, J.D. (1986) Iodoazomycin riboside (1-(5′-iodo-5′-deoxyribofuranosyl)-2-nitroimidazole): a hypoxic cell marker. Radiat. Res. 105, 169–179.

Knapp, W.H., Debatin, J., Layer, K., Helus, F., Altmann, A., Sinn, H.J. and Ostertag, H. (1985) Selective drug induced reduction of blood flow in tumour transplants. Int. J. Radiat. Oncol. Biol. Phys. 11, 1357–1366.
Maxwell, R.J., Workman, P. and Griffiths, J.R. (1989) Demonstration of tumour-selective retention of fluorinated nitroimidazole probes by ^{19}F magnetic resonance spectroscopy in vivo. Int. J. Radiat. Oncol. Biol. Phys. 16, 925–930.
Mohindra, J.K. and Rauth, A.M. (1976) Increased cell killing by metronidazole and nitrofurazone of hypoxic compared to aerobic mammalian cells. Cancer Res. 36, 930–936.
Nunn, G.R., Dance, G., Peters, J., Cohn, L.H. (1983) Effect of fluorocarbon exchange transfusion on myocardial infarction size in dogs. Am. J. Cardiol. 52, 203–205.
Overgaard, J., Hansen, S.H., Anderson, A.P., Hjelm-Handsen, M., Jorgensen, K., Sandberg, K., Rygard, J., Jensen, R.H. and Petersen, M. (1987) Misonidazole as an adjuct to radiotherapy in the treatment of invasive carcinoma of the larynx and pharynx, *in*: Progress in Radio-Oncology III. (Kärcher, K.H., Kogelnik, H.D. and Szepesi, T., eds.), pp. 137–147, Proceedings of the 3rd International Meeting on Progress in Radio-Oncology, March 1985, ICRO, Vienna.
Overgaard, J., Hansen, S.H., Jorgensen, K. and Hjelm-Handsen, M. (1986) Primary radiotherapy of larynx and pharynx carcinoma – an analysis of some factors influencing local control and survival. Int. J. Radiat. Oncol. Biol. Phys. 12, 515–521.
Raleigh, J.A., Franko, A.J., Treiber, E.O., Lunt, J.A. and Allen, P.S. (1986) Covalent binding of a fluorinated 2-nitroimidazole to EMT tumours in BALB/c mice: Detection by F-19 nuclear magnetic resonance of 2.35T. Int. J. Radiat. Oncol. Biol. Phys. 12, 1243–1245.
Rasey, J.S., Grunbaum, Z., Magee, S., Nelson, N.J., Olive, P.L., Durand, R.E., Krohn, K.A. (1987) Characterization of radiolabelled fluoromisonidazole as a probe for hypoxic cells. Rad. Res. 111, 292–304.
Roberts, J.T., Bleehen, N.M., Workman, P. and Walton, M.I. (1984) A phase I study of the hypoxic cell radiosensitizer Ro 03-8799. Int. J. Radiat. Oncol. Biol. Phys. 10, 1755–1758.
Rose, C.M., Lustig, R., McCintosh, N. and Teicher, B.A. (1986) A clinical trial of Fluosol-DA (20%) in advanced squamous cell carcinoma of the head and neck. Int. J. Radiat. Oncol. Biol. Phys. 12, 1325–1327.
Rose, C.M., Millar, J.L., Peacock, J.H., Phelps, T.A. and Stephens, T.C. (1980) Differential enhancement of melphalan cytotoxicity in tumour and normal tissue by misonidazole, *in*: Radiation Sensitizers: Their Use in the Clinical Management of Cancer, Cancer Management Vol. 5, pp. 250–256, Masson, New York.
Saunders, M.I., Anderson, P.J., Bennett, M.H., Dische, S., Minchinton, A., Stratford, M.R.L. and Tothill, M. (1984) The clinical testing of Ro 03-8799: pharmacokinetics, toxicology, tissue and tumour concentrations. Int. J. Radiat. Oncol. Biol. Phys. 10, 1759–1763.
Siemann, D.W., Alliet, K., Maddison, K. and Wolf, K. (1985) Enhancement of the anti-tumour efficacy of lomustine by the radiosensitizer RSU 1069. Cancer Treat. Rep. 69, 1409–1414.
Siemann, D.W., Hill, R.P., Bush, R.S. and Chabra, P. (1979) The in vivo radiation response of an experimental tumour: the effect of exposing mice to a reduced oxygen environment prior to but not during irradiation. Int. J. Radiat. Oncol. Biol. Phys. 5, 61–68.
Stratford, I.J., Adams, G.E., Godden, J., Howells, N., Nolan, J. and Timpson, N. (1988) Potentiation of the anti-tumour effect of melphalan by the vaso-active drug, hydralazine. Br. J. Cancer 58, 122–127.
Stratford, I.J., Godden, J., Howells, N., Embling, P. and Adams, G.E. (1987) Manipulation of tumour oxygenation by hydralazine increases the potency of bioreductive radiosensitizers and enhances the effect of melphalan in experimental tumours, *in*: Radiation Research, Vol. 2. (Fielden, E.M., Fowler, J.F., Hendry, J.H. and Scott, D., eds.), Taylor and Francis, London.
Stratford, I.J. and Stephens, M.A. (1989) The differential hypoxic cytotoxicity of bioreductive agents determined in vitro by the MTT assay. Int. J. Radiat. Oncol. Biol. Phys. 16, 973–976.

Teicher, B.A. and Holden, S.A. (1987) Survey of the effect of adding Fluosol-DA (20%) plus oxygen to treatment with various chemotherapeutic agents. Cancer Treat. Rep. 71, 173–177.

Urtasun, R.C., Chapman, J.D., Raleigh, J.A., Franko, A.J. and Kock, C.J. (1986) Binding of [^{3}H]misonidazole to solid human tumours as a measure of tumour hypoxia. Int. J. Radiat. Oncol. Biol. Phys. 12, 1263–1267.

Walling, J.M., Deacon, J., Holliday, S. and Stratford, I.J. (1989) High uptake of RSU 1069 and its analogues into melanotic melanomas. Cancer Chemother. Pharmacol., in press.

Wardman, P. (1982) Molecular structure and biological activity of hypoxic cell radiosensitizers and hypoxic-specific cytotoxins, in: Advanced Topics on Radiosensitizers of hypoxic cells. (Breccia, A., Rimondi, C. and Adams, G.E., eds.), NATO Advanced study institute series A. Life Sci. 43, 49–75.

Watts, M.E. and Jones, N.R. (1985) The effect of extracellular pH on radiosensitization by misonidazole and acidic or basic analogues. Int. J. Radiat. Biol. 47, 645–653.

Wood, P.J. and Hirst, D.G. (1988) Cinnarizine and flunarizine as radiation sensitizers in two murine tumours. Br. J. Cancer 58, 742–745.

CHAPTER 12

Radiobiology of human tumour cells

G. GORDON STEEL

Radiotherapy Research Unit, The Institute of Cancer Research, Cotswold Road, Sutton, Surrey SM2 5NG, England

---

12.1	Introduction	163
12.2	Experimental cell system	164
	12.2.1 In vitro cell lines	164
	12.2.2 Multicellular spheroids	165
	12.2.3 Xenografts of human tumours	165
12.3	The range of radiosensitivity among human tumour cells	166
	12.3.1 The initial slope of cell-survival curves	168
	12.3.2 Correlation with clinical response	169
	12.3.3 The radiobiology of xenografts	171
12.4	Recovery processes in human tumour cells	172
	12.4.1 Recovery of potentially lethal damage	172
	12.4.2 Implications of the linear-quadratic model for recovery in human tumour cell lines	173
12.5	Overview: The importance of the linear component of cell killing	174

12.1 Introduction

For many years it was not appreciated that tumour cells differ widely in radiosensitivity and that this is an important reason for success or failure in clinical radiotherapy. Although a few cell lines derived from human tumours have been available for many years (particularly the HeLa cell line which came from a human cervix carcinoma), it was not until the 1970s that data on a variety of human tumour types began to appear. There were two reasons for this. Firstly, early work on the radiosensitivity of mouse tumour cells (see Berry, 1974, for review) seemed to indicate that radiosensitivity did not vary widely with tumour type: radiation appeared to be a relatively non-specific killing agent. Secondly, human tumour cells are not easy to clone in vitro, and it was not until around 1975 that widely applicable techniques became available. As a result, the search for reasons for failure in clinical radiotherapy has for many years focused mainly on hypoxic cells and on methods to reduce their impact (see Chapters 9, 10 and 11).

The picture now is very different. It is clear that differences in the inherent radiosensitivity of tumour cells may play a decisive part in clinical success or failure. This is indicated particularly in Section 12.3 below, and also by the wide range of sensitivity seen among human tumour cells irradiated at low dose rate (Section 15.2).

12.2 Experimental cell systems

The radiobiology of human tumours has been studied in the laboratory using a variety of cell systems which can be grouped in the following categories: tissue culture cell lines (exponentially-growing or in plateau-phase), multicellular spheroids, and xenografts of human tumours in immune-deficient mice.

12.2.1 In vitro cell lines

The clonal growth of human tumour cells in tissue culture is technically difficult, probably because of their often low growth rate and particular growth requirements. The problem is made more difficult by the need to suppress the in vitro growth of connective-tissue cells, for instance by keeping the cells in suspension in soft agar. The approach described by Courtenay and Mills (1978) has been particularly successful, emphasizing the need for meticulous attention to obtaining a single-cell suspension, adequate duration of growth in culture, the consequent need to replenish the growth medium, the requirement for added growth factors, and the common benefit of incubating under low oxygen concentration (say 2–5%). This method has been used in a number of other laboratories with success (e.g., Tveit et al., 1981). Growth in soft agar seems to be satisfactory for many cell types but not for others. Some tumour cells have a degree of anchorage dependence; a recent successful assay for human cervix carcinoma cells was based on the use of a feeder layer of mouse 3T3 cells (Kelland and Steel, 1988a).

Other investigators have sought to develop simpler and quicker assays for cloning tumour cells directly from patients, and the so-called Tumour Stem-cell Assay (Salmon, 1980) has been widely used. Unfortunately, the criteria for lack of cell clumps in the cell suspensions and for what constitutes a growing colony are so weakened in this procedure that the method is unreliable.

More recently, there have been claims that an assay based on a colorimeric assay for viable cells can achieve both a high success rate and reliable evaluation of cell survival (Section 21.2; Cole, 1986). This is not a true clonogenic assay but it may be sufficiently reliable for practical purposes. A further development has been the production of coatings for plastic tissue-culture dishes that allow tumour cells to be grown in monolayer with minimal contamination by the growth of fibroblasts. It is known that some cultured cells normally produce such a coating and this has now been made artificially and called Cell Adhesive Matrix or CAM (Baker et al., 1986). No doubt the original formulation of CAM is not unique and variants will continue to appear.

12.2.2 Multicellular spheroids

Spheroids are small cell clumps that are grown in tissue culture under conditions in which the aggregates remain intact and may grow in a roughly spherical form to a size of perhaps half a millimetre. They retain some types of intracellular communication whilst being easy to handle in vitro. A variety of human tumours have been grown in this way. Under well-oxygenated conditions, small spheroids are fully oxic but central hypoxia tends to appear when the diameter exceeds about 100 μm. A number of studies have shown evidence for a 'contact effect': the radiosensitivity of cells in small fully-oxic spheroids is slightly less than when cells are irradiated as a cell suspension. Spheroids have been used as models for radiation studies on tumours (Yuhas et al., 1984; Rofstad et al., 1986).

12.2.3 Xenografts of human tumours

A wide variety of human tumours can be grown in immune-deficient mice. Immune deprivation of conventional animals can be carried out in a number of ways (Steel et al., 1982). These are only partially successful, however, and although they may allow human tumour grafts to take there is usually a residual immune response which may recover during a period of months following the immune-suppressive treatment. Perhaps the most successful technique is to depress immunity using a supra-lethal dose of whole body irradiation. The animals are kept alive either by giving an immediate bone marrow graft or better by making use of the radioprotective action of cytosine arabinoside (Ara-C) (Steel et al., 1978; 1980).

The alternative approach is to use the congenitally immune-deficient athymic 'nude' mouse. There is an extensive literature on the growth of human tumours in nude mice (see Fogh and Giovanella, 1982; Sordat, 1984). A wide range of tumour types can be grown in these animals. The proportion of patients giving successful grafts can be over 50% in some tumour types (e.g., melanoma, colo-rectal carcinoma) but with other types the take-rate is much lower (e.g., around 10% in breast tumours). Seminoma is an example of a tumour that has so far not been successfully grown in xenograft, in spite of repeated tests. The reasons for this variation in engraftment rate are not known. What is clear is that nude mice are not completely non-reactive hosts. Although they lack T-cell response they still possess responses mediated by the so-called natural killer cells (NK cells). This response tends to increase with the age of the mice and seems to be variable from one mouse colony to another, perhaps depending on exposure to micro-organisms.

The existence of rejection mechanisms both in immune-suppressed and in nude mice has important implications for their use in therapeutic cancer research. By the time a xenograft has grown to a size at which it can be treated, it may well have produced a host reaction which, though perhaps not strong enough to cause spontaneous tumour regression, will nevertheless influence regrowth after the number of viable cells within the tumour has been greatly reduced by irradiation or chemotherapy. A particular danger is that chemotherapy may modify the host response and therefore perhaps influence the outcome of treatment by a process that is unconnected with the cytotoxic effect on tumour cells. The appropriate choice of end-point is therefore essential: tumour-cure experiments will be highly vulnerable to this artefact; growth-delay experiments less so; best of all is to remove the tumour cells shortly after treatment and assay for colony-forming tumour cells (Courtenay, 1984).

When tumour cells are transferred from man to mouse, changes in biological characteristics no doubt occur. Selection pressures are considerable and artificial. Thus it is not surprising that the growth of xenografts tends to be faster than metastases in patients (Steel et al., 1983): rapidly proliferating cell clones may tend to outgrow the slow ones. In spite of this, histological appearance is often well maintained, as are many other biological properties. Xenografting has therefore provided a valuable method of maintaining human tumour cell lines in the laboratory and for therapeutic studies.

12.3 The range of radiosensitivity among human tumour cells

The older radiobiological literature described radiosensitivity in terms of the parameters of the multitarget equation: n and D_o. Current interest in the linear-quadratic model requires formulation in terms of new parameters (α and β). Figure 12.1 shows survival curves for four human tumour cell lines, selected from over 20 cell lines that have been studied in this laboratory. The figure illustrates the range of sensitivities that have been found among human tumour cells irradiated with low LET radiation under oxic conditions. Although these four cell lines come from different tumour types, they are not claimed to be representative of them: within each tumour type there is a wide range of sensitivity.

For a larger range of tumour cell lines, Figure 12.2 shows the two parameters of sensitivity, α and β. These parameters can be obtained by fitting cell-survival data at a single high dose rate (panel A); however, values obtained in this way are not very precise (a steeper α can often be traded off against a shallower β). More robust values

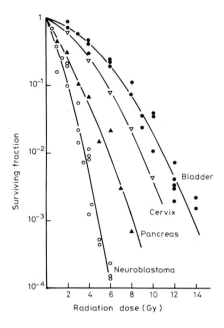

Figure 12.1. Illustrating the range of radiation cell-survival curves that are observed for human tumour cells. Data are shown for four selected cell lines: neuroblastoma HX142 (Holmes, unpublished data); ca. pancreas HX58; cervix HX156 (Kelland and Steel, 1986); ca. bladder RT112 (Peacock, unpublished data).

are obtained by experimental data at a range of dose rates fitted with the 'incomplete repair' model (Sections 4.2.6 and 15.3). These are shown in panel B. The shaded areas show regions where data are unlikely. To the right is a region in which the combined effect of the parameter values is to produce a survival curve which is steeper than HX138 (Figure 12.1) and which at a survival level of 10^{-3} has an equivalent D_o value that is less than 0.5 Gy. Curves steeper than this have not been observed for human tumour cells. To the left is a shaded area where the curve is shallower than that shown in Figure 12.1 for the bladder line, RT112, which is the most resistant human tumour cell line that we have found. The area between these shaded regions seems to encompass most data on human tumour cell lines. There is evidence in panel B that the more precisely determined values fall in the region where the α/β ratio is between 5 and 15. Recent work by J.H. Peacock using split-dose experiments at a range of dose levels (Section 12.4.2) has defined even better values for β. When combined with α values obtained by low dose-rate irradiation these are found to cluster closely around an α/β ratio of 12.

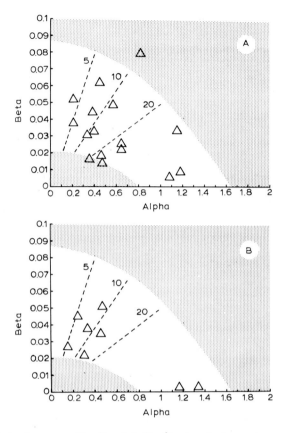

Figure 12.2. Correlation between α (Gy^{-1}) and β (Gy^{-2}) values for human tumour cell lines. (A) The values were obtained by fitting a linear-quadratic curve to data at high dose rate. (B) The values come from fitting data at a range of dose-rates using the 'incomplete repair' model. The broken lines show constant values of α/β ratio. The shaded regions show areas where the survival curves would be unusually shallow or steep. (Data from Steel et al., 1987.)

12.3.1 The initial slope of cell-survival curves

The way in which cell inactivation increases with dose in the low-dose region (up to say 5 Gy) is important both from a mechanistic and a practical point of view. The choice between models of cell killing (Section 4.2) depends heavily on data in this region. The doses per daily fraction in clinical radiotherapy are also often in the region of 2 Gy. It has been found that cell lines derived from individual human tumours may differ in low-dose radiosensitivity and this may reflect considerable intratumour heterogeneity among clonogenic cells (Leith et al., 1982). Evidence that the initial slope of cell-survival curves correlates with clinical response to radiotherapy has helped to focus attention on this aspect of radiosensitivity.

12.3.2 Correlation with clinical response

The first convincing evidence of a clinical correlation came from the work of Fertil and Malaise (1981). They surveyed the available published data on survival curves for human tumour cells irradiated under oxic conditions. Fifty-nine data sets were included, 16 of them on HeLa cells, and exclusions reduced this number to 26 different cell lines. The authors fitted each data set with a linear-quadratic equation and evaluated the initial slope either by the parameter α or by the attractively simple procedure of reading off the surviving fraction at a dose of 2 Gy (which we term SF_2). They ranked the tumour types in terms of clinical response to radiotherapy by reference to published estimates of the 'prescribed 95% tumour control dose'. An excellent correlation between SF_2 and this crude estimate of clinical responsiveness was obtained. Subsequent publications by this group proposed the concept of Mean Inactivation Dose as a measure of initial slope (Fertil et al., 1984), extended their review of human tumour cell lines with similar conclusions (Fertil and Malaise, 1985), and carried out the same type of analysis on human fibroblast cell strains (Malaise et al., 1987).

The analysis of published data on the initial slope in human tumour cells was repeated by Deacon et al. (1984). The number of cell lines was increased to 51 non-HeLa lines and clinical responsiveness to radiotherapy was more cautiously included by placing the tumour types in five response categories (Table 12.1). Such a classification is neither easy nor entirely reliable; there are many factors that complicate the comparison of radioresponsiveness between different tumour types and anatomical sites (patient selection, tumour bulk, dose prescription, etc.). It was found that within each of the five categories the SF_2 values ranged widely (by a factor of 5 in survival) but that in spite of this there was evidence for a correlation with response category. The result of a more recent update of this study is shown in Figure 12.3, covering a total of 76 human tumour cell lines. The results are now plotted as the mean and standard error of the SF_2 values within each response category. They show that groups C, D and E did not differ in initial slope, but that for groups A and B the curves were significantly steeper.

Are these differences in initial slope large enough to be clinically important? The mean SF_2 values are: group A (0.15), group B (0.27) and groups C–E (0.49). If

TABLE 12.1
Classification of human tumours according to clinical radioresponsiveness

A.	Neuroblastoma, lymphoma, myeloma
B.	Medulloblastoma, teratoma, small-cell lung carcinoma
C.	Breast, bladder, cervix carcinoma
D.	Pancreas, colorectal, adeno- and squamous lung carcinoma
E.	Melanoma, osteosarcoma, glioblastoma, renal carcinoma

Based on Deacon et al., 1984.

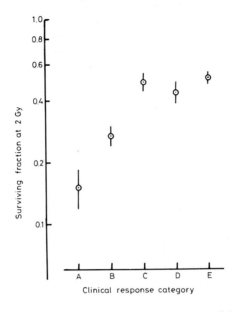

Figure 12.3. Correlation between the surviving fraction at 2 Gy and the clinical response categories set out in Table 12.1. The points show mean values for 76 data sets, with standard errors.

we assume that these in vitro values are realistic for cell killing in vivo and that they are constant throughout a course of fractionated radiotherapy then it is possible to calculate the overall surviving fraction. Such a calculation involves some further very big assumptions, especially that hypoxia does not distort the results and that cell contact effects (Malaise et al., 1986) can be ignored. But in very simple terms, the overall effect of say 30 daily 2 Gy fractions is SF_2 raised to the power 30. Figure 12.4 shows the results of such calculations using the above values for SF_2. The survival curves differ substantially in slope. Comparing horizontally, the total radiation dose required for a survival of 10^{-12} ranges from 28 Gy in group A to 80 Gy in groups C–E. Comparing vertically, the surviving fraction for a total dose of 50 Gy ranges from 10^{-21} to $2 \cdot 10^{-8}$. The former would be expected to be curative, the latter probably not. Although these calculations are crude and ignore known factors that modify SF_2, they do indicate that the magnitude of the initial slope could be a critical determinant of success or failure in clinical radiotherapy and that the range of SF_2 values that have been determined can easily explain experience in local tumour control by radiotherapy.

An alternative way of obtaining a clinically important measure of radiosensitivity is to determine cell survival at low dose rate (Chapter 15). Such studies confirm that among human tumour cell lines there is a wide range of radiosensitivity (see Figure 15.2).

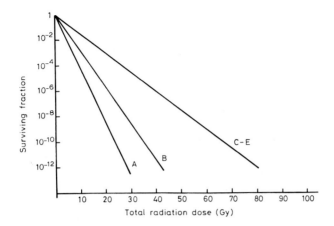

Figure 12.4. Theoretical cell survival curves for fractionated irradiation with 2 Gy per fraction. The SF_2 values are assumed to be A, 0.15; B, 0.27; and C–E, 0.49.

12.3.3 The radiobiology of xenografts

Studies of radiation response in human tumour xenografts have been extensively pursued at the Norwegian Cancer Hospital in Oslo and the Institut Gustave-Roussy, Paris, with additional contributions from a number of other laboratories. Rofstad and his colleagues have published mainly on the radiobiology of a group of human melanomas which they established themselves and have investigated in terms of combined modality treatment (Rofstad et al., 1977), radiosensitization (Rofstad and Brustad, 1978), cell kinetics (Rofstad et al., 1980), adaptation to tissue culture (Rofstad and Brustad, 1983), vascular changes (Solesvik et al., 1984), hyperthermia (Rofstad and Brustad, 1983), and fractionation (Rofstad and Brustad, 1987). The group in Paris have mainly employed well-established human cell lines (which are more likely to have diverged from the original tumours), including melanomas and colo-rectal tumours. They have studied radiosensitization (Guichard et al., 1979), hypoxia and repair (Chavaudra et al., 1981), and cell–cell contact phenomena (Guichard et al., 1983; Dertinger et al., 1984). Cell kinetic changes in human melanoma xenografts have been studied by Spang-Thomsen and co-workers (1981; 1986), and studies of response to fractionated irradiation have been made in a squamous carcinoma by Lindenberger et al. (1986).

Although the range of tumour types used in these studies has been small, a wide variety of radiobiological processes have been examined. There have been no great surprises. The results have broadly been similar to earlier observations on rodent tumours. This perhaps provides reassurance that rodent tumour data are relevant (Kallman, 1987), but does not by itself justify the wider study of xenograft radiobiology.

12.4 Recovery processes in human tumour cells

The earlier radiobiological literature envisaged three principal ways of judging the capacity of cells to recover from radiation damage: the size of the shoulder on the acute radiation survival curve, the recovery seen when a fixed radiation dose is split into two fractions separated by a few hours (i.e., split-dose or Elkind recovery), and the recovery seen when non-dividing cells are held in that state for some hours after irradiation (i.e., delayed-plating or Potentially Lethal Damage recovery, PLD).

Recent considerations of the implications of the linear-quadratic model for cellular recovery suggest not only that shoulders are less clearly defined than has been supposed, but also that the shoulder size may be a poor indicator of recovery. This will be dealt with in Section 12.4.2 below. There have been few careful attempts to compare recovery between human tumour cell lines on the basis of split-dose recovery; it has been assumed that radioresistant cell lines tend to give a larger degree of recovery than sensitive lines (but as we will indicate below, this assumption is also now in question). Much more attention has been given to the PLD recovery phenomenon.

Split-dose and PLD recovery are defined on the basis of the type of experiment by which they are detected. They do not always go together: for instance, split-dose recovery is shown to a varying degree by most cell types, but PLD recovery tends to be shown only by non-proliferating cells. Nevertheless, they should be thought of as operationally defined measures of a single underlying repair process (Pohlit and Heyder, 1981). The LPL model of Curtis (1986) is an example of a cell-survival model that seeks to describe both of these manifestations of recovery in terms of a single repair process (Section 4.2.5). As indicated in Section 3.5, it is a useful convention to use the term 'repair' to describe processes by which radiation-induced DNA lesions are successfully dealt with, and to use 'recovery' for situations where we describe an increase in cell survival after irradiation.

12.4.1 Recovery from potentially lethal damage

PLD recovery has been extensively studied in human tumour cell lines by Weichselbaum and his co-workers (1976; 1982; 1984). Some of the data have indicated a positive correlation between the extent of PLD recovery and clinical radioresistance, but some have not supported this conclusion. Other work has also failed to find such a correlation (Marchese et al., 1987). Recently it has been claimed that cells derived from tumours that have recurred following radiotherapy are less sensitive than those from untreated tumours (Weichselbaum et al., 1988), a result that supports the view that inherent cellular radiosensitivity varies either within or between tumours and can therefore lead to cell selection as a result of treatment.

12.4.2 Implications of the linear-quadratic model for recovery in human tumour cell lines

It has been thought that, provided radiation dose levels off the shoulder of the cell-survival curve are employed, the amount of recovery seen in a split-dose experiment is a good measure of recovery capacity (Hall, 1978). This would be true if the multitarget model of cell survival were valid. If, however, the survival curve is continuously bending, the recovery ratio will increase with the radiation dose employed. In the case of the linear-quadratic model, the survival recovery ratio (*RR*) for an equal-split experiment is given by:

$$RR = \exp(2\beta d^2)$$

where the split is $d + d$ (Thames, 1985). Recovery is thus a very steep function of the dose at which it is determined. To compare recovery between cell lines it is important to use identical dose levels, or better to employ a range of dose levels, to plot log (*RR*) against $2d^2$, and thus from the slope to obtain a reliable value for β (Peacock et al., 1988). On this model it is the value of β that is the best measure of the extent of cellular recovery. The above equation shows that *RR* is a function only of β, not α, and according to the 'incomplete repair' model (Section 4.2.6) lowering the dose rate allows the β-component of cell killing to recover, leaving the residual effect of the α-component. This aspect of the model seems to be supported by experimental data (Section 15.3).

If we take β as the measure of recovery, what can we say about its variation among human tumour cell lines? On the basis of previous radiobiological thinking, we would expect that radioresistant tumours would have large β values, this being a reason why they are resistant. As indicated above, values for β that are determined solely by fitting acute irradiation cell-survival data are not very precise. It can be seen in Figure 12.2 (panel A or B) that there is little tendency for β values to be large in the radioresistant tumours (i.e., those with small α values). The new approach described in the previous Section, using split-dose experiments at a number of dose levels, has shown a clear positive correlation between α and β values for human tumour cells, with a mean α/β ratio of 12.

Our conclusion at the present time is that the data do not support the traditional view that the reason why some cell lines are resistant to radiation is because they have a large capacity for recovery from radiation damage (as indicated by split-dose experiments). Far more important is the magnitude of α, i.e., the steepness of the linear component of cell killing. Radiosensitive cell lines have large α values, radioresistant lines have low α values. This can also be seen clearly in Figure 15.2. At low dose rate the survival curves are close to the pure α-components of cell killing, they show a wide range of sensitivities, and cell lines that are resistant at high dose rate also tend to be so at low dose rate.

12.5 Overview: the importance of the linear component of cell killing

The conclusion reached in the previous Section has wider implications, both for the mechanisms of radiation cell killing and for attempts to increase the radiosensitivity of tumour cells. First, is it true that radiation cell killing can be divided into two components, one linear, the other bending (quadratic in the case of the L-Q model)? The basis for this lies not only in the shape of acute cell-survival curves (which tolerate a variety of models) but in the success of the 'incomplete repair' model (which is based on an underlying L-Q model) to fit cell-survival data over a wide range of dose rates, similar to the LPL model (Section 4.2). Other quite different models also require a 'non-repairable' component in order to simulate the initial slope of the cell-survival curve (for instance repair saturation models, Section 4.2.4).

A further illustration of the importance of the linear component is shown in Figure 12.5. For 17 human tumour cell lines, representing the full range of radiosensitivity shown in Figure 12.1, we have calculated α and β values from the fit to the acute cell-survival curves. These values have then been used to calculate the contribution to the total effect of the two separate components: 'α survival' = $\exp(-\alpha D)$; 'β survival' $\exp(-\beta D^2)$. This is done at four dose levels. For doses of 1 or 2 Gy the points lie down the right-hand side of the diagram: the contribution of the β-component is very small. As dose is increased, the β-component increases more rapidly and begins to have a significant effect. The broken lines show where the two components are equal.

What this indicates is that for doses of 2 Gy or less the dispersion in radiosensitivity

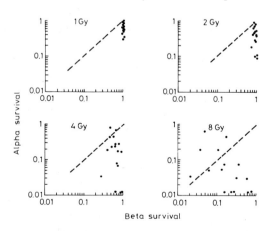

Figure 12.5. Relationship between the surviving fraction due to the α component and that due to the β component, calculated at four dose levels. The dashed lines indicate equal values. At 4 Gy and 8 Gy the points at the bottom of the diagram indicate a survival of 0.01 or less. (From Steel and Peacock, 1989.)

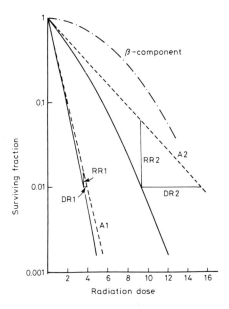

Figure 12.6. The addition of a fixed β-component to a steep α-component (A1) leads to an almost straight survival curve (full line) and to low estimates for recovery (*RR*1 is the maximum recoverable survival; *DR*1 the maximum dose-rate sparing effect). When the α-component is less steep by a factor of 4 (A2) the survival curve is recognisably curved and recovery is greater.

between these cell lines is entirely due to the linear component of cell killing. The effect of many fractions of this size will even more be dominated by the α-component, because when the separate contributions are raised to a large power the differences become greater. Thus the cell-survival curves for fractionated irradiation with low fraction sizes (as with those for low dose-rate irradiation, Figure 15.2) are almost entirely determined by the steepness of the linear component.

What are the implications of this for the evaluation of repair capacity among human tumour cell lines? We now realise that when the α-component is steep there is a tendency for recovery capacity to be underestimated. This is shown in Figure 12.6. A constant β-component is combined either with a steep α-component (A1) or with a shallow one (A2). The result in the first case is an acute survival curve that appears almost straight. The maximum amount of recovery that can occur is the complete disappearance of damage due to the β-component, as is the case at very low dose rate or for many small dose fractions. This can be judged either by the survival recovery ratio (*RR*) or by the amount of dose recovery (*DR*). When α is large, both *RR*1 and *DR*1 are smaller than when α is smaller (*RR*2, *DR*2). Split-dose recovery values would be less than *RR*, but the same argument applies. As indicated in the previous section, it would seem that on the L-Q model the most satisfactory measure of recovery capacity (independent of α) by which to compare cell lines is the β-value itself. In Figure 12.6 this is the same for the two hypothetical cell lines.

The nature of the linear component of radiation cell killing thus becomes an important aspect of the biological basis of radiosensitivity. A linear and non-repairable component has often been described as due to 'single-hit' killing, i.e., to a process by which single events lead directly and inevitably to cell death. This could arise in two general ways. Firstly, the presence within the cell of hypersensitive regions within which a single ionisation event will kill the cell. This could be a single isolated target; more plausibly, there could be a number of small regions within the genome that are so vital to the reproductive integrity of the cell that if any one of them is damaged the cell will die. The second hypothesis is that the single-hit component derives more from the nature of the energy deposition by low LET radiation. Ionisations due to X- or γ-radiation are not produced randomly. Most of the dose is due to well-separated ionisations but in addition there are 'spurs', 'blobs' and 'tracks' (Figure 17.4; Goodhead and Brenner, 1983) within which multiple ionisations occur within a distance of a few nanometres. If such an event impinged upon a DNA strand (diameter 2 nm) it could lead to a group of lesions, multiple strand breaks (ssb and dsb) and damaged bases within the span of say 10 base pairs. The cell might be easily capable of repairing single breaks, but when faced with this degree of local damage there would inevitably be failure to correctly repair, loss of some bases, and thus permanent damage. Ward (1986) has termed such lesions Local Multiply Damaged Sites (LMDS).

These two hypotheses are not mutually exclusive. A single-hit component could arise predominantly from LMDS produced within critically important parts of the genome. The importance of non-repairable damage in the effects of high LET radiation is considered in Section 17.2.1.

It is important to stress that the claim that cellular response to low radiation doses, fractionated irradiation, and low dose-rate irradiation is dominated by a non-repairable component does not diminish the importance of repair. The reason why the above statement may be true is because under these conditions repair is allowed to go to completion. The residual damage is then largely non-repairable. It is well known that irradiation in the presence of exogenous repair inhibitors leads to a steepening of the cell-survival curves and recent data have shown that this often occurs by increasing α and decreasing β (Kelland and Steel, 1988b). This can be understood if the mechanism of the inhibitor is to convert a repairable lesion into a non-repairable one. Furthermore, the fact that the initial slope of the cell-survival curve critically determines the overall therapeutic effect, and that it can be modified, holds out the hope that if an inhibitor could be found that is selective against tumour cells, it should have significant therapeutic potential.

Acknowledgement

This work was supported in part by NCI grant No. RO1 CA 26059.

References

Baker, F.L., Spitzer, G., Ajani, J.A., Brock, W.A., Lukeman, J., Pathak, S., Tomasovic, B., Thielvoldt, D., Williams, M., Vines, C. and Tofilon, P. (1986) Drug and radiation sensitivity measurements of successful primary monolayer culturing of human tumor cells using cell-adhesive matrix and supplemented medium. Cancer Res. 46, 1263–1274.

Barendsen, G.W. (1980) Variations in radiation responses among experimental tumors, in: Radiation Biology in Cancer Research. (Meyn, R.E. and Withers, R.H., eds.), pp. 333–343, Raven Press, New York.

Barranco, S.C., Romsdahl, M.M. and Humphrey, R.M. (1971) The radiation response of human malignant melanoma cells grown in vitro. Cancer Res. 31, 830–833.

Berry, R.J. (1974) Population distribution in tumors and normal tissues; a guide to tissue radiosensitivity, in: The Biological and Clinical Basis of Radiosensitivity (Freidman, M., ed.), pp. 141–155, Charles C. Thomas, Dundee.

Chavaudra, N., Guichard, M. and Malaise, E.P. (1981) Hypoxic fraction and repair of potentially lethal radiation damage in two human melanomas transplanted into nude mice. Radiat. Res. 88, 56–68.

Cole, S.P.C. (1986) Rapid chemosensitivity testing of human lung tumor cells using the MTT assay. Cancer Chemother. Pharmacol. 17, 259–263.

Courtenay, V.D. (1984) A replenishable soft agar colony assay for human tumour sensitivity testing, in: Predictive Drug Testing in Human Tumor Cells. pp. 17–34. Recent Results in Cancer Research, Vol. 94, (Hofmann, V., Berens, M.E. and Martz, G., eds.), Springer-Verlag, Berlin.

Courtenay, V.D. and Mills, J. (1978) An in vitro colony assay for human tumours grown in immune-suppressed mice and treated in vivo with cytotoxic agents. Br. J. Cancer 37, 261–268.

Curtis, S.B. (1986) Lethal and potentially lethal lesions induced by radiation – unified repair model. Radiat. Res. 106, 252–270.

Deacon, J., Peckham, M.J. and Steel, G.G. (1984) The radioresponsiveness of human tumours and the initial slope of the cell-survival curve. Radiother. Oncol. 2, 317–323.

Dertinger, H., Guichard, M. and Malaise, E.P. (1984) Relationship between intercellular communication and radiosensitivity of human tumour xenografts. Eur. J. Cancer Clin. Oncol. 20, 561–566.

Fertil, B., Dertinger, H., Courdi, A. and Malaise, E.P. (1984) Mean inactivation dose: a useful concept for intercomparison of human cell survival curves. Radiat. Res. 99, 73–84.

Fertil, B. and Malaise, E.P. (1981) Inherent cellular radiosensitivity as a basic concept for human tumor radiotherapy. Int. J. Radiat. Oncol. Biol. Phys. 7, 621–629.

Fertil, B. and Malaise, E.P. (1985) Intrinsic radiosensitivity of human cell lines is correlated with radioresponsiveness of human tumors. Analysis of 101 published survival curves. Int. J. Radiat. Oncol. Biol. Phys. 9, 1699–1707.

Fogh, J. and Giovanella, B.C. (eds.) (1982) The Nude Mouse in Experimental and Clinical Research, Vol. 2., Academic Press, New York.

Goodhead, D.T. and Brenner, D.J. (1983) Estimation of a single property of low LET radiations which correlates with biological effectiveness. Phys. Med. Biol. 28, 485–492.

Guichard, M., De Langen-Omri, F. and Malaise, E.P. (1979) Influence of misonidazole on the radiosensitivity of a human melanoma in nude mice: time-dependent increase in surviving fraction. Int. J. Radiat. Oncol. Biol. Phys. 5, 487–489.

Guichard, M., Dertinger, H. and Malaise, E.P. (1983) Radiosensitivity of four human tumour xenografts: influence of hypoxia and cell–cell contact. Radiat. Res. 95, 602–609.
Hall, E.J. (1987) Lethal, potentially lethal, and sublethal radiation damage, and the dose-rate effect, in: Radiobiology for the Radiologist, pp. 129–169, 2nd Edn., Harper and Row, London.
Kallman, R.F. (ed.) (1987) Rodent Tumour Models in Experimental Cancer Therapy, Pergamon Press, London.
Kelland, L.R. and Steel, G.G. (1988a) Differences in radiation response among human cervix carcinoma cell lines. Radiother. Oncol. 12, 1–8.
Kelland, L.R. and Steel, G.G. (1988b) Modification of radiation dose-rate sparing effects in a human carcinoma of the cervix cell line by inhibitors of DNA repair. Int. J. Radiat Biol. 54, 229–244.
Leith, J.T., Dexter, D.L., DeWyngaert, J.K., Zeman, E.M., Chu, M.Y., Calabresi, P. and Glicksman, A.S. (1982) Differential responses to X-irradiation of subpopulations of two heterogeneous human carcinomas in vitro. Cancer Res. 42, 2556–2561.
Lindenberger, J., Hermeking, H., Kummermehr, J. and Denekamp, J. (1986) Response of human tumour xenografts to fractionated X-irradiation. Radiother. Oncol. 6, 15–27.
Malaise, E.P., Fertil, B., Chavaudra, N. and Guichard, M. (1986) Distribution of radiation sensitivities for human tumor cells of specific histological types: comparison of in vitro to in vivo data. Int. J. Radiat. Oncol. Biol. Phys. 12, 617–624.
Malaise, E.P., Fertil, B., Deschavanne, P.J., Chavaudra, N. and Brock, W.A. (1987) Initial slope of radiation survival curves in characteristic of the origin of primary and established cultures of human tumour cells and fibroblasts. Radiat. Res. 111, 319–333.
Marchese, M.J., Zaider, M. and Hall, E.J. (1987) Potentially lethal damage repair in human cells. Radiother. Oncol. 9, 57–65.
Peacock, J.H., Cassoni, A.M., McMillan, T.J. and Steel, G.G. (1988) Radiosensitive human tumour cell lines may not be recovery deficient. Int. J. Radiat. Biol. 54, 945–954.
Pohlit, W. and Heyder, I.R. (1981) The shape of dose-survival curves for mammalian cells and repair of potentially lethal damage analyzed by hypertonic treatment. Radiat. Res. 87, 613–634.
Rofstad, E.K. and Brustad, T. (1978) The radiosensitizing effect of metronidazole and misonidazole (Ro 07-0582) on a human malignant melanoma grown in the athymic mutant nude mouse. Br. J. Radiol. 51, 381–38.
Rofstad, E.K. and Brustad, T. (1983) Radiation and heat sensitivity of cells from human melanoma xenografts: lack of correlates with tumour-growth parameters. Eur. J. Cancer Clin. Oncol. 19, 427–432.
Rofstad, E.K. and Brustad, T. (1983) Radiosensitivity of the cells of an established human melanoma cell line and the parent melanoma xenograft. Int. J. Radiat. Biol. 44, 447–454.
Rofstad, E.K. and Brustad, T. (1987) Radioresponsiveness of human melanoma xenografts given fractionated irradiation in vivo: relationship to the initial slope of the cell-survival curves in vitro, in press.
Rofstad, E.K., Brustad, T., Johannessen, J.V. and Mossige, J. (1977) Effect of cobalt-60 gamma-rays and DTIC (5-(3,3-dimethyl-1-triazeno)-imidazole-4-carboxamide) on human malignant melanomas grown in athymic nude mice. Br. J. Radiol. 50, 314–320.
Rofstad, E.K., Lindmo, T. and Brustad, T. (1980) Effect of single-dose irradiation on the proliferation kinetics in a human malignant melanoma in athymic nude mice. Acta Radiol. Oncol. 19, 261–269.
Rofstad, E.K., Wahl, A. and Brustad, T. (1986) Radiation response of human melanoma multicellular spheroids measured as single cell survival, growth delay, and spheroid cure: comparisons with the parent tumor xenograft. Int. J. Radiat. Oncol. Phys. 12, 975–982.
Salmon, S.S. (ed.) (1980) Cloning of human tumor stem cells. Progress in Clinical and Biological Research, Vol. 48, Alan R. Liss, New York.
Solesvik, O.V., Rofstad, E.K. and Brustad, T. (1984) Vascular changes in a human malignant melanoma xenograft following single-dose irradiation. Radiat. Res. 98, 115–128.
Sordat, B. (ed.) (1984) Immune-deficient animals. Proceedings 4th International Workshop on Immune-

Deficient Animals in Experimental Research, Chexbres, S. Karger, London.
Spang-Thomsen, M., Clerici, M., Engelholm, S.A. and Vindelov, L.L. (1986) Growth kinetics and in vivo radiosensitivity in nude mice of two subpopulations derived from a single human small-cell carcinoma of the lung. Eur. J. Cancer Clin. Oncol. 22, 549–556.
Spang-Thomsen, M., Visfeldt, J. and Nielsen, A. (1981) Effect of single-dose X-irradiation on the growth curves of a human malignant melanoma transplanted into nude mice. Radiat. Res. 85, 184–195.
Steel, G.G., Courtenay, V.D. and Peckham, M.J. (1982) The immune-suppressed mouse as an alternative host for heterotransplantation, in: The Nude Mouse in Experimental and Clinical Research, Vol. 2 (Fogh, J. and Giovanella, B.C., eds.), pp. 207–227, Academic Press, New York.
Steel, G.G., Courtenay, V.D. and Peckham, M.J. (1983) The response to chemotherapy of a variety of human tumour xenografts. Br. J. Cancer 47, 1–13.
Steel, G.G., Courtenay, V.D., Phelps, T.A. and Peckham, M.J. (1980) The therapeutic response of human tumour xenografts. in: Symposium on Immune-Deficient Animals in Cancer Research (Sparrow, S., ed.), pp. 179–189, McMillan, London.
Steel, G.G., Courtenay, V.D. and Rostom, A.Y. (1978) Improved immune-suppression techniques for the xenografting of human tumours. Br. J. Cancer 37, 224–230.
Steel, G.G., Deacon, J.M., Duchesne, G.M., Horwich, A., Kelland, L.R. and Peacock, J.H. (1987) The dose-rate effect in human tumour cells. Radiother. Oncol. 9, 299–310.
Steel, G.G. and Peacock, J.H. (1988) Why are some human tumours more radiosensitive than others? Radiother. Oncol. 15, 63–72.
Thames, H.D. (1985) An 'incomplete-repair' model for survival after fractionated and continuous irradiations. Int. J. Radiat. Biol. 47, 319–339.
Tveit, K.M., Endresen, L., Rugstad, H.E., Fodstad, O. and Pihl, A. (1981) Comparison of two soft-agar methods for assaying chemosensitivity of human tumours in vitro: malignant melanomas. Br. J. Cancer 44, 539–544.
Ward, J.F. (1986) Mechanisms of DNA repair and their potential modification for radiotherapy. Int. J. Radiat. Oncol. Biol. Phys. 12, 1027–1032.
Weichselbaum, R.R., Beckett, M.A., Schwartz, J.L. and Dritschilo, A. (1988) Radioresistant tumor cells are present in head and neck carcinomas that recur after radiotherapy. Int. J. Radiat. Oncol. Biol. Phys. 15, 575–579.
Weichselbaum, R.R., Dahlberg, W., Little, J.B., Ervin, T.J., Miller, D., Hellman, S. and Rheinwald, J.G. (1984) Cellular X-ray repair parameters of early passage squamous cell carcinoma lines derived from patients with known responses to radiotherapy. Br. J. Cancer 49, 595–601.
Weichselbaum, R.R., Epstein, J., Little, J.B. and Kornblith, P. (1976) Inherent cellular radiosensitivity of human tumors of varying clinical curability. Am. J. Roentgenol. 127, 1027–1032.
Weichselbaum, R.R. and Little, J.B. (1982) The differential response of human tumours to fractionated radiation may be due to a post-irradiation repair process. Br. J. Cancer 46, 532–537.
Yuhas, J.M., Blake, S. and Weichselbaum, R.R. (1984) Quantitation of the response of human tumor spheroids to daily radiation exposures. Int. J. Radiat. Oncol. Biol. Phys. 10, 2323–2327.

CHAPTER 13

Fractionation and therapeutic gain

JACK F. FOWLER

Department of Human Oncology K4/336, University of Wisconsin Clinical Cancer Center, 600 Highland Avenue, Madison, WI 53792, USA

13.1 Introduction 182
     13.1.1   The new radiobiological bases 182
     13.1.2   Hyperfractionation and accelerated fractionation 182

13.2 Overall time 183
     13.2.1   Proliferation in normal tissues 183
     13.2.2   Proliferation in tumours 183
     13.2.3   Flow cytometry measurement of T_{pot} in human tumours 184
     13.2.4   Accelerated fractionation 184

13.3 Dose per fraction 185
     13.3.1   Difference between late and early reactions 185
     13.3.2   Advantages of hyperfractionation 187
     13.3.3   Linear-quadratic formula 187
     13.3.4   Multiple fractions 189
     13.3.5   Biologically effective doses; calculations of effect 189
     13.3.6   Clinical values of α/β for human tissues 193
     13.3.7   Calculations of total doses in new schedules 194

13.4 Linear-quadratic formula with time factors 195
     13.4.1   Time factors in general 195
     13.4.2   Time factors to allow for proliferation 195
     13.4.3   Comparisons of various fractionation schedules 197
     13.4.4   Intervals between multiple fractions per day 203

13.5 Conclusions 203

13.1 Introduction

13.1.1 The new radiobiological bases

When the new aspects of fractionated radiotherapy described in the previous edition of this book became well known in the early 1980s, many new fractionation protocols were designed (Withers et al., 1988; Peters et al., 1988a). The clinical results tend to confirm these principles. The field of fractionation is an active one. The two main thrusts were first on *hyperfractionation* and later on *accelerated fractionation*, and these developments still continue.

The radiobiological bases were that time factors were negligible for late effects but large for tumours (and early-reacting normal tissues); and that late effects decreased more rapidly than early (and tumour) effects if smaller doses per fraction were used. The linear-quadratic formula for describing the effects of changes in dose per fraction has held up extremely well both in animal experiments designed to test it and in clinical data.

13.1.2 Hyperfractionation and accelerated fractionation

Hyperfractionation is the use of larger numbers of smaller fractions than the usual 30 or 35 fractions of 1.8–2 Gy. The strategy is to increase the total dose by using small doses per fraction which are significantly less effective for late reactions than for early or tumour effects. Accelerated fractionation is the use of shorter overall times. The strategy here is simply to circumvent proliferation in the tumour. Some protocols combine the advantages of both by using several fractions per day.

Hyperfractionation has already yielded good results in at least one randomised clinical trial. Two fractions per day of 1.15 Gy × 70F totalling 80.5 Gy in 7 weeks (with a 6–8 hour interval between the two) was compared with 35F × 2 Gy totalling 70 Gy, also in 7 weeks, in an EORTC trial of patients with T_2–T_3 squamous carcinoma of the larynx which closed in 1985. The radiobiological prediction from linear-quadratic theory was that about 10% extra log cell-kill should be obtained, leading to 10–15% better local control with no increase in late complications. This is just what has been found clinically (Horiot et al., 1988); a significant therapeutic gain has thus been achieved by hyperfractionation alone. The same result was also reported from a rather similar but non-randomised trial carried out at Gainesville, Florida (64F × 1.2 Gy = 76.8 Gy/6.5 weeks, given as 2F per day with a 4 hour interval; Parsons et al., 1988). Wendt and Peters (personal communication) also report good results from a trial of twice-daily treatments of laryngeal and hypopharyngeal cancer begun at Houston in 1982. It is satisfying that modern radiobiological predictions do seem to work in the field of fractionated radiotherapy.

Trials using accelerated fractionation have started later, although the experience of

Svoboda (1978) using overall times of 10 to 14 days and 2 or 3 fractions per day goes back into the 1970s.

These and other clinical trials will be critically compared in this chapter, using the linear-quadratic formula with an optional time factor added to deal with proliferation in tumours.

13.2 Overall time

13.2.1 Proliferation in normal tissues

Late reactions do not depend greatly on overall time, because compensatory proliferation usually does not begin until after the end of radiotherapy. Late reactions occur, by definition, in slowly or non-proliferating tissues. The important point is that late reactions are not made worse by shortening overall time, nor can they be spared by prolongation.

Early effects in normal tissues and tumours are, however, significantly reduced by proliferation occurring within the weeks of radiotherapy. Therefore, shortening overall time will make early reactions worse unless the total dose is reduced by at least 50 cGy per day. Accelerated proliferation begins in human oral mucosa at 2–3 weeks and in human skin at 3–4 weeks after the start of fractionated radiotherapy. These starting times are approximately equal to the normal, preirradiation, turnover time of the epithelium and are not much altered by the type of fractionation. Towards the end of standard radiotherapy, proliferation in skin or mucosa can be fast enough to keep up with the depopulation by successive fractions, i.e., more than 100 cGy per day.

13.2.2 Proliferation in tumours

Proliferation in tumours may or may not begin until a few weeks after the start of treatment: there are two schools of thought. Withers et al. (1988), from a review of doses required to control 50% of head and neck tumours, presented evidence for no significant proliferation until 3 weeks after the start of treatment and then for rapid proliferation requiring an average of 60 cGy per day to overcome it, which corresponds to a doubling time of the tumourigenic cells of 3 or 4 days. Others, including the present author, consider that tumour cells will be brought closer to the nutritional supply as soon as the tumour shrinks, i.e., after only a few fractions in some tumours, especially carcinomas. There is now ample evidence from clinical radiotherapy schedules where the total dose has to be increased to control tumours if the overall time is increased, that proliferation can in practice equal these fast doubling times of 3 to 7 days in many types of human tumour, at least in the latter half of a 6-week treatment (Parsons et al., 1980; Maciejewski et al., 1983; Trott and

Kummermehr, 1985; Fowler, 1986; Withers et al., 1988; and Overgaard et al., 1988). These practical doubling times are closer to the potential doubling times of tumour cells than to the cell-cycle times of 1 or 2 days or – especially – than to the volume doubling times of several weeks or months.

Potential doubling time, T_{pot}, was defined by Steel (1977) as a combination of cell-cycle time and growth factor, and it represents the rate of increase of the cell population *if there were no cell loss* (see Chapter 6). A cell-loss factor of 90 or 95% means that the volume doubling time is 10 or 20-times greater than the potential doubling time – a common occurrence in human tumours. Further, experiments with mouse tumours have shown that the volume doubling times can indeed shorten to approach the potential doubling times during treatment. In these cases the cell-loss factor fell to zero.

13.2.3 Flow cytometry measurements of T_{pot} in human tumours

These facts have increased our interest in T_{pot}, which can be measured before treatment in human tumours using flow cytometry of a biopsy taken after in situ labelling with tracer doses of the DNA precursor BUdR or IUdR (Begg et al., 1985; see Chapter 21). It is not yet possible to interpret such kinetic measurements during treatment, although we need to know the proliferation rates. Interest is centred on pretreatment values of T_{pot} for two reasons (a) that we can measure them and (b) that they do match the values estimated from real radiotherapy when overall time is changed. The values of T_{pot} obtained from flow cytometry do not differ greatly from earlier values obtained using tritiated thymidine (Steel, 1977), but interest is greatly sharpened because results from individual tumour biopsies are obtained within a day. There is agreement from different groups that median values of T_{pot} are as short as 4 to 6 days for tumours in several sites (head and neck, breast, lung, rectum, bladder, cervix and malignant melanoma) with a range from 2 to 25 days (Wilson et al., 1988; Begg et al., 1988). The coefficients of variation for repeated biopsies from the same tumour are 25 to 30%. Prostate tumours usually have longer T_{pot} values, as do some breast carcinomas; but there are large and overlapping ranges of individual values for each type of tumour, and labelling indices ranging from 1 to 50%. Values of T_{pot} for individual patients are required, so that ultimately patients can be selected for accelerated fractionation or conventional (6–7 week) treatment on the basis of their own tumour's measured proliferation rate.

13.2.4 Accelerated fractionation

A reduction in overall time by 21 days corresponds to seven doublings if T_{pot} is 3 days. Two to the power 7 is 128, i.e., more than 2 logs to base 10. If 9 or 10 logs of cells must be killed to obtain local control, the shortening by 3 weeks would in effect increase the cell kill by more than 2/10 (i.e. 20%). This is the obvious advantage of shorter overall times.

It was calculated (Thames et al., 1983) that accelerated fractionation would give better local control than hyperfractionation (using 2 or 3 fractions per day) if the doubling time of the tumourigenic cells was shorter than about 5 days. There is no reason to revise this rough estimate, but more precise comparisons will be presented below, for accelerated hyperfractionation too. From recent flow-cytometry studies a potential doubling time of 5 days corresponds to a labelling index of 10 to 15% (Wilson et al., 1988).

It is the stronger realisation of these short doubling times that encourages radiotherapists to design schedules with shorter overall times.

13.3 Dose per fraction

13.3.1 Difference between late and early reactions

The most obvious way of shortening overall time, the use of a few big fractions, is not open to us for curative radiotherapy. It leads to severe late complications, but not because of any shortening of overall time. It is because the dose-response curves for late reactions (which are usually considered to be the cell-survival curves for the critical stem cells of the tissue concerned, Chapter 5) are curving significantly in the clinically used range of 1 to 4 Gy per fraction (Figure 13.1). However, the dose-response curve for proliferating tissues, both for acutely reacting normal tissues and tumour cells, curves much less until doses of 8 to 10 Gy are reached (Figure 13.1). It is not known why these are different but one suggestion has been that slowly proliferating cells have more time to repair; however, after higher doses they can

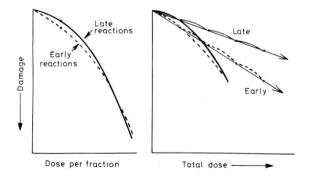

Figure 13.1. Relative shapes of the dose-response curves to individual dose fractions of late- and early-reacting tissues. Those for late reactions bend significantly within the dose per fraction range used in radiotherapy schedules. Those for early reactions are straighter.

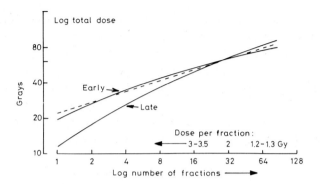

Figure 13.2. Total dose to give equal biological reactions versus number (and size) of fractions in radiotherapy.

misrepair more than cells which are proliferating fast.

The practical result of this difference has the effect of giving steeper 'Strandqvist-like' curves of total isoeffect dose versus number of fractions for late than for early reactions (Figure 13.2). Strictly, these curves would be better if plotted against size of dose per fraction but in Figure 13.2 the size is also shown approximately on the bottom axis. Figure 13.3 indicates the same difference when the dose per fraction is changed: a large change in total dose for the late reacting tissues but a small change for tumours or early reactions.

Figure 13.2 shows the two most important features of this essential difference. The two curves are normalized at 64 Gy given in 32 fractions of 2 Gy. That is,

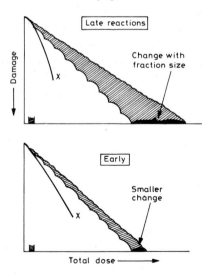

Figure 13.3. Effect of changing fraction size (shown as the small block at the bottom left) on total dose to give equal effects. Upper: late reactions. Lower: early and tumour reactions. X = Single dose response curve.

the proportion of late to early complications and of tumour control is assumed to be acceptable for this 'standard' treatment. If the number of fractions is reduced to say 5 or 6, it is clear that the total dose should be reduced much more in order to keep late reactions constant than to keep early reactions constant. Failure to appreciate this has led to clinical disasters. Singh (1978) changed from 20 fractions to only 5 in treating cancer of the cervix, adjusting his total dose using NSD (TDF or CRE would have been the same). The result was similar to the 'early' curve in Figure 13.2: the early reactions (and local control) were the same, but there was a very high incidence of late complications. Such a difference has been documented by Arcangeli et al. (1974) and by Turesson and Notter (1984) and well reviewed (Withers et al., 1982; Thames et al., 1982; Fowler, 1984). A recent example is the change from 5 weekly fractions of 2 Gy to 4 weekly fractions of 2.5 Gy, both totalling 70 Gy (Thomas et al., 1988). The early reactions and tumour control were not significantly different, but the late reactions were significantly worse. The calculated differences are 4% and 10% extra effect, assuming $\alpha/\beta = 10$ and 3 Gy, respectively.

13.3.2 Advantages of hyperfractionation

Figure 13.2 also shows the potential advantage of hyperfractionation, if we move to the right of the crossover point, to a larger number of smaller fractions. If we choose doses along the upper curve, i.e., to keep late reactions constant, we shall then overdose the early reacting tissues. Provided the acute reactions do not become intolerable, we then can expect a therapeutic gain consisting of more tumour cell kill for no extra late complications. It can be seen that changing from 2 to 1.2 Gy per fraction provides an increased dose of approximately 10% to the tumour, as mentioned in the Introduction. This is the essential advantage of hyperfractionation, which has now been realised in practical radiotherapy (Horiot et al., 1988; Parsons et al., 1988), so it is no longer just 'potential'.

In addition, there is a more subtle advantage that may work with more than one fraction per day, called reassortment, redistribution (in the phases of the cell cycle), or self-sensitization (Withers, 1975). This depends on the fact that cells are at their most sensitive when in mitosis and at the G_1/S interface. There is a better chance that survivors will move into such a sensitive phase if more fractions are used than the usual 30 or so, and given more often than daily. There would of course be no such enhancement of effect on late-reacting tissues or slowly proliferating tumours.

13.3.3 The linear-quadratic formula

It is convenient, and has been found remarkably reliable, to represent the difference in response between late and early-reacting tissues in terms of a linear-quadratic shape for their underlying dose-response curves. Figure 13.4 presents the animal evidence

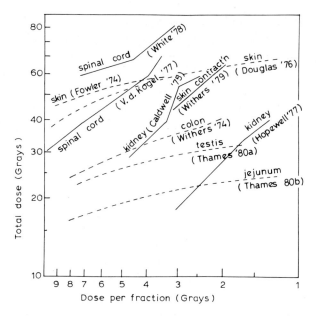

Figure 13.4. Total dose to give equal biological effects versus size of dose per fraction for several experimental animal systems (redrawn from Withers et al., 1982). Late effects (full lines) require larger changes of total dose than early effects (broken lines) as in Figure 13.2.

that enabled Withers et al. (1982) to perceive this distinction. This is a vital point which NSD, TDF and SRE etc. did not reveal (Ellis, 1969).

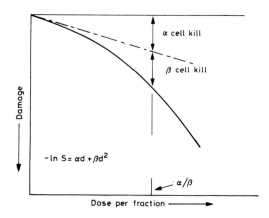

Figure 13.5. Representation of dose-response curves like those in Figure 13.1 using the linear-quadratic formula. The ratio α/β has the dimensions of dose and is that dose at which the log cell-kill from the linear process equals that from the dose-squared process. At this dose per fraction the curve has bent very significantly away from the initial slope. At 0.1 α/β (the 'flexure dose'), the response has deviated by 10% and might just detectably be different.

This difference between early and late response can conveniently be described as the difference in shape, between the dose-response curves, or underlying cell-survival curves of the critical cells in the tissue. It is convenient, but not essential, to describe these shapes in terms of a linear term with coefficient α and a dose-squared term with coefficient β (Figure 13.5):

$$S = e^{-E}$$

where $E = \alpha D + \beta D^2$ for single doses,

and $E = n(\alpha d + \beta d^2)$ for n fractions of d each.

There is no need to assume biophysical significance in this linear-quadratic formula. It is simply the first two terms of a polynomial expansion (Curtis, 1986). Alpha is the initial slope, in units of log to base e of cells killed per gray. Beta defines the rate at which the curve falls away from this initial slope, perhaps as a result of saturation or gradual failure of repair as the dose (in any one session) is increased. This relationship holds well between 1 and 8 or 10 Gy per fraction. The ratio α/β has the dimensions of dose and is, in fact, the dose at which the α-type damage is equal to the β-type damage, i.e., when the dose-response curve has deviated by rather a large amount from the initial slope. This ratio has a particular importance because it characterises the shape of the curve for each tissue.

Table 13.1 summarises α/β values for various animal tissues. It can be seen that late-reacting tissues have low values (below about 6 Gy) while early-reacting tissues have values above 7 or 8 Gy, often about 10 Gy. Tumours have values similar to, or even above, those for early-reacting normal tissues (Williams et al., 1985).

13.3.4 Multiple fractions

The results of multiple equal fractions are illustrated by joining up the chords of the dose-response curve, i.e., the slope of the line from the origin to the log cell-kill at the dose-per-fraction used, and extending this n times for n fractions (Figure 13.6). In several animal experiments it has been found that successive fractions do indeed have identical effects, in spite of some in vitro experiments which have failed to confirm this; perhaps because it is more difficult to maintain the correct physiological conditions over many fractions in vitro than in animals (Joiner and Denekamp, 1986).

13.3.5 Biologically effective doses: calculations of effect

Figure 13.6 illustrates the convenient way of calculating Biologically Effective Doses which has replaced the use of NSD, TDF and CRE (Barendsen, 1982; Fowler, 1989).

TABLE 13.1
Ratio of linear to quadratic coefficients from multi-fraction experiments on animals

	Source	α/β (Gy)
EARLY REACTIONS:		
Skin		
Desquamation	Douglas and Fowler (1976)	9.1–12.5
	Joiner et al. (1983)	8.6–10.6
	Moulder and Fischer (1976)	9–12
Jejunum		
Clones	Withers et al. (1976)	6.0–8.3
	Thames et al. (1981)	6.6–10.7
Colon		
Clones	Tucker et al. (1983)	8–9
Weight loss	Terry and Denekamp (1984)	9–13
Testis		
Clones	Thames and Withers (1980)	12–13
Mouse lethality		
30d	Kaplan and Brown (1952)	7–10
30d	Mole (1957)	13–17
30d	Paterson et al. (1952)	11-26
Tumour bed		
45d	Begg and Terry (1984)	5.6–6.8
LATE REACTIONS:		
Spinal cord		
Cervical	Van der Kogel (1979)	1.8–2.7
Cervical	White and Hornsey (1978)	1.6–1.9
Cervical	Ang et al. (1983)	1.5–2.0
Cervical	Thames et al. (1988)	2.2–3.0
Lumbar	Van der Kogel (1979)	3.7–4.5
Lumbar	White and Hornsey (1978)	4.1–4.9
	Leith et al. (1981)	3.8–4.1
	Amols and Yuhas (quoted by Leith et al., 1981)	2.3–2.9
Colon		
Weight loss	Terry and Denekamp (1984)	3.1–5.0
Kidney		
Rabbit	Caldwell (1975)	1.7–2.0
Pig	Hopewell and Wiernik (1977)	1.7–2.0
Rats	Van Rongen et al. (1988)	0.5–3.8
Mouse	Williams and Denekamp (1984)	1.0–3.5
Mouse	Stewart et al. (1984a)	0.9–1.8
Mouse	Thames et al. (1988)	1.4–4.3
Lung		
LD_{50}	Wara et al. (1973)	4.4–6.3
LD_{50}	Field et al. (1976)	2.8–4.8
LD_{50}	Travis et al. (1983)	2.0–4.2
Breathing rate	Parkins et al. (1985)	1.9–4.4
Bladder		
Frequency, capacity	Stewart et al. (1984b)	5–10

Values before 1984 are recalculated from references in Fowler 1984. Values after 1984 are as quoted in the references listed in the present paper.

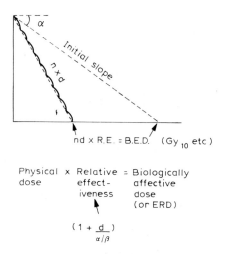

Figure 13.6. The total effect of n fractions is represented by extending the line joining the origin to the survival (or damage) caused by the dose per fraction d. The total effect (level of damage) is the same as if the *initial* slope had been extended to the Biologically Effective Dose, equal to actual dose multiplied by $(1 + \frac{d}{\alpha/\beta})$ (Barendsen, 1982). The Biologically Effective Dose is thus a useful measure of the effectiveness of any schedule, depending only upon d and α/β (and the total dose).

As in Section 13.3.3, the total effect is:

$$E = nd(\alpha + \beta d)$$

for n fractions of d each. To use the ratio α/β as if it were a single parameter, we must divide through by α (Barendsen, 1982) or by β (Thames and Hendry, 1987). Here we shall divide by α, because it gives E/α in dimensions of dose, as a useful measure of effect called Biologically Effective Dose, BED (Barendsen called it extrapolated response dose, ERD):

$$\frac{E}{\alpha} = nd\left(1 + \frac{d}{\alpha/\beta}\right) \qquad \text{(Eqn. 13.1)}$$

$$\text{Biologically Effective Dose (BED in grays)} = \text{total dose} \times \left(\begin{array}{c}\text{relative}\\\text{effectiveness}\end{array}\right)$$

For example, if we calculate the *BED* doses for late and early damage for the 'standard' schedule of 30F × 2 Gy = 60 Gy we obtain:

late damage $BED = E/\alpha = 60(1 + 2/3) = 60 \times 1.667 = 100 \text{ Gy}_3$
early damage $BED = E/\alpha = 60(1 + 2/10) = 60 \times 1.20 = 72 \text{ Gy}_{10}$

The subscripts 3 or 10 are used to indicate that the value of $\alpha/\beta = 3$ Gy (late effects) or 10 Gy (early effects) was assumed in calculating that Biologically Effective Dose. *BED* is in fact the dose which would produce the same effect if it could be delivered at enormously low dose-rate or as ultimate hyperfractionation, i.e., along the initial slope of the dose response curve (Figure 13.6). Values of *BED* in Gy_{10} units can be compared with any other values of Gy_{10} from other schedules or parts of schedules, as representing tumour effects or early reactions. They cannot be compared with Gy_3 values. Values of *BED* in Gy_3 units can be compared with any other Gy_3 values but not with *BED* values calculated with any value of α/β other than $\alpha/\beta = 3$ Gy. The *BED* values of 100 Gy_3 and 72 Gy_{10} just calculated can be remembered and used as 'standard' values, if 30F × 2 Gy can be regarded as a standard schedule. A 'stronger standard' consisting of 35F × 2 Gy would yield values of 116.7 Gy_3 and 84 Gy_{10}, respectively. These values illustrate perhaps an upper limit of acceptable normal values.

Different fractionation schedules can be compared using this method, but only the late effects are truly valid because they do not need any time factor. For example, the Concomitant Boost schedule of Knee et al. (1975) consists of 30F × 1.8 Gy = 54

TABLE 13.2
Total doses for radiotherapy schedules calculated to keep late effects constant, as a function of dose per fraction. Standardised to 200 cGy per fraction

Dose per fraction (cGy)	Total dose					
	30F × 200 = 6000 cGy			35F × 200 = 7000 cGy		
	α/β = 2 Gy	3 Gy	4 Gy	2 Gy	3 Gy	4 Gy
120	7500	7143	6923	8750	8333	8080
140	7059	6818	6667	8235	7955	7778
160	6667	6522	6429	7778	7609	7500
180	6316	6250	6207	7368	7292	7241
200	6000	6000	6000	7000	7000	7000
220	5714	5769	5807	6667	6731	6774
240	5455	5556	5625	6364	6482	6563
260	5217	5357	5455	6087	6250	6364
280	5000	5172	5294	5833	6035	6177
300	4800	5000	5143	5600	5833	6000
350	4364	4615	4800	5091	5385	5600
400	4000	4286	4500	4667	5000	5250
450	3692	4000	4235	4308	4667	4941
500	3429	3750	4000	4000	4375	4667
600	3000	3333	3600	3500	3889	4200
700	2667	3000	3273	3111	3500	3818
800	2400	2727	3000	2800	3818	3500

This table is only a guide. It should not be used to pre-empt clinical judgement. Calculated from $E/\alpha = nd(1 + d\beta/\alpha)$ = constant: e.g. 100 Gy_3 for 30F × 2 Gy; 116.7 Gy_3 for 35F × 2 Gy.

Gy in 6 weeks with a second fraction of 1.5 Gy given to a smaller volume on some of the same days, to add 12F × 1.5 Gy = 18 Gy, so that the total dose to the tumour is 72 Gy in 6 weeks. The resulting values of *BED* are:

late damage E/α = 54 (1 + 1.8/3) + 18 (1 + 1.5/3)
$\qquad\qquad\qquad$ = 54 × 1.6 + 18 × 1.5 = 110.4 Gy$_3$

early damage E/α = 54 (1 + 1.8/10) + 18 (1 + 1.5/10)
$\qquad\qquad\qquad$ = 54 × 1.18 + 18 × 1.15 = 84.4 Gy$_{10}$

It is obvious that the late damage is not as great as in the 'strong standard' of 35F × 2 Gy (*BED* was 116.7 Gy$_3$), whilst the early (and tumour) effects are equally strong (*BED* is 84 Gy$_{10}$ for both). This illustrates the advantage of the concomitant boost method.

These calculations depend critically on the choice of α/β for late reactions and it is recommended that several calculations should be made, using a set of values of α/β such as 2, 3 and 4 Gy, as in Table 13.2. Early or tumour effects do not depend so critically on the choice of α/β, but for them the question of proliferation, i.e., overall time, has to be faced, which does not apply to late effects.

13.3.6 Clinical values of α/β for human tissues

It should not be thought that the values of α/β mentioned above are restricted to mice, rats or pigs. Values of α/β that have been derived for human tissues, where changes of fractionation schedule combined with careful observations have been made, agree well with the animal results. If two schedules give the same biological effects then:

$\alpha/\beta = (D_1 \cdot d_1 - D_2 \cdot d_2)/D_2 - D_1)$ $\qquad\qquad\qquad$ (Eqn. 13.2)

TABLE 13.3
α/β ratios for early and late endpoints in different human tissues (Overgaard, 1985; 1988)

Tissue	Endpoint	α/β (Gy)
Skin	Erythema	10.5–11.3
	Moist desquamation	10.0
	Late fibrosis	1.9–2.3
	Telangiectasia	5.7
	(Telangiectasia*	3–5)
Lung	Pneumonitis	4.4–6.9
	Fibrosis (later)	3.0–3.6
Bone	Rib fractures	1.8–2.5

* Turesson and Notter (1985).

where d and D are the dose-per-fraction and the total dose, respectively. The confidence limits are difficult to calculate.

Table 13.3 lists some of the values that have been obtained from clinical data where isoeffect doses were available for defined levels of normal tissue reaction. Values of α/β for human tumours appear to be mostly high, 10 Gy to 25 or 30 Gy; although some of the more radioresistant tumours may have values as low as 5 or 6 Gy (Williams et al, 1985; Lindenberger et al., 1986; Suit et al., 1988).

13.3.7 Calculations of total dose in new schedules

It is easy to calculate the total dose required to deliver a certain Biologically Effective Dose, whether for a full course of radiotherapy or for a part of a course. BED values are simply additive, provided that they are for the same value of α/β. For example, if half of a treatment intended to consist of 30F × 2 Gy has been given (15 × 2 Gy) and then the schedule is changed to one using 3 Gy fractions, what should the remaining half consist of? Presumably late effects will be dose-limiting. The remaining half is equivalent to $E/\alpha = 30 \, (1 + d/(\alpha/\beta)) = 30 \, (1 + 2/3)$ for late effects, i.e., 50 Gy$_3$ is still to be given. Putting this into the fractionation formula with the new d of 3 Gy we obtain:

$$BED = n \cdot d \, (1 + 3/3) = 50 \text{ Gy}_3$$

Hence, $n \times 3 \times 2 = 50$; i.e., $n = 8.33$ fractions. A total dose of 25 Gy is required using the 3 Gy fractions (8.33F × 3 Gy), to give the same chance of late complications.

When there is simply a change of dose-per-fraction from a well known schedule $n_1 \cdot d_1$ to a new one $n_2 \cdot d_2$, the estimate of the new total dose is particularly simple. For equal effects the two values of E or E/α are of course equal:

$$n_1 d_1 \, (1 + d_1/(\alpha/\beta)) = n_2 \cdot d_2 \, (1 + d_2/(\alpha/\beta))$$

Therefore $\dfrac{n_2 \cdot d_2}{n_1 \cdot d_1} = \dfrac{(1 + d_1/(\alpha/\beta))}{(1 + d_2/(\alpha/\beta))}$

The ratio of total doses is the inverse ratio of the Relative Effectiveness (Section 13.3.5).

If the number of fractions is altered instead of the dose-per-fraction, the same equations can be used but the result is the solution of a quadratic equation:

$$n_2 \cdot d_2 + \dfrac{n_2 \cdot d_2^2}{\alpha/\beta} = BED \text{ (obtained from the standard schedule)}$$

Rearranging this, $d_2^2 + d_2 (\alpha/\beta) - (\alpha/\beta) BED/n_2 = 0$

So that $d_2 = -\dfrac{(\alpha/\beta)}{2} \pm \sqrt{\dfrac{(\alpha/\beta)^2}{4} + \dfrac{(\alpha/\beta) BED}{n_2}}$ (Eqn. 13.3)

Only the positive root is meaningful.

All the calculations so far have ignored overall time, which is correct for late-reacting tissues. If effects in tumours or early-reacting normal tissues have to be estimated, either the overall times should be similar in the schedules being compared or – much better – some of the effect of the n fractions has to be subtracted because of proliferation. The next section presents a simple way of doing this, within the obvious limitations of our knowledge of starting times for proliferation and of doubling times of the tumourigenic or tissue-rescuing cells.

13.4 Linear-quadratic formula with time factors

13.4.1 Time factors in general

The linear-quadratic formula was at first criticised because it has no time factor whilst the NSD formula had one (Ellis, 1969). The NSD time factor was too large for late reactions and too small for tumour proliferation or for early reactions; it is curious why people should hanker after wrong factors long after it became clear that they were wrong. It is *correct* that there should be no time factor for *late* effects. This is the main application of the linear-quadratic (L-Q) formula so it is well that no time factor should be applied. Calculations for comparing late effects are therefore straightforward.

13.4.2 Time factors to allow for proliferation

It is now possible to add a time factor to take account of proliferation in tumours or early-reacting tissues, with potentially high precision but in practice with useful accuracy only if four parameters are known. Even so, this time factor is only a simple one. It assumes exponential proliferation at a constant rate γ from the starting time of proliferation (T_k, which might not coincide with the starting time of treatment, as discussed in Section 13.2.2) to the end of treatment of time T. γ is the proliferation constant:

$N = N_0 \, e^{\gamma t}$

This assumption requires a linear increase in total dose to keep the biological effect the same. If we assume values for α and β we can relate this daily increment of dose to γ, the daily proportional increase in cell number. It will be assumed that γ is simply constant, after proliferation begins. We saw in Section 13.2.2 that proliferation in tumours can require an average of about 60 cGy per day. We do not know enough about changes in proliferation rate during treatment to propose any more complicated pattern of proliferation. We then have:

$$\text{effect} = E = nd(\alpha + \beta d) - \gamma(T - T_k).$$

The proliferation constant γ is the increase in proportion of cells occurring per day between the starting time T_k and the overall time T. It is equal to $(\log_e 2)/T_p$ where T_p is the average doubling time for regrowth of the tumourigenic (or normal-tissue-rescuing) cells. This doubling time might equal T_{pot}, but it is wise to keep these two quantities separate because we cannot be sure of this. The condition for T_p to equal T_{pot} is that the cell loss factor (Steel, 1977) should be zero. If we divide this equation through by α, we obtain the Biologically Effective Dose:

$$BED = \frac{E}{\alpha} = nd\left(1 + \frac{d}{\alpha/\beta}\right) - \frac{0.693}{\alpha}\frac{(T - T_k)}{(T_p)} \quad \text{(Eqn. 13.4)}$$

This is the L-Q formula with the time factor term added (Travis and Tucker, 1987; Wheldon and Amin, 1988; Fowler, 1989; Dale, 1989).

It is, unfortunately, now necessary to specify four disposable parameters: α, β, average doubling time T_p, and starting time of proliferation T_k. They are, however, all real biological parameters, not abstractions like the slope of a log–log graph. This multiplicity makes the 'L-Q with time factor' formula of little use for an individual patient's calculation, unless measurements both of cell survival at say 2 Gy (Brock et al., 1986) and of T_{pot} (Wilson et al., 1988) have been made on that patient. Even then T_p might not be the same as T_{pot}. Equation 13.4 is, however, useful for comparing the effectiveness of various fractionation schedules when new protocols are being designed. The same values for the parameters must be assumed for all the protocols to be compared.

For example, $\alpha/\beta = 10$ Gy is reasonable for tumours (Williams et al., 1985; Lindenberger et al., 1986; Suit et al., 1988); it could be higher but the resulting difference would be small. Malaise (1988) has pointed out that values of α of 0.2 to 0.3 Gy^{-1} are often found for primary explants from human tumours, whereas cells from established lines of culture often give values of 0.4 to 0.5 Gy^{-1}. However, many values are obtained outside these ranges (see Figure 12.2). If α is below about 0.3 Gy^{-1} no local control is possible and if it is above about 0.4 Gy^{-1} all tumours would be cured. For simple calculations comparing different schedules, values of α

between 0.3 and 0.4 Gy^{-1} are usually used, with $\alpha/\beta = 10$ Gy or sometimes 25 Gy for tumour cells.

13.4.3 Comparisons of various fractionation schedules

It is easiest to compare the effects on *late-reacting tissues* because only one parameter has to be chosen: α/β. Table 13.4 shows the comparison of various currently used fractionation schedules. Some of them use other levels of total dose in addition to the level indicated in the table. Several values of α/β are assumed for these comparisons. Values of 1.5 Gy would probably apply best for spinal cord or brain, in order to be safe in calculating for fewer and larger fractions. Values of 3 Gy are often taken as applying to generalised late connective-tissue damage such as fibrosis, ulceration or necrosis. Values of 2–3 Gy would be appropriate for kidneys and 3–4 Gy for lungs. The ranking order of intensity of these schedules changes slightly if different values of α/β are assumed, by up to 5 or 6% of effective damage (E or E/α) for a change of 1 Gy in α/β (Table 13.4).

For *tumour effects* we have assumed here $\alpha = 0.35$ Gy^{-1}, $\alpha/\beta = 10$ Gy, and proliferation occurring at a constant rate with doubling times of 2, 3, 5, 7 and 20 days. Figure 13.7 shows the log cell-kill calculated for two 'standard' schedules: 30F

TABLE 13.4
List of radiotherapy schedules ranked[b] in decreasing order of 'hotness' of late effects.

Radiotherapy schedule	Biologically Effective Dose (*BED*)		
	$\alpha/\beta = 3$ Gy	2 Gy	4 Gy
Strong standard 35F × 2 Gy = 70 Gy	116.7	116.7	116.7
Manchester 16F × 3.38 Gy = 54 Gy	114.8	120.9	110.6
RTOG HypF 68F × 1.2 Gy = 81.6 Gy	114.2	108.8	117.9
Concom boost 72 Gy[d]	113.4	111.8	114.5
EORTC HypF 70F × 1.15 Gy = 80.5 Gy	111.4	105.7	115.2
Pipard SAI 70 Gy[e]	111.1	109.7	112.0
EORTC AccHF 45F × 1.6 Gy = 72 Gy[c]	110.4	107.5	112.0
Standard 33F × 2 Gy = 66 Gy	110.0	110.0	110.0
RTOG HypF 65F × 1.2 Gy = 78 Gy[c]	109.2	104.0	112.7
Scotland 20F × 2.8 Gy = 56 Gy	108.3	112.0	106.8
CC Wang 42F × 1.6 Gy = 67.2[c]	103.4	100.8	104.5
Standard 30F × 2 Gy = 60 Gy	100.0	100.0	100.0
CHART 36F × 1.56 Gy = 56 Gy	85.0	83.0	86.4
CHART 36F × 1.5 Gy = 54 Gy	81.0	78.8	82.5

[a] Compared with 30F × 2 Gy as 100%.
[b] Ranking on the basis of column 1 ($\alpha/\beta = 3$ Gy). Note different ranking in other columns.
[c] 4-hour intervals. Late effects could be 5 to 9% stronger than listed.
[d] Concomitant boost: 30F × 1.8 Gy + 12F × 1.5 Gy = 72 Gy in 39 days.
[e] Pipard Swiss Accel Irrad: 10F × 2 Gy + 30F × 1.67 Gy = 70 Gy in 32 days.

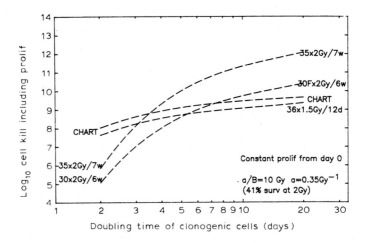

Figure 13.7. Calculated log cell kill for a range of doubling times of tumourigenic cells from 2 to 20 days. α is assumed to be 0.35 Gy^{-1} and α/β = 10 Gy. The steep curves are for 'standard' schedules of 30F × 2 Gy in 6 weeks and 35F × 2 Gy in 7 weeks. The flatter curves are for the CHART schedule (Saunders et al., 1988) consisting of 36F × 1.5 Gy in 12 days prescribed but 36F × 1.56 Gy at the ICRU-defined point in the tumour. Constant proliferation throughout the treatment is assumed.

× 2 Gy = 60 Gy in 6 weeks, and a stronger standard of 35F × 2 Gy = 70 Gy in 7 weeks. Also shown are two dose levels for the highly accelerated Continuous Hyperfractionated Accelerated Radiation Therapy (CHART) schedule consisting of 36F × 1.5 Gy = 54 Gy in 12 days, given 3 times a day with 6 hour intervals (Saunders et al., 1988). For any value of doubling time, the highest curves represent the most cell kill and the best probability of local control. Reference to Table 13.4 indicates how severe the late effects are expected to be from any of these schedules.

Figure 13.7 shows that the 7-week schedule loses 6 logs of cell kill, i.e., about half its total effect, if tumour cells proliferate as fast as 2 days doubling time instead of 20 days. The shorter schedule (CHART) loses less than 2 logs by the same comparison. This calculation assumes constant proliferation throughout the treatment. If, however, proliferation did not start until about 3 weeks after the beginning of treatment (Withers et al., 1988), then these curves would be about half as steep for the longer treatments and simply flat for the shorter schedule.

Figure 13.7 shows the large loss in cell kill in the tumour as the doubling time becomes shorter, for the 6 week and 7 week schedules. There is, by contrast, little loss of effectiveness for the short, 12-day, CHART schedule with faster proliferation in the tumours. Although the total doses have to be kept lower in the 12-day schedule (to avoid severe early reactions), it is more effective than the 30F and 35F × 2 Gy schedules for tumours which double in less than 5–6 and 3 days, respectively. The late reactions are expected to be low in the CHART schedule (Table 13.4).

Figure 13.8 illustrates the relative effects of intrinsic radiosensitivity and prolifer-

Fractionation and therapeutic gain 199

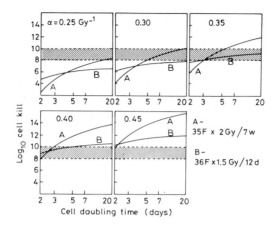

Figure 13.8. As in Figure 13.7 but for (A) the 35F × 2 Gy in 7 weeks schedule and (B) the 36F × 1.5 Gy in 12 days schedule, showing the effect of changes in intrinsic radiosensitivity (α) from 0.25 to 0.45 Gy^{-1}. α/β is 10 Gy throughout. As the radiosensitivity increases, the gain from the avoidance of proliferation provided by the short schedule becomes less important: it occurs only for tumours proliferating faster than 2.2 days where $\alpha = 0.45$ Gy^{-1}. Proliferation throughout is assumed with the average doubling time shown.

ation rate on such comparisons. For simplicity only the strong standard (35F × 2 Gy = 70 Gy in 7 weeks) and a single level of dose of the CHART schedule (36F × 1.5 Gy = 54 Gy in 12 days) are shown. They represent opposite ends of the spectrum of long and short schedules, respectively. Results are shown for five values of α ranging from 0.25 to 0.45 Gy^{-1}; α/β is assumed to be 10 Gy as usual for tumours. The

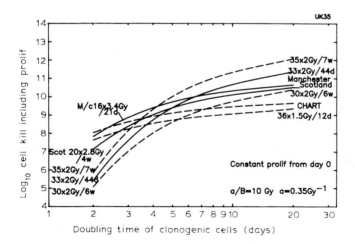

Figure 13.9. As in Figure 13.7: the same four curves are reproduced as dashed lines here. The three full curves are for three schedules used in the UK: a 'standard' 33F × 2 Gy in 6.5 weeks; Manchester 16F × 3.375 Gy = 54 Gy in 21 days; and Scotland/Canada 20F × 2.8 Gy = 56 Gy in 4 weeks.

200 J.F. Fowler

major effect is that both schedules pass from below the arbitrary shaded level of cell kill to above it over this range, i.e., from very ineffective to very effective. There is another result concerning their relative effectiveness which is not so obvious at first sight. The crossover point, or doubling time below which the CHART schedule is more effective than even the strong 35F standard, changes from 4.2 to 2.2 days as the tumour becomes more radio-sensitive. This means that accelerated fractionation is more helpful in cases where the tumour cells are radioresistant.

Figure 13.9 shows these same four curves as dashed lines, together with several schedules used in the U.K. Starting from the right-hand side, the upper full line is for 33F × 2 Gy given 'daily' (5F/week) in 6.5 weeks. This schedule loses effectiveness rapidly as proliferation rate increases, becoming less effective than the CHART schedule for doubling times less than about 4 days. The middle full line is for Manchester's 3 week treatment, 54 Gy in 16 fractions (to small fields). This is predicted to be better than CHART until proliferation is faster than a 2-day doubling time, and better than 30F × 2 Gy throughout. However, the late damage is relatively severe, as listed in Table 13.4; so the relative therapeutic gains of the schedules are probably not very different. The third full line, for the 4-week schedule of 20 fractions totalling 56 Gy (for small fields) as used in Scotland and Canada, is similar to the Manchester schedule, except for the fastest proliferating tumours.

Figure 13.10 shows the corresponding calculated values for three recently designed European schedules. Reading from the right, the upper full line is for the EORTC randomised trial of hyperfractionation completed in 1985, for which favourable results

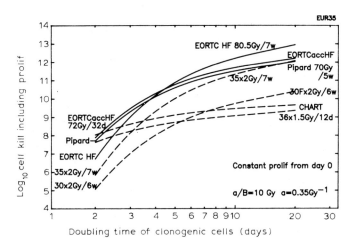

Figure 13.10. As in Figure 13.9 but the three full lines represent three recently designed European schedules: EORTC HF (hyperfractionation) 70F × 1.15 Gy b.i.d. = 80.5 Gy in 7 weeks; EORTC accelerated hyperfractionation 45F × 1.6 Gy t.i.d. with a planned gap after 28.8 Gy then on to 72 Gy in 5 weeks; and Pipard's Swiss Accelerated Irradiation totalling 70 Gy in 5 weeks with no gap.

Fractionation and therapeutic gain 201

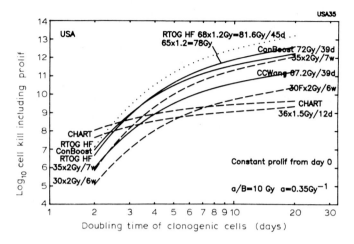

Figure 13.11. As in Figure 13.10 but the three full lines represent three currently used USA schedules: RTOG HF (hyperfractionation) 65 or 68F × 1.2 Gy b.i.d. = 78 or 81.6 Gy (full and dotted curves, respectively) in 44 or 45 days; concomitant boost totalling 72 Gy in 39 days; and C.C. Wang's 42F × 1.6 Gy b.i.d. with a gap after 38.4 Gy and then on to 67.2 Gy in 6 weeks.

are reported as mentioned in the introduction (Horiot et al., 1988; 70F × 1.15 Gy given b.i.d to 80.5 Gy in 7 weeks). This is one log higher than its control arm, which was 35F × 2 Gy = 70 Gy in 7 weeks. It corresponds to a 10% increase in log cell-kill (at the middle of Figure 13.10) which would lead to a 10–15% increase in local control, just as has been observed clinically. The other two full lines are for two schedules which give 72 or 70 Gy, respectively, in an overall time as short as 5 weeks. They do not lose effectiveness with decreasing doubling time as rapidly as the 6 or 7 week schedules. The EORTC Accelerated Hyperfractionation protocol gives 3 fractions per day of 1.6 Gy and differs also from Wang's twice daily protocol (see next paragraph) by starting the planned gap after only 28.8 Gy in less than 2 weeks (6 treatment days, 8 real days). The acute reactions are then less severe and the gap can be shorter; the whole overall time is 1 week shorter. The Pipard Swiss Accelerated Irradiation gives an initial boost (to a small volume) of 10F × 2 Gy in 2 weeks, followed with no gap by 30F × 1.667 Gy given twice daily to a total of 70 Gy in 5 weeks to the full volume. These two protocols were designed to shorten the overall times from 6 or 7 weeks by a modest amount, whilst maintaining a high total dose of at least 70 Gy. The calculated relative late effects are shown in Table 13.4. They are all rather effective schedules compared with those previously discussed.

Figure 13.11 shows three schedules currently used in the USA, as the full lines, with the same four dashed curves. The upper dotted curve is for the current escalation to 81.6 Gy of the RTOG Hyperfractionation trial of 1.2 Gy given b.i.d., although this looks hot. The upper full line is for the same protocol when escalated to 78 Gy;

favourable results were reported from this level (Parsons et al., 1988). This is rather similar to the Concomitant Boost schedule of Knee et al. (1985) which, however, is in a shorter overall time of 6 instead of 7 weeks. The lowest full line is for the split course b.i.d. schedule of Wang (1988). Here 1.6 Gy fractions are given twice daily to a total of 38.4 Gy (12 treatment days, 2.5 weeks) then a gap of 2 weeks followed by the same fractionation, up to a total of 67.2 Gy in 6 weeks. Because the interval was only 4 instead of 6 hours, the cell kill (and the damage to early reacting tissues) would be greater than shown here by 2 to 4%. The excess damage to late reaching tissues would be 5 to 9%.

Figure 13.11 shows that the upper two of these US protocols would be expected to be better than the strong standard of 35F × 2 Gy throughout, and better than CHART for tumours with cells proliferating faster than a doubling time of 2.5 days. Such modern schedules can be significantly better than the previous standard treatments simply using 1.8 or 2 Gy 'daily' on 5 days per week.

TABLE 13.5
Percent extra effective dose for interfraction intervals of 4, 6 and 8 hours

Schedule (& half-time of repair)	Late effects			Early and tumor effects		
	4 h	6 h	8 h	4 h	6 h	8 h
2 fractions per day						
2 × 2 Gy						
(2 h)	10.0	5.0	2.5	4.2	2.1	1.0
(1.5 h)	6.3	2.5	1.0	2.6	1.0	0.4
2 × 1.6 Gy						
(2 h)	8.7	4.4	2.2	3.5	1.0	0.9
(1.5 h)	5.5	2.2	0.9	2.2	0.9	0.3
2 × 1.2 Gy						
(2 h)	7.1	3.6	1.8	2.7	1.3	0.7
(1.5 h)	4.5	1.8	0.7	1.7	0.7	0.3
3 fractions per day						
3 × 1.6 Gy						
(2 h)	13.0	6.5	3.3	5.2	5.2	1.3
(1.5 h)	8.2	3.3	1.3	3.3	3.3	0.5
3 × 1.2 Gy						
(2 h)	10.7	5.4	2.7	4.0	4.0	1.0
(1.5 h)	6.8	2.7	1.1	2.5	2.5	0.4
3 × 1.0 Gy						
(2 h)	9.4	4.7	2.3	3.4	3.4	0.9
(1.5 h)	5.9	2.3	0.9	2.2	2.2	0.3

13.4.4 Intervals between multiple fractions per day

It is important that intervals between fractions should be long enough to allow full repair of the repairable component of radiation damage, or else some of the advantage of accelerated or hyperfractionation can be lost. Since there is a higher proportion of repairable injury per gray in late than early-reacting tissue (because the dose-response curves are more curvy), it takes longer for this to fade to an undetectable level for late than early damage (Fowler, 1988). An interval of 4 or 5 hours might be adequate for early reactions but this interval would not be sufficient for late effects. It is not clear whether any human tissues or tumours have half-times of repair less than an hour and a half, as in some tissues in mice; but it is not safe to assume that they do. It is clear from clinical results that intervals of 4.5 hours are not long enough (Marcial et al., 1987). Any schedules that use less than 6-hour intervals could be producing more damage than would be expected assuming complete repair; and this will be worse for late than early (or tumour) damage. Thames and Hendry (1987) provide a table with incomplete repair factors which can be added to the β term in the Relative Effectiveness bracket (Equation 13.1) to take account of various fraction intervals in relation to the half-time of repair.

It is not safe to assume half-times of repair of less than 1.5 hours. Although shorter times than this have been measured in mice, it is possible that human cells repair sublethal radiation damage slightly more slowly, just as their cell-cycle times are 1.5 or 2-times longer than in mice. Table 13.5 lists the percentage extra effect of incomplete repair between 2 or 3 fractions per day, calculated from Thames and Hendry (1987).

13.5 Conclusions

Withers (1988) has summed up the strategy of fractionated radiotherapy by saying 'Give as high a dose as you can without causing severe late effects; using smaller doses per fraction than 1.8–2 Gy to keep the late effects moderate compared with tumour cell kill; and give the dose as fast as you can without causing severe acute effects'.

'As fast as you can' is something we are still learning about. Three doses per day of 2 Gy is too fast to be acceptable. Three doses per day of 1.6 Gy are being used, and experience will accumulate. It appears at present that no more than about 5 Gy per day can be delivered, no matter how it is fractionated (except for very low dose rates). Multiple fractions per day are a feature of all of the recently designed, radiobiologically based, high-performance schedules.

No more than about 55 Gy can be given within 2 weeks, no matter how it is fractionated. Even that level can only be obtained with small fields or shrinking fields.

If doses of about 70 Gy are to be given, a gap may have to be allowed, preferably planned *before* half the total dose has been given, so as to keep the gap short; even then the overall times cannot be less than about 5 weeks. However, the Swiss Accelerated Irradiation technique achieves 70 Gy in 5 weeks without a gap, although it delivers the boost fields (to small volumes) first instead of at the end. These high-dose schedules appear at present to be probably better than the 12-day ultra accelerated approach, using lower doses, for tumours which proliferate less rapidly than with a 2–2.5 day doubling time. A minority of tumours have potential doubling times as fast as this when measured before treatment. It is not known whether a substantial proportion of tumours can accelerate their proliferation to become faster than this during the course of radiotherapy. If so, the results of the CHART studies will come out better than expected. We do not know whether such extreme acceleration occurs. We cannot yet interpret cell kinetic measurements made in tumours during non-equilibrium conditions, i.e., during treatment. It is to be hoped that ways will be found to obtain this information.

It is obvious that good clinical results can be obtained with schedules as long as 6 weeks or so. The point of the highly accelerated schedules is to prevent some of the failures which still occur. This could best be achieved by an individual measurement of T_{pot} by flow cytometry of a biopsy before the start of treatment. In this way the most rapidly growing tumours could be selected for accelerated schedules.

It is even more important to develop individual assays of tumour cell radiosensitivity to doses of about 2 Gy; for example, by the method of Brock et al. (1986) or other methods (See Chapter 21). That would identify resistant tumours which would require extra measures such as concomitant chemotherapy or high LET radiation, and relatively sensitive tumours which should, when sufficient correlations with outcome have been obtained, be treatable by ordinary schedules.

Acknowledgements

I should like to acknowledge many fruitful discussions with colleagues including Drs. Ang, Barendsen, Begg, Curtis, Dale, Denekamp, Dische, Douglas, Dutreix, Ellis, Field, Fletcher, Glatstein, Hendry, Holsti, Horiot, Joiner, Liversage, Notter, Orton, Parkins, Peters, Saunders, Steel, Stewart, Thames, Tubiana, Turesson, Williams and Withers. My thanks also to Karen Blomström for converting my script to legibility.

References

Arcangeli, G., Friedman, M. and Paoluzi, R. (1974) A quantitative study of the radiation effect on normal skin and subcutaneous tissues in human beings. Br. J. Radiol. 47, 44–50.

Barendsen, G.W. (1982) Dose fractionation, dose rate and iso-effect relationships for normal tissue responses. Int. J. Radiat. Oncol. Biol. Phys. 8, 1981–1997.

Begg, A.C. and Terry, N.H.A. (1984) The sensitivity of normal stroma to fractionated radiotherapy measured by a tumor growth rate assay. Radiother. Oncol. 2, 333–341.

Begg, A.C., McNally, N.J., Shrieve, D.C. and Kärcher, H. (1985) A method to measure the duration of DNA synthesis and the potential doubling time from a single sample. Cytometry 6, 620–626.

Begg, A.C., Moonen, L., Hofland, E., Desseng, M. and Bartelink, H. (1988) Human tumor cell kinetics using a monoclonal antibody against IUdR: intra-tumor sampling variations. Radiother. Oncol. 11, 337–347.

Brock, W.A., Maor, M.M. and Peters, L.J. (1986) Predictors of tumor response to radiotherapy. Radiat. Res. 104 (Suppl.), S290–296.

Curtis, S.B. (1986) Lethal and potentially lethal lesions induced by radiation – a unified repair model. Radiat. Res. 106, 252–270.

Dale, R.G. (1989) Time-dependent tumour repopulation factors in linear quadratic evaluations. Radiother. Oncol., in press.

Douglas, B.G. and Fowler, J.F. (1976) The effect of multiple small doses of X-rays on skin reactions in the mouse and a basic interpretation. Radiat. Res. 66, 401–426.

Ellis, F. (1969) Dose, time and fractionation: a clinical hypothesis. Clin. Radiol. 20, 1–7.

Fowler, J.F. (1984) What next in fractionated radiotherapy? Br. J. Cancer 49 (Suppl. VI), 285–300.

Fowler, J.F. (1986) Potential for increasing the differential response between tumors and normal tissues: can proliferation rate be used? Int. J. Radiat. Oncol. Biol. Phys. 12, 641–645.

Fowler, J.F. (1988) Intervals between multiple fractions per day; differences between early and late reactions. Acta Oncol. 27, 181–183.

Fowler, J.F. (1989) What do we need to know to predict the effectiveness of fractionated radiotherapy schedules? in: Proceedings 3rd International Symposium on Time Dose and Fractionation, Madison, Wisconsin, September 1988. AAPM Conference Series.

Horiot, J.C., Lefur, R., Nguyen, T., Schraub, S., Chenal, C., DePauw, M. and Van Glabbeke, M. (1988) Two fractions per day versus a single fraction per day in the radiotherapy of oropharynx trial. Int. J. Radiat. Oncol. Biol. Phys. 15 (Suppl. 1), p. 178, Abstract.

Joiner, M.C. and Denekamp, J. (1986) Evidence for a constant repair capacity over 20 fractions of X-rays. Int. J. Radiat. Biol. 49, 143–150.

Knee, R., Fields, R. and Peters, L. (1985) Concomitant boost radiotherapy for advanced squamous cell carcinoma of the head and neck. Radiother. Oncol. 4, 1–7.

Lindenberger, J., Hermeking, H., Kummermehr, J. and Denekamp, J. (1986) Response of human tumor xenografts to fractionated X-irradiation. Radiother. Oncol. 6, 15–17.

Maciejewski, B., Preuss-Bayer, G. and Trott, K.R. (1983) The influence of the number of fractions and of overall treatment time on local control and late complication rate in squamous cell carcinoma of the larynx. Int. J. Radiat. Oncol. Biol. Phys. 9, 321–328.

Malaise, E.P., Fertil B., Chavaudra, N., Brock, W.A., Rofstad, E.K. and Weichselbaum, R.R. (1989) The influence of technical factors on the in vitro measurements of intrinsic radiosensitivity of cells derived from human tumours, in Proceedings 3rd International Symposium on Time Dose and Fractionation, Madison, Wisconcin, September 1988. AAPM Conference Series.

Marcial, V.A., Pajak, T.F., Chang, C., Tupchong, L. and Stetz, J. (1987) Hyperfractionated photon radiation therapy in the treatment of advanced squamous cell carcinoma of the oral cavity, pharynx, larynx and sinuses, using radiation therapy as the only planned modality: (preliminary report) by the Radiation Therapy Oncology Group (RTOG)). Int. J. Radiat. Oncol. Biol. Phys. 13, 41–47.

Overgaard, M. (1985) The clinical implications of non-standard fractionation. Int. J. Radiat. Oncol. Biol. Phys. 11, 1225–1229.

Overgaard, J., Hjelm-Hansen, M., Vendelbo, J.L. and Andersen, A.P. (1988) Comparison of conventional and split-course radiotherapy as primary treatment in carcinoma of the larynx. Acta Oncol. 27, 147–161.

Parkins, C.S. and Fowler, J.F. (1985) Repair in mouse lung of multifraction X-rays and neutrons: extention of 40 fractions. Br. J. Radiol. 58, 1097–1103.
Parsons, J.T., Bova, F.J. and Million, R.R. (1980) A re-evaluation of split-course technique for squamous cell carcinoma of the head and neck. Int. J. Radiat. Oncol. Biol. Phys. 6, 1645–1652.
Parsons, J.T., Mendenhall, W., Cassisi, N., Isaacs, J. and Million, R.R. (1988) Accelerated hyperfractionation for head and neck cancer. Int. J. Radiat. Oncol. Biol. Phys. 14, 649–658.
Pipard, G., Guillemin, E. and Stepanian, E. (1988) High-dose accelerated irradiation for head and neck carcinoma. 7th Annual meeting ESTRO at Den Haag, Abstract p. 233.
Peters, L.J., Ang, K.K. and Thames, H.D. (1988a) Accelerated fractionation in the treatment of head and neck cancer: a critical comparison of different strategies. Acta Oncol. 27, 185–194.
Peters, L.J., Brock, W.A., Chapman, D.J., Wilson, G.D. and Fowler, J.F. (1988b) Response predictors in radiotherapy: a review of research into radiobiologically based assays. Br. J. Radiol. (Suppl. 22), 96–108.
Van Rongen, E., Kuijpers, W.C., Madhuizen, H.T. and Van der Kogel, A.J. (1988) Effects of multifraction irradiation of the rat kidney. Int. J. Radiat. Oncol. Biol. Phys. 15, 1161–1170.
Saunders, M., Dische, S., Fowler, J.F., Denekamp, J., Dunphy, E., Grosch, E., Fermont, D., Ashford, R., Maher, J. and Des Rochers, C. (1988) Radiotherapy with three fractions per day for twelve consecutive days for tumors of the thorax, head and neck, *in*: Frontiers of Radiation Therapy and Oncology, Vol. 22 (Vaeth, J. and Meyer, J., eds.), pp. 99–104.
Singh, K. (1978) Two regimens with the same TDF but differing morbidity used in the treatment of stage III carcinoma of the cervix. Br. J. Radiol. 51, 357–362.
Steel, G.G. (1977) Growth Kinetics of Tumours, pp. 191 and 202, Clarendon Press, Oxford.
Stewart, F.A., Soranson, J., Alpen, E.L., Williams, M.V. and Denekamp, J. (1984a) Radiation-induced renal damage: the effects of hyperfractionation. Radiat. Res. 98, 407–420.
Stewart, F.A., Randhawa, V.S. and Michael, B.D. (1984b) Multifraction irradiation of mouse bladders. Radiother. Oncol. 2, 131–140.
Suit, H.D., Zietman, A., Miralbell, R. and Sedlacek, R. (1988) Human tumour xenografts as models for the study of the radiation response of human tumors, *in*: Proceedings 3rd International Symposium on Time Dose and Fractionation, Madison, Wisconsin, September, 1988. AAPM Conference Series.
Svoboda, V.H.J. (1978) Further experience with radiotherapy by multiple daily sessions. Br. J. Radiol. 51, 363–369.
Terry, N.H.A. and Denekamp, J. (1984) RBE values and repair characteristics for colorectal injury after caesium-137 γ-ray and neutron irradiation. II. Fractionation up to ten doses. Br. J. Radiol. 57, 617–629.
Thames, H.D., Withers, H.R., Peters, L.J. and Fletcher, G.H. (1982) Changes in early and late radiation responses with altered dose fractionation: implications for dose-survival relationships. Int. J. Radiat. Oncol. Biol. Phys. 8, 219–226.
Thames, H.D., Peters, L.J., Withers, H.R. and Fletcher, G.H. (1983) Accelerated fractionation versus hyperfractionation: rationales for several treatments per day. Int. J. Radiat. Oncol. Biol. Phys. 9, 127–138.
Thames, H.D. and Hendry, J.H. (1987) Fractionation in radiotherapy, 297 pp., Taylor and Francis, London.
Thames, H.D., Ang, K.K., Stewart, F.A. and Van der Schueren, E. (1988) Does incomplete repair explain the apparent failure of the basic L-Q model to predict spinal cord and kidney responses to low doses per fraction? Int. J. Radiat. Biol. 54, 13–19.
Thames, H.D., Peters, L.J. and Ang, K.K. (1989) Time-dose considerations for normal-tissue tolerance, *in*: Frontiers of Radiation Therapy and Oncology, Vol. 23 (Vaeth, J. and Meyer, J., eds.), in press.
Thomas, F., Ozanne, F., Mamelle, G., Wibault, P. and Eschwege, F. (1988) Radiotherapy alone for oropharyngeal carcinomas: the role of fraction size (2 Gy vs. 2.5 Gy) on local control and early and late complications. Int. J. Radiat. Oncol. Biol. Phys. 15, 1097–1102.
Travis, E.L. and Tucker, S.L. (1987) Iso-effect models and fractionated radiation therapy. Int. J. Radiat.

Oncol. Biol. Phys. 13, 283–287.
Trott, K.R. and Kummermehr, J. (1985) What is known about tumour proliferation rates to choose between accelerated fractionation or hyperfractionation? Radiother. Oncol. 3, 1–9.
Turesson, I. and Notter, G. (1984) The influence of fraction size in radiotherapy on the late normal tissue reaction. I. Comparison of the effects of daily and once-a-week fractionation on human skin. Int. J. Radiat. Oncol. Biol. Phys. 10, 593–598.
Wang, C.C. (1988) Local control of oropharyngeal cancer after two accelerated hyperfractionation radiation therapy schemes. Int. J. Radiat. Oncol. Biol. Phys. 14, 1143–1146.
Wheldon, T.E. and Amin, A.E. (1988) The linear quadratic model. Br. J. Radiol. 61, 700–702.
Williams, M.V. and Denekamp, J. (1984) Radiation-induced renal damage in mice: Influence of fraction size. Int. J. Radiat. Oncol. Biol. Phys. 10, 885–893.
Williams, M.V., Denekamp, J. and Fowler, J.F. (1985) A review of α/β ratios for experimental tumours: implications for clinical studies of altered fractionation. Int. J. Radiat. Oncol. Biol. Phys. 11, 87–96.
Wilson, G.D., McNally, N.J., Dische, S., Saunders, M.I., Des Rochers, C., Lewis, A.A. and Bennett, M.H. (1988) Measurement of cell kinetics in human tumours in vivo using bromodeoxyuridine incorporation and flow cytometry. Br. J. Cancer 58, 423–431.
Withers, H.R. (1975) Cell cycle redistribution as a factor in multifraction irradiation. Radiology 114, 199–202.
Withers, H.R., Thames, H.D. and Peters, L.J. (1982) Differences in the fractionation response of acutely and late-responding tissues, in: Progress in Radio-Oncology, Vol. II. (Kärcher, K.H., Kogelnik, H.D. and Reinartz, G., eds.), pp. 287–296, Raven Press, New York.
Withers, H.R., Taylor, J.M.G. and Maciejewski, B. (1988) The hazard of accelerated tumor clonogen repopulation during radiotherapy. Acta Oncol. 27, 131–146.

CHAPTER 14

Radiotherapy with multiple fractions per day

WALTER VAN DEN BOGAERT[1], JEAN-CLAUDE HORIOT [2] and
EMMANUEL VAN DER SCHUEREN[1]

[1]*Department of Radiotherapy, University Hospital St. Rafaël, Kapucijnenvoer 33, 3000 Leuven, Belgium and* [2]*Centre G.F. Leclerc, Département de Radiothérapie, Rue du Prof. Marion, 21034 Dijon, France.*

14.1   Historical background 210

14.2   Current concepts 213
      14.2.1   Recovery capacity 213
      14.2.2   Repopulation 213

14.3   Multiple fractions per day 214
      14.3.1   Hyperfractionation 215
      14.3.2   Accelerated fractionation 217

14.4   Conclusions 220

Interaction between radiobiologists and clinical radiotherapists occurs in two ways: radiobiologists seeking to explain clinical observations, and clinicians seeking to test radiobiological predictions. Hitherto the first of these has predominated, but now the second is becoming more common. When a dose is not given in a single session but divided over several fractions, the effect on tissues is decreased and a higher total dose has to be given to obtain the same effect. This is due to recovery of these tissues during the overall time the irradiation is given.

This recovery consists of two different phenomena:

(i) Recovery from sublethal damage during intervals between irradiations (see Section 12.4). Sublethal damage recovery takes place immediately after irradiation and is completed in a few hours (Elkind, 1959; Withers, 1974).

(ii) Increased proliferation or repopulation of surviving cells. The radiation damage is recognised by some tissues, and compensatory accelerated proliferation of the surviving cells can take place (see Section 7.4). The time of onset is usually several days or even weeks after the start of irradiation and differs among dose-limiting normal tissues. Accelerated proliferation in response to radiation damage can also take place in tumours (Sections 6.3.4 and 13.2).

The therapeutic success of radiotherapy depends on the radiation sensitivity of the cells in tumours and normal tissues (Section 12.3). It has also widely been thought that differences in recovery capacity are important, although the newer ideas set out in Section 12.4 may call this in question. The ability of acute-reacting normal tissues to proliferate more rapidly following cell depletion is also recognised as an important contribution to therapeutic success.

14.1 Historical background

In the first years of radiation therapy, high doses were given in single or a few fractions, resulting in serious reactions, a high incidence of necrosis and a relatively low therapeutic efficiency.

The work of Regaud (1921 and 1927) and Coutard (1932) demonstrated that the delivery of dose over a longer time-span in many fractions could have a profound effect upon the importance of radiation injury to normal tissues and tumours. The famous experiment on ram testicles, showing that sterilisation was possible without scrotal skin necrosis when the dose was given in four fractions rather than in one, and the clinical investigations it initiated, gave a strong impulse to the pragmatic development of fractionated radiation therapy. These clinical studies explored the possibility of increasing the dose and the anti-tumour effect by decreasing the incidence of acute tissue reactions.

Various time schedules were explored and a number of remarkable therapeutic successes were obtained by trial and error, mainly in head and neck tumours (Coutard 1932). Subsequently, Baclesse (1949) succeeded in administering very high total doses without prohibitive acute reactions by extending the total time to 12 weeks or more, resulting in significant control of breast cancer. Such very long overall treatment times were abandoned later on as new insights in the proliferation rate of tumours made people aware of possible negative repercussions of prolonging treatment time and also since awareness grew that, past a certain overall time, tolerance limits do shift from acute to late reactions.

Interestingly, Coutard (1932) investigated also the use of low dose rate, delivering the dose over several hours, a technique he called 'protraction', mimicking brachytherapy dose rates for tissue sparing. The technique was later on abandoned, as it was thought that increasing overall treatment time was more important than prolonging irradiation time (Baclesse 1949).

While the work of the French school defined to a large extent the influence of total time on acutely-reacting tissues, this concept of fractionation did not yet distinguish clearly the influence of repopulation and repair and the role of the fraction size, by itself, remained obscure. The arrival of high-energy machines changed the scope of research in radiotherapy. The important advances in dose distribution received most of the interest, and for a while clinical development of time-dose-fractionation studies became of secondary interest. Much information was gathered on 'absolute' tolerance of tissues and organs, resulting in detailed, practical guidelines (Rubin and Casarett, 1968).

There is a wide range of tolerance doses for different organs due to the different radiosensitivity of the tissues. The tolerance of a number of normal connective tissues was considered in the 1960s and 1970s to be about 60 Gy in 6 weeks.

The importance of two factors was, however, only very slowly realized. The effect of changes in fraction size, by themselves, was still mostly disregarded, and the general idea was that one remained on the safe side of tolerance as long as an irradiation rhythm of 10 Gy per week was respected (Buschke and Parker, 1972). It is striking to see, as late as in the 1960s and 1970s in two major Radiotherapy Centers, MD Anderson (Houston) and IGR (Villejuif), that dose fractionation was changed from 5 to 3 fractions per week without any adjustment for the increase in fraction size: the weekly dose and the total dose remained the same, leading to clearly increased normal tissue sequelae as demonstrated in their subsequent analyses (Fletcher, 1966; Gallez-Marchal, 1984).

A second idea was that the severity of late reactions was directly related to the importance of acute reactions (Lederman, 1961; Buschke, 1972) and many clinicians considered these acute reactions as a valuable guideline and safeguard for avoiding late complications (Buschke, 1972). While this is true within certain limits for the 'classical' fractionation schedules, it was not always realised that in some fractionation schedules this association would prove to be a false security. Indeed, protraction and split-course do selectively favour repopulation, which occurs mainly in tissues responsible for early reactions. Also, changes in fraction size were shown to affect to a much larger extent slowly proliferation tissues than tissues with a rapid turnover. Changes in time and fractionation could thus selectively reduce acute reactions while leaving late reactions unchanged or even increased.

Until 1969, the relation of dose and time, and how mathematically to compare different fractionation schedules, was based upon the Strandqvist formula, dating from 1944. In this formula, a relation was established between dose and time, expressing the amount of recovery with increasing protraction. No consideration was given to the number of fractions and according to this formula one was 'allowed' to divide the dose into as many fractions as one wished as long as the total time was respected. The belief in '1000 a week' is consistent with this concept.

Another erroneous motivation to use large fraction sizes came in the 1960s, paradoxically from radiobiological data. The cell-survival curves published by Elkind and Sutton (1959) and Lajtha and Oliver (1961) showed relatively more cell killing with increasing fraction size and the significance of this was not fully understood. It is not so much the absolute amount of cell killing but the difference in cellular damage between tumour and normal tissues which creates therapeutic gain. Some clinicians citing 'the relative inefficiency of radiation, given in small fractions' started to use large fractions, resulting in horrendous complications (Atkins and Tretter, 1966; Andrews, 1965).

A giant step forward in the understanding of the phenomena underlying the effect of irradiation on biological tissues resulted from the Ellis formula (1969) and the NSD concept (Nominal Standard Dose) the unit of which is the ret (Roentgen Equivalent Therapy). In this formula the number of fractions in relation to the total treatment time was taken into account. The effect of fraction size was also implicit in this formula.

In the same period a number of warnings appeared in the literature against the use of large fraction sizes (Fletcher, 1966; Kok, 1971), and it was soon demonstrated that the Ellis formula was not satisfactory for large changes in fraction size nor for all tissues. For instance, in the larynx it was demonstrated by Loeffler (1971) that the incidence of late complications was more related to fraction size by itself than to the NSD.

At the present time the limits of the Ellis formula are well known (Byhardt et al., 1977; Dische et al., 1981). Already in the original paper, Ellis (1969) expressed a firm warning against extrapolating the equation towards effects in tissues other than skin, since the formula was obtained from data on erythema and skin cancer. This advice was not followed: the NSD concept fulfilled a tremendous need of radiotherapists who started being aware of the role of fraction number and who were now able to calculate equivalent doses for different schedules. The great differences in impact of the exponents of T and N for different tissues were not yet realised. While the general concept of Ellis was valid between certain limits, the formula did not take into account differences in recovery capacity of different tissues. The availability of a mathematical model led to a false sense of security and even encouraged the use of fewer (larger) fractions to gain machine time, with the idea that the biological effects were 'equivalent' anyway. It is now known to what disasters this led (Singh, 1978; Hatlevoll et al., 1983).

The difficulties encountered in the clinical application of the NSD formula and others derived from it, TDF (Orton and Ellis, 1973) and CRE (Kirk, 1971), have two reasons (Thames and Hendry, 1987). The first is the power-law nature of the models, which implies that recovery is maximal in the first weeks of irradiation, which is not consistent with biological data on repopulation. The second reason is the fact that tissues differ in their fractionation sensitivity, so no single exponent can describe their relation to dose-time factors.

Recently, a more biologically orientated model has become of general use, the linear-quadratic formula (Douglas and Fowler, 1976; Barendsen, 1982). This formula describes the survival of irradiated tissues by assuming a double mechanism for cell killing, non-repairable (α) and repairable (β) damage, the ratio of these components being a measure for fractionation sensitivity (see Section 4.2.3 and Chapter 13). This model covers only cellular recovery. Repopulation has to be accounted for separately (Section 13.4).

At the present time there is much more quantitative information available on normal tissues than on tumours, and most investigations of altered fractionation schedules aim at improved tolerance. As progressively more data are obtained on tumours, new fractionation schedules will also be aimed more specifically at greater anti-tumour efficacy.

14.2 Current concepts

14.2.1 Recovery capacity

It has become gradually evident that recovery capacity varies widely between tissues: slowly-proliferating tissues usually have a large recovery capacity as compared to rapidly-proliferating tissues. Consequently, the use of many small fractions will spare these slowly-proliferating tissues (responsible for late effects) relatively more than rapidly-proliferating tissues (responsible for acute reactions). Conversely, with large fraction sizes, the tolerance of slowly-renewing tissues will be lowered to a larger extent than in rapidly-renewing tissues. As the recovery capacities of tumours are assumed to be in range of those of rapidly-proliferating tissues it is assumed that conditions in which optimal recovery can take place would relatively increase late tolerance, while leaving the anti-tumour effect less affected. The higher dose which can then be given should result in better tumour control for equal late sequelae. Such an aim is pursued in 'hyperfractionation' in which fraction sizes significantly below 2 Gy are applied. The critical questions which remain are the lack of information on the recovery capacity of individual tumours and the ultimate limit of recovery in normal tissues, which will define the lowest fraction size that should practically be applied.

'Hypofractionation', or the use of large fractions could only advantageously be used in tumours that have a larger recovery capacity than normal tissues, of which the tolerance in such situations is known. Presently, this is only suggested to be the case for melanoma (Overgaard, 1986) while in most other cases no advantage was demonstrated (Cox, 1985).

14.2.2 Repopulation

After cell depletion, increased proliferation of surviving cells will take place in most tissues. The extent of this repopulation is related to the cell kinetics of these tissues: rapidly-renewing tissues will start off repopulation after a few days and will usually be able to ultimately replace the total cellular deficit.

The tremendous impact of repopulation on tolerance of tissues such as skin and gastro-intestinal mucosae was established decades ago. Better insight into the kinetics of these processes, which were thought for a long time to occur at constant rates, now allow for an even more effective exploitation of this phenomenon. Slowly-renewing tissues show little evidence of repopulation, although some slow recovery may occur over a long period (Field et al., 1976).

It has not yet been established whether tumours react to radiation injury with increased proliferation, although some indications for this are present in the literature (Van Peperzeel, 1970; Maciejewski, 1983). Evidence on the proliferation rate of tumour cells in presented in Section 13.2 and Chapter 6.

Increased efficacy of accelerated treatment has been clearly demonstrated in many animal tumours which are known to have much shorter doubling times than human tumours. Also in a few rare tumours in humans, rapid irradiation schedules have been shown to yield better results and in a few tumour types the deleterious influence of very long or interrupted treatment schedules has been hinted at. Accelerated irradiation can only be carried out, if one does not want to increase the fraction size, by giving several irradiations per day. In such conditions it becomes critically important to know how rapidly recovery is complete after an irradiation. While this may be so after about 4 hours in many tissues, it may require 6 hours or more in tissues where relatively more recovery takes place (Ang et al., 1987).

'Accelerated irradiation' can be defined as a schedule in which significantly more than 10 Gy (in 2 Gy/fraction) or biologically equivalent doses are given per week.

14.3 Multiple fractions per day

Until some years ago, nearly all fractionation schedules were based on a single fraction per day. Initially this was six times per week, then, due to social reasons, five times; sometimes, for technical reasons such as accelerator maintenance, four times per week has been used. Better understanding of the importance of fraction size has led to the avoidance of this last practice, and in most departments standard practice is again based on five irradiations per week.

A few years ago, studies of multiple fractions per day were initiated. This was based on investigations using both 'hyperfractionation' and 'accelerated irradiation'. Daily irradiation using fraction sizes much less than 2 Gy leads to significant prolongation of overall treatment time. This results in treatment regimens which, in intensity, are below acute tolerance, and have an unfavourable therapeutic effect on tumours where proliferation constitutes a significant factor. In order to avoid this, two or more irradiations are given per day, thus keeping the overall treatment time similar to conventional fractionation schedules. In such studies the aim is to take advantage of the better recovery capacity of some critical normal tissues, usually those determining late tolerance.

A second group of studies aims at keeping the fraction size at a conventional level and by giving several irradiations per day to shorten the overall treatment time. The objective here is to counteract tumour repopulation. It must be expected that this will lead to greater damage in early-reacting normal tissues, within which cell proliferation makes a substantial contribution to tolerance.

A new and very important question which results from this policy of irradiating several times per day has been the critical importance of the kinetics of recovery from sublethal damage. As long as intervals of 24 hours were used, a large safety margin existed and recovery could always be assumed to be totally complete at the time of a subsequent irradiation. However, in the normal working hours of a department, intervals between irradiations cannot be greater than 7–8 hours when two treatments are given in a single day, and can be as low as 4 hours for three sessions per day. In a few studies where even more fractions were given per day, intervals as small as 2 hours were used (Nguyen et al., 1988).

For the moment, little experimental information is available on the time necessary to complete recovery when fraction sizes of around 2 Gy are applied. It appears that there are differences between tissues and those where more extensive recovery takes place apparently require longer recovery times. Whether this is simply related to the fact that they recover larger amounts of damage or whether different processes play a role in not yet clear.

In mouse lip mucosa, recovery is essentially complete within 3 hours after fractions of 2–4 Gy. For rat spinal cord 10–15% of repair remains still unfinished 4 hours after irradiation with 4 Gy. Further experiments are required to assess repair kinetics in spinal cord after 2 Gy fractions.

Also in clinical practice there have been some indications that short intervals between irradiations could result in increased toxicity to late-reacting tissues, but not for early reactions (Nguyen et al., 1988). Great caution is therefore recommended in such studies and minimum intervals of 4 hours are now to be respected, where possible even 6 hours, until more data are available.

14.3.1 Hyperfractionation

The anticipated therapeutic benefit of hyperfractionation lies mainly in the higher total dose that can be given for equivalent normal tissue tolerance. Thames et al. (1983) mentions also a possible role of redistribution and less dependence on efficiency of reoxygenation. A number of such studies have been carried out, initially mainly with the aim of investigating feasibility and tolerance. Unfortunately, in many instances, other parameters were also changed at the same time, obscuring the interpretation of results (Wang, 1988). The experience in the clinic with these schedules is growing and in some departments (mainly in the U.S.A.) hyperfractionation is used routinely in head and neck cancer.

The evidence for hyperfractionation to have a higher therapeutic ratio than conventional schemes mainly derives from non-randomised treatment of head and neck cancer (Parsons et al., 1984; Meoz et al., 1984; Medini et al., 1985). The data from Wang (1988) show a remarkable improvement in comparison to historical controls. The data would be much more convincing if from a randomised study, since we are all aware of the pitfalls of comparisons with historical controls.

The most important clinical experience in hyperfractionation is the EORTC study in oropharyngeal cancer (Horiot et al., 1988). In this trial a conventional schedule of 70 Gy at 2 Gy/day is compared with a schedule in which two irradiations of 1.15 Gy are given per day, in the same overall treatment time of 7 weeks, to a total dose of 80.5 Gy. This correction of 15% for total dose was pragmatically defined, based on a number of pilot studies in which tolerance was investigated. Using the presently available information on fractionation sensitivity, the application of an α/β ratio of 3 would suggest a possible total dose of 83.5 Gy. There may thus be a reasonably good correlation between clinical tolerance studies and calculated values based on biologically available information. The patients included in the study had squamous cell carcinoma of the oropharyngeal region, T_2 and T_3, N_o or N_+ with nodes less than 3 cm in diameter. The trial was activated in February 1980 and closed in April 1987. This trial is the first to show a benefit for hyperfractionation in a randomised setting.

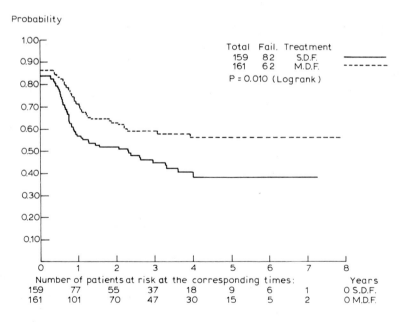

Figure 14.1. Locoregional control in patients with oropharyngeal tumours treated with conventional irradiation (S.D.F.) or hyperfractionated irradiation (M.D.F.). Study of the Radiotherapy Group of the EORTC.

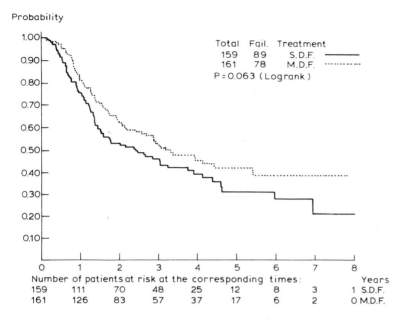

Figure 14.2. Survival results for patients treated with conventional (S.D.F.) and hyperfractionated radiotherapy (M.D.F.).

A clear, statistically significant, advantage was obtained in locoregional control for the patient group treated with hyperfractionation (Figure 14.1). Benefit is not yet seen in survival (Figure 14.2). The trial also showed a trend to increased acute reactions in the hyperfractionated treatment while there was no clinically significant difference between late reactions, specifically fibrosis, for patients treated with regular fraction sizes and hyperfractionation.

Other studies are currently underway (for instance in the RTOG) and further data are still needed before one can conclude that hyperfractionation represents a real therapeutical benefit.

14.3.2 Accelerated fractionation

Accelerated fractionation schedules have a reduced overall time – 2, 3 (or more) fractions per day – while the number of fractions, the fraction size and the total dose can be left unchanged. When reducing overall treatment time, the critical question is the possible loss of tolerance occurring in normal tissues. This would be least important in treatments where the critical tissues have little or no proliferation, for instance in the treatment of glioblastomas where the tolerance is determined by the brain. In an early study, the overall treatment time was reduced from 6 to 4 weeks. For this, three fractions of 2 Gy were given per day, to a dose of 30 Gy in a week.

After a rest period of two weeks this was repeated, coning the irradiated volume down for the last 20 Gy. A split-course schedule was selected for fear of excessive reaction in the irradiated skin in which a drastic drop in tolerance was expected. This sharp divergence from the then existing concept of tolerance for the brain of 10 Gy per week was not generally accepted in 1979. For more than a year the study was carried out in a single institution and only following the first analysis of tolerance was it expanded to a number of additional centres in the Radiotherapy Group of the EORTC (Ang et al., 1983).

Subsequently, a large prospective study was carried out, including over three hundred patients. No difference in results was found between the conventionally treated patients (60 Gy/6 weeks) and the accelerated regimen (60 Gy in 4 weeks, split course). It is interesting to see that at the time of analysis the use of accelerated fractionation was an acceptable treatment; lack of improvement was thought to be related to the loss of efficiency associated with the split course.

After a number of pilot studies in single institutions (Svoboda, 1975; Gonzalez et al., 1980; Cappellini et al., 1978) several multicentre studies were done in the EORTC Radiotherapy Group in advanced head and neck cancer (Van den Bogaert et al., 1983). In these studies it became clear that it is possible to give up to 48 Gy in 2 weeks. However, it was not possible to administer the full total doses usually given in such cases (65 to 72 Gy) without inserting a rest period, since the acute reactions became prohibitive. In head and neck cancer the treatment schedule consisted of an initial 2 weeks treatment period in which a dose of 48 Gy was given (three times 1.6 Gy per day, ten times, in 2 weeks). After 3 to 4 weeks of rest, another week of treatment followed in which about 24 Gy was added. Overall treatment time was thus left unchanged compared to conventional schedules.

No differences in survival or local control were seen between conventional radiotherapy and the schedule studied (Van den Bogaert et al., 1986), though it was shown that it is possible to use such very concentrated schedules.

Many different possibilities exist in the way the total dose can be divided over the treatment time. Several such schedules have been tested in head and neck cancer in Leuven (van der Schueren et al., 1983). In all these schedules, the total time was kept unchanged and irradiation was administered in several blocks, using 3 or 4 fractions per day. Various doses and also different time intervals between these blocks (split-course regimens) were studied. Two blocks of 30 Gy in 4 weeks, three of 22.4 Gy in 7 weeks and four of 16 Gy in 6 weeks were given (Figure 14.3). It is interesting to compare the mucosal reactions of conventional continuous daily irradiation to such discontinuous split-course treatments for their effects on mucosal reactions. The conventional 65–70 Gy always led to confluent mucositis developing around the fourth week and persisting until about 2–3 weeks after the end of the irradiation. The first study on accelerated fractionation used the highest possibly tolerable dose in the initial block (48 Gy) leaving a smaller block of about 24 Gy for the second 'top-up'

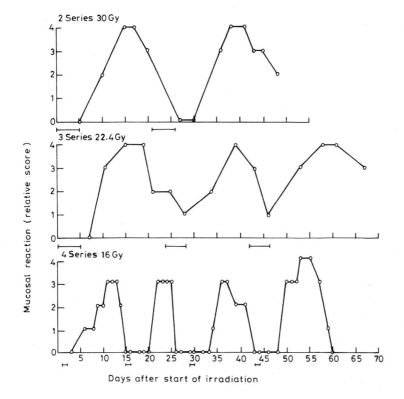

Figure 14.3. Mucosal reactions in patients irradiated with accelerated multiple fractions per day. The days of irradiation are indicated with horizontal bars below the time scheme.

irradiation. Due to the very heavy mucosal reactions after the 48 Gy in 2 weeks, a rest period of 3 and often 4 weeks was necessary before the second block could be given leading to an overall treatment time of about 7 weeks. So, while the initial part of the irradiation was very concentrated, very little gain was obtained in overall treatment time.

From the split-course studies (Figure 14.3) it could be demonstrated that the threshold for punctiform mucositis is around 20 Gy in fractions of 2 Gy and that repopulation is extremely rapid and effective when doses are around this value. Intervals of 14 days for 22.4 Gy and of 12 days for 16 Gy were sufficient to restore completely the integrity of the irradiated mucosa, allowing subsequent irradiation without cumulative toxicity. These data were used to develop the new randomised study of the Radiotherapy Group of the EORTC on accelerated fractionation for head and neck tumours. In order to keep overall irradiation time as short as possible, it is necessary to be able to keep the rest period short; it was therefore decided to start treatment with a short irradiation 'burst' of 28.8 Gy, 18 fractions in 1 week, with which treatment was concluded in the first trial. This has the great advantage that therapy can easily be resumed 2 weeks later resulting in an overall treatment time of 5 weeks for a total dose of 72 Gy.

This study was activated in 1985 and preliminary results show the feasibility of the schedule at least in terms of acute reactions (Horiot et al., 1988). Concurrently with this study, the proliferation rate of the tumours prior to treatment is investigated on biopsy specimens by measuring IUDR labelling index with flow cytometry. It is the aim to relate this parameter to treatment results, since it is suggested that accelerated fractionation would be most efficient in rapidly growing tumours (Withers, 1985).

14.4 Conclusions

A large number of fractionation studies are now complete or underway both in the USA and in Europe, both randomised and non-randomised. These studies are largely inspired by new concepts and deeper insights in radiobiology (Chapter 13). At the present time it is not yet known whether these new schedules will become incorporated into standard radiotherapy practice. Fletcher (1988) has expressed his personal doubts about this.

These are, however, only the first steps, and future studies will be needed to investigate the specific indications of fractionation schedules for tumours in different sites and in specific clinical situations.

References

Andrews, J.R. (1965) Dose-time relationships in cancer radiotherapy, a clinical radiobiology study of extremes of dose and time. Am. J. Roentgenol. 93, 56–74.

Ang, K.K., Van der Schueren, E., Notter, G., Horiot, J.G., Chenal, C., Fauchon, F., Raps, J., Van Peperzeel, H., Goffin, J.C., Vessiere, M. and Van Glabbeke, M. (1983) Split-course multiple daily fractionated radiotherapy schedule combined with misonidazole for the management of grade III and IV gliomas. Int. J. Radiat. Oncol. Biol. Phys. 8, 1657–1664.

Ang, K.K., Thames, H.D., Van der Kogel, A.J. and Van der Schueren, E. (1987) Is the rate of repair of radiation induced sublethal damage in rat spinal cord dependent on the size of dose per fraction? Int. J. Radiat. Oncol. Biol. Phys. 13, 557–562.

Atkins, H.L. and Tretter, P. (1966) Time-dose considerations in radiation myelopathy. Acta Radiol. Ther. Phys. Biol. 5, 79–94.

Baclesse, F. (1949) Roentgen therapy as the sole method of treatment for cancer of the breast. Am. J. Roentgenol. Radium Ther. Nucl. Med. 62, 311–319.

Baclesse, F. (1949) Carcinoma of the Larynx. Br. J. Radiol. 3 (Suppl.), 1–63.

Barendsen, G.W. (1982) Dose fractionation, dose rate and iso-effect relationships for normal tissue responses. Int. J. Radiat. Oncol. Biol. Phys. 8, 1981–1999.

Buschke, F. and Parker, R.G. (1972) in: Radiation therapy in Cancer Management, p. 37, Grune and Stratton, New York.

Byhardt, R.W., Greenberg, M. and Cox, J.D. (1977) Local control of squamous carcinoma of oral cavity and

oropharynx with 3 versus 5 treatment fractions per week. Int. J. Radiat. Oncol. Biol. Phys. 2, 415–420.
Cappellini, M., Chiavacci, A. and Olmi, P. (1978) Radioterapia con frazionamento multiple giornaliere: reazioni cutanee e mucose. Estratto da: radiobiologia dei Tumori. Ed. Med. Sci. Int. Rome, 197–208.
Cox, J.D. (1985) Large-dose fractionation. Cancer 55, 2105–2111.
Coutard, H. (1932) Roentgen therapy of epitheliomas of the tonsillar region, hypopharynx, and larynx from 1920 to 1926. Am. J. Roentgenol. 28, 313–331.
Dische, S., Martin, W.M.C. and Anderson, P. (1981) Radiation myelopathy in patients treated for carcinoma of the bronchus using a six fraction regime of radiotherapy. Br. J. Radiol. 54, 29–35.
Douglas, B.G. and Fowler, J.F. (1976) The effect of multiple small doses of X-rays on skin reactions in the mouse and a basic interpretation. Rad. Res. 66, 401–26.
Elkind, M.M. and Sutton, H. (1959) X-ray damage and recovery in mammalian cells in culture. Nature 184, 1293–5.
Ellis, F. (1969) Dose time and fractionation; a clinical hypothesis. Clin. Radiol. 20, 1–7.
Field, S.B., Hornsey, S. and Kutsutani, Y. (1976) Effects of fractionated irradiation on mouse lung and a phenomenon of slow repair. Br. J. Radiol. 49, 700–707.
Fletcher, G.H. (1966) *in*: Textbook of Radiotherapy. p. 344, Lea and Febiger, Philadelphia.
Fletcher, G.H. (1988) Regaud Lecture Perspectives on the History of Radiotherapy. Radiother. Oncol. 12, 253–271.
Gallez-Marchal, D., Fayolle, M., Henry-Amar, M., Le Bourgeois, J.P., Rougier, P. and Cosset, J.M. (1984) Radiation injuries of the gastrointestinal tract in Hodgkin's disease: the role of exploratory laparotomy and fractionation. Radiother. Oncol. 2, 93–99.
Gonzalez-Gonzalez, D., Breur, K. and Van der Schueren, E. (1980) Preliminary results in advanced head and neck cancer with radiotherapy by multiple fractions a day. Clin. Radiol. 31, 417–421.
Hatlevoll, R., Host, H. and Kaalhus, O. (1983) Myelopathy following radiotherapy of bronchial carcinoma with large single fractions: a retrospective study. Int. J. Radiat. Oncol. Biol. Phys. 9, 41–44.
Horiot, J.C., Van den Bogaert, W., Ang, K.K., Van der Schueren, E., Bartelink, H., Gonzalez, D., De Pauw, M. and Van Glabbeke, M. (1988) European Organization for Research on Treatment of Cancer Trials Using Radiotherapy with Multiple Fractions per Day, *in* Front. Radiat. Ther. Oncol. pp. 149–161.
Kirk, J., Gray, W.M. and Watson, E.R. (1971) Cumulative radiation effect. Part I. Fractionated treatment regimes. Clin. Radiol. 22, 145–155.
Kok, G. (1971) Influence of the size of the fraction dose on normal and tumor tissue in ^{60}Co radiation treatment of carcinoma of the larynx and inoperable carcinoma of the breast. Radiol. Clin. Biol. 40, 100–115.
Lajtha, L.G. and Oliver, R. (1961) Some radiobiological considerations in radiotherapy. Br. J. Radiol. 34, 252–257.
Lederman, M. (1961) Place of radiotherapy in treatment of cancer of the larynx. Br. Med. J. 5240, 1639–1949.
Loeffler, R.K. (1974) Influence of fractionation on acute and late reactions in vocal cord carcinoma. Am. J. Roentgenol. 121, 748–753.
Maciejewski, B., Gunhild, P.B. and Trott, K.R. (1983) The influence of the number of fractions and of overall treatment time on local control and late complication rate in squamous cell carcinoma of the larynx. Int. J. Radiat. Oncol. Biol. Phys. 9, 321–328.
Medini, E., Rao, Y., Kim, T., Levitt, S.H. (1985) Radiation therapy for advanced head and neck squamous cell carcinoma using twice-a-day fractionation. Am. J. Clin. Oncol. 8, 65–68.
Meoz, R.T., Fletcher, G.H., Peters, L.J., Barkley, H.T., Jr. and Thames, H.D., Jr. (1984) Twice-daily fractionation schemes for advanced head and neck cancer. Int. J. Radiat. Oncol. Biol. Phys. 10, 831–836.
Nguyen, T.D., Panis, X., Froissart, D., Legros, M., Coninx, P. and Loirette, M. (1988) Analysis of late complications after rapid hyperfractionated radiotherapy in advanced head and neck cancers. Int. J. Radiat. Oncol. Biol. Phys. 14, 23–25.

Orton, C.G. and Ellis, F. (1973) A simplification in the use of the NSD concept in practical radiotherapy. Br. J. Radiol. 46, 529–537.

Overgaard, J. (1986) The role of radiotherapy in recurrent and metastatic malignant melanoma: a clinical radiobiology study. Int. J. Radiat. Oncol. Biol. Phys. 12, 867–872.

Parsons, J.T., Cassisi, N.J. and Million, R.R. (1984) Results of twice-a-day irradiation of squamous cell carcinoma of the head and neck. Int. J. Radiat. Oncol. Biol. Phys. 10, 2041–2051.

Regaud, C. (1921) Sur la radio-immunisation des tissus cancéreux et sur le mécanisme de l'action des rayons X et des rayons gamma de radium sur les cellules et les tissus vivants en géneral. Bull. Acad. Paris 91, 604.

Regaud, C. and Ferroux, R. (1927) Discordance des effets de rayons X, d'une part dans le testicule, par le fractionnement de la dose. C.R. Soc. Biol. 97, 431.

Rubin, P. and Casarett, G.W. (1968) Clinical Radiation Pathology, Saunders, Philadelphia.

Singh, K. (1978) Two regimes with the same TDF but differing morbidity used in the treatment of stage III carcinoma on the cervix. Br. J. Radiol. 51, 357–362.

Svoboda, V. (1975) Radiotherapy by several fractions a day. Br. J. Radiol. 48, 131–133.

Thames, H.D. and Hendry, J.H. (1987) *in*: Fractionation in Radiotherapy, p. 163, Taylor and Francis, London.

Thames, H.D. Jr., Peters, L.J., Withers, H.R. and Fletcher, G.H. (1983) Accelerated fractionation vs. hyperfractionation: rationales for several treatments per day. Int. J. Radiat. Oncol. Biol. Phys. 9, 127–138.

Van den Bogaert, W., Van der Schueren, E., Horiot, J.C., Chaplain, G., Arcangeli, G., Gonzalez, D. and Svoboda, V. (1983) The feasibility of high-dose multiple daily fractionation (MDF) and its combination with anoxic cell sensitizers in the treatment of advanced head and neck cancer. Int. J. Radiat. Oncol. Biol. Phys. 8, 1649–1656.

Van den Bogaert, W., Van der Schueren, E., Horiot, J.C. et al. (1986) Early results of the EORTC randomized clinical trial on multiple fractions per day (MFD) and misonidazole in advanced head and neck cancer. Int. J. Radiat. Oncol. Biol. Phys. 12, 587–591.

Van der Schueren, E., Van den Bogaert, W. and Ang, K. (1983) Radiotherapy with multiple fractions per day, *in*: The Biological Basis of Radiotherapy, pp. 195–208, Taylor and Francis, London.

Van Peperzeel, H.A. (1970) Patterns of tumor growth after irradiation: a comparative study in men, dogs and mice. Ph. D. Thesis, University of Amsterdam.

Wang, C.C. (1988) Local control of oropharyngeal carcinoma after two accelerated hyperfractionation radiation therapy schemes. Int. J. Radiat. Oncol. Biol. Phys. 14, 1143–1146.

Withers, H.R. and Mason, K.A. (1974) The kinetics of recovery in irradiated colonic mucosa of the mouse. Cancer 34, 896–903.

Withers, H.R. (1985) Biological basis for altered fractionation schemes. Cancer 55, 2086–2095.

CHAPTER 15

The dose-rate effect

G. GORDON STEEL

Radiotherapy Research Unit, The Institute of Cancer Research, Cotswold Road, Sutton, Surrey SM2 5NG, England

---

15.1 Biological mechanisms underlying the dose-rate effect 223

15.2 The dose-rate effect in human tumour cells 226

15.3 Models of the dose-rate effect 227

15.4 Dose-rate effects in normal tissues 229

15.5 Fractionated low dose-rate irradiation 230

15.6 Concept of curative zones in implant radiotherapy 232

15.7 Therapeutic implications 233

15.1 Biological mechanisms underlying the dose-rate effect

At the acute dose rates of a few grays per minute that are usually employed in radiobiology and radiotherapy, the initial subcellular processes of damage infliction take place and free-radical reactions go to completion (Section 1.1). These processes occur so quickly that within an exposure time of a few minutes they will be finished. Dose rate must be increased (and exposure time thus decreased) very considerably in order to prevent this happening; there is therefore little effect of dose rate within this high dose-rate region.

If, however, the dose rate is reduced much below 1 Gy/min, then the exposure time becomes long enough for further processes to take place during irradiation and thus to influence response. These consist of the '4 Rs of radiobiology': Recovery, Reassortment, Repopulation and Reoxygenation (Withers, 1975). Each of these processes modifies the response of a tissue to a second dose or increment in dose. The dose rate

TABLE 15.1
Recovery half-times[a] in tumour-cell systems

Designation	Type	IR model	LPL model	Split-dose experiment
Human Tumour Cells				
HX34	Melanoma	0.11	0.09	0.97
HX118	Melanoma	0.16	0.23	0.36
HX58	Pancreas	0.82	0.80	1.3
HX32K	Pancreas	_[b]	_[b]	1.7
HX156	Cervix	0.54	0.54	
RT112	Bladder	0.86	0.85	0.93
GCT27	Testis	0.31	0.34	0.46
HX99	Breast	_[b]	_[b]	1.0
WX67	Bladder	_[c]	_[c]	0.23
HX144	Lung AdCa.			2.3
HX148	Lung AdCa.			2.1
HX147	Lung, LC			1.8
HC12	Lung, SC			0.6
HX138	Neuroblastoma	_[b]	_[b]	1.0
HX142	Neuroblastoma	0.54	0.54	1.6
HX143	Neuroblastoma	_[c]	_[c]	0.74
Murine Tumour Cells				
MT		0.094	0.10	0.19
Lewis lung		0.092	0.069	0.61
B16		0.13	0.12	0.16

[a] In hours.
[b] Data incompatible with IR and LPL models.
[c] No significant dose-rate effect.
Data mostly from Steel et al. (1987) and Stephens et al. (1987).

at which any of them will modify response depends upon the speed of the process in question. A fast process will take place during a short exposure time, and thus influence response at high dose rate. A slower process cannot compete with a high rate of infliction of damage, and it will modify response only at a lower dose rate.

Of the 4 Rs, recovery is the fastest, with half-times in the region of an hour (Table 15.1). If the exposure time becomes a significant part of an hour, then some recovery will take place and cells will become less sensitive. Reassortment is somewhat slower: cells would have to move through a few hours of the cell cycle in order to change their radiosensitivity significantly. Repopulation is slower still, for the maximum increase in cell number that can occur within one cell-cycle time is one doubling. Cell-cycle times for human cells are around 2–3 days, a factor of 50 longer than the typical recovery half-time. Furthermore, under continuous irradiation both cell-cycle progression and proliferation will be inhibited. Little is known about the speed of reoxygenation in human tumours, but it is to be expected that a few hours to some days may be required.

The implications of this argument are illustrated in Figure 15.1. This indicates the dependence of duration of irradiation on dose rate, for different end-points. The

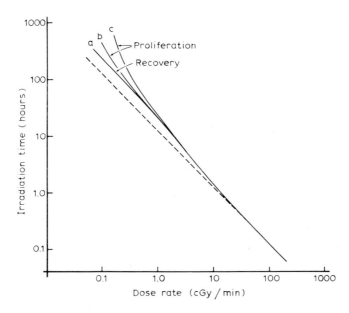

Figure 15.1. Exposure time as a function of dose rate in four theoretical situations. The broken line shows times required to give a dose of 7.5 Gy. Curve (a) shows the effect of cellular recovery according to the IR model with parameters typical of human tumours. The other two curves show the additional effect of assuming that surviving cells proliferate with a doubling time of 3 days (curve b) or 1 day (curve c).

full line shows the time required to deliver a *dose* of 7.2 Gy. This time is strictly proportional to the reciprocal of the dose rate: duration of irradiation = dose/dose rate. This is mathematics, not biology. The biology comes in when we ask: 'What duration of exposure is required to produce *the same effect* as say 7.2 Gy at high dose rate?'. Reassortment or reoxygenation, if they occur, will tend to bend the curve down; these mechanisms make cells more sensitive and the irradiation time will therefore be less. Cellular recovery or repopulation will bend the curve up, because these tend to make cells more resistant. The broken and dotted lines show, for a typical human tumour cell line, roughly the extent and range of dose rates over which this will occur.

The conclusion, therefore, is that recovery will be the main process that modifies radiosensitivity within the dose-rate range from a few grays per minute down to a few centigrays per minute. Below about 2 cGy/min, the response may be complicated by cell-cycle progression. Below about 0.5 cGy/min, the dose required for an isoeffect will increase rapidly in proliferating cell systems as a result of cell multiplication. The basis of this picture of the dose-rate effect lies in the extensive experimental work carried out on in vitro cell lines at Colorado State University (Mitchell, Bedford and Bailey, 1979; Wells and Bedford, 1983).

The effect of hypoxia on the dose-rate effect in tumours is not well understood in quantitative terms. At high dose rate, the response will be that of a mixture of oxic and hypoxic cells. As the dose rate is reduced, the prolongation of exposure will begin to allow some reoxygenation of hypoxic cells, thus tending to counteract the dose-sparing effects of recovery from potentially lethal damage.

15.2 The dose-rate effect in human tumour cells

The current picture of radiosensitivity in human tumour cells at high dose rate is described in Section 12.3. There is considerable variation in the steepness and curvature of cell-survival curves, and the initial slope is steeper in the more radiocurable tumour types. Figure 15.2 shows a comparison for a representative group of human tumour cell lines between the high-dose-rate curves and those observed at about 2 cGy/min. These data come from a detailed study on 12 human tumour cell lines (Steel et al., 1987). At the lower dose rate, the differences in sensitivity between the cell lines are magnified. The survival curves have in most cases become straight and linearly extrapolate the initial slope of the high dose-rate curves. Since the survival for 2 Gy at high dose rate is also close to the initial slope (Figure 15.3), a succession of 2 Gy doses with full recovery between would also produce similar survival curves to those in panel B of Figure 15.2. This is therefore a dramatic illustration of the fact that human tumour cells do differ greatly in radiosensitivity, especially when, as is the case in most clinical treatments, there is ample opportunity for recovery to occur. Any

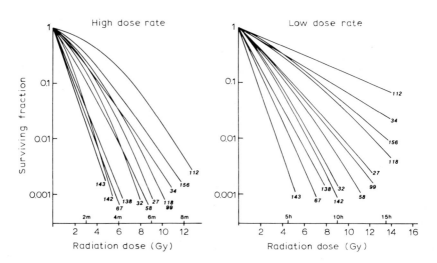

Figure 15.2. Cell-survival curves for 12 human tumour cell lines irradiated at high dose rate (approx. 150 cGy/min) or at low dose rate (approx. 1.6 cGy/min). The duration of exposure has been marked on the abscissa. A variety of human tumour types are represented: bladder (HX67, 112), cervix (HX156), melanoma (HX34, 118), breast (HX99), pancreas (HX32, 58), teratoma (GCT27), neuroblastoma (HX138, 142, 143). From Steel et al. (1987).

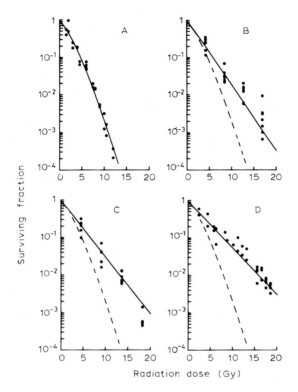

Figure 15.3. The dose-rate effect in human melanoma cells (HX34). The dose rates (in cGy/min) are: A (150), B (14), C (7.6), C (1.6). Full lines show the best fit using the LPL model. From Stephens et al. (1987).

attempt to discriminate between human tumours in terms of radiosensitivity would be best done at low dose rate, though this has not so far been exploited in work on predictive testing (Section 21.2).

Some of the curves in Figure 15.2 are almost as steep at low dose rate as at high. But those that are least sensitive and have the greatest apparent curvature at high dose rate become much shallower. This is shown in Figure 15.3 which shows the results of a detailed study on the human melanoma cell line (HX34). These data have been simultaneously fitted using the Lethal–Potentially Lethal model (Section 4.2.5) which simulates the data well. The melanoma cells require about twice the dose to produce a few decades of cell killing, comparing low and high dose rate.

15.3 Models of the dose-rate effect

To what extent can the data shown in the previous section be simulated by current models of radiation cell killing? Most cell-survival models are static, in the sense that whilst they indicate how cell survival may depend on dose, they say nothing about the duration of exposure. Two dynamic models have been described in Section 4.2. The Lethal–Potentially Lethal (LPL) model of Curtis (1986) is based on the idea that irradiation induces two types of cellular lesion: lethal lesions and potentially lethal lesions. The fate of potentially lethal lesions depends upon competing processes of repair and binary fixation, and it is assumed that these processes occur exponentially with time. The model thus has four basic parameters: two describing sensitivity, and two time constants. It allows survival to be calculated for any given dose rate or for any series of fractions. A fifth parameter fixes the length of time after exposure for which repair is allowed to proceed.

The Incomplete Repair (IR) model described by Thames (1985) is not based on putative mechanisms of cell killing. It assumes a linear-quadratic equation at high dose rate; time is introduced by making the assumption that the dose-equivalent of damage decays exponentially with time to a limiting value; a similar approach was used by Szechter and Schwartz (1977). The basic equation for continuous exposure is:

$$S = \exp(-\alpha D - \beta g D^2)$$

where $\quad g = 2[\mu t - 1 + \exp(-\mu t)] / (\mu t)^2$

(μ is the time-constant for recovery, i.e., $\ln(2)$/half-time). When the exposure time, t, is very short, $g \to 1$ and survival is as given by the linear-quadratic equation. As the duration of exposure increases, $g \to 0$ and survival approaches that given by the linear term in the equation. As shown in Figure 4.6, the model thus simulates a bending survival curve at high dose rate, and it asymptotically approaches a straight survival curve at low dose rate. The LPL model produces very similar results down to a survival of about 10^{-2}, below which the IR model continues to bend while the LPL model becomes straight.

The value of these models is that when fitted to data at a number of dose rates they allow response over a wider range of dose rates to be calculated and they also enable values for the speed of recovery to be deduced. The full lines through the data in Figure 15.3 were calculated by the LPL model. A useful method of displaying the form of the dose-rate effect is as an isoeffect curve. This is shown in Figure 15.4. For each of five human tumour cell lines, survival data at three or more dose rates have been fitted with the IR model. The model is then used to calculate the dose to give a surviving fraction of 10^{-2} at any dose rate. The full lines in the Figure show the results down to a dose rate of 2 cGy/min (the range within which the data were obtained); they are continued as broken lines in order to show the predictions of the model down to very low dose rates. It can be seen that recovery by itself (the only process built into the model) continues to influence response down to about 0.1 cGy/min. As described above, cell proliferation normally prevents this effect from being observed.

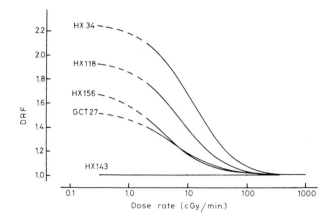

Figure 15.4. DRF (i.e., ratio of doses to give survival of 0.01 at low and high dose rate) as a function of dose rate for five human cell lines. Curves were calculated by the LPL model. HX34 and 118, melanomas; HX156, cervix ca.; GCT27, testicular teratoma; HX143, neuroblastoma. From Steel et al. (1987).

The modelling approach has been used to obtain values for the half-time for recovery from potentially lethal damage. Some of these are given in Table 15.1; they vary from roughly 0.1 to 1.0 hour. Also shown in the table are values of recovery half-time obtained by fitting a rising exponential to split-dose recovery data; for each cell line the split-dose value is longer than the dose-rate value. The reason for this is not known. It has been postulated (Steel et al., 1987) that it may be due to recovery being a multi-component process, the dose-rate experiments tending to emphasize the faster component, but this idea has not been substantiated by detailed modelling.

To return to the question at the start of this Section, how good are these models in simulating the available data? In broad terms they do well, but a number of data sets show significant deviations. A not uncommon problem is that the data at low dose rate describe a bending survival curve when the theoretical line is almost straight (Kelland and Steel, 1986). Some data sets show a dose-rate effect on the initial slope of the survival curve, which the models cannot follow. For dose rates below 5 cGy/min, it has sometimes been found that lowering the dose rate *increases* sensitivity slightly, perhaps as a result of cell-cycle progression.

15.4 Dose-rate effects in normal tissues

The fact that lowering the dose rate also spares normal tissues has been shown in many experimental studies. There is evidence that the amount of sparing varies considerably from one tissue to another, for instance with a large sparing effect in lung (Down et al., 1986) and very little in bone marrow (Glasgow et al., 1983).

The results that are summarised in Figure 15.5 were obtained on mice by two

230   G.G. Steel

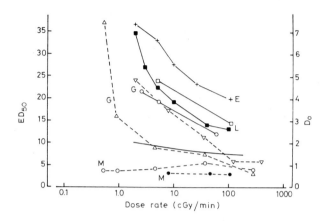

Figure 15.5. Dose-rate effect in normal tissues of the mouse: L = lung, G = intestine, E = epilation, M = marrow, further described in the text. (From Steel et al., 1986.)

types of experiment. By performing a dose-response curve at any chosen dose rate it is possible to find the dose at which 50% of animals reach some selected threshold of normal tissue damage. This is termed the ED_{50} dose and in the figure these values are plotted (full lines) on the same logarithmic dose-rate scale as is used in Figures 15.1 and 15.4. The full line without points summarises a great deal of data on mouse lethality (from Hall and Bedford, 1964). Other studies have made use of cell-cloning techniques. Such data on the small intestine and bone marrow are included in the figure by plotting D_o values (the broken lines). This collection of data shows that in the dose-rate region down to say 2 cGy/min the amount of sparing varies considerably. In the lung and hair follicle it is comparable with that seen in the most recovery-proficient human tumour cells. In the marrow, there is little or no dose-rate effect. The upward sweep in the curve for intestine below 2 cGy/min (Fu et al., 1975) is presumably due to proliferation.

15.5 Fractionated low-dose-rate irradiation

There are a number of clinical situations in which low-dose-rate radiotherapy is used, normally in a single exposure or small number of dose fractions. How does this affect the amount of dose sparing that may be expected?

Figure 15.6 shows calculations of the total radiation dose that can be tolerated by a hypothetical normal tissue for an isoeffect of 0.01 survival. The calculations have been based on parameters for acute pneumonitis in the mouse (data shown in Figure 15.5; Down et al., 1986). In this study the Incomplete Repair model gave parameter values as follows: $\alpha = 0.0774$ Gy^{-1}; $\beta = 0.0207$ Gy^{-2}; half-time = 50.8 min. The

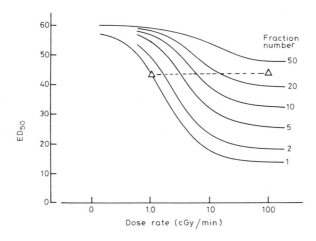

Figure 15.6. Isoeffect curves for fractionated irradiation of a hypothetical tumour cell population at various dose rates. Curves are calculated on the Thames IR model using an α/β ratio of 3.7 Gy. ED_{50} is the dose in Gy to give a survival of 0.01. The triangles joined by a broken line indicate the comparison of 30 fractions at high dose rate with continuous treatment at 1 cGy/min.

α/β ratio was thus 3.7 Gy. The line that fitted the experimental data is shown as the single-fraction curve in Figure 15.6. The other lines in the figure are calculated for various fraction numbers.

The vertical displacement of the six curves at high dose rate reflects the steep dependence of total dose on fraction number. The IR model embodies a linear relationship between the reciprocal of the ED_{50} and the dose per fraction (Thames et al., 1982). All the curves in Figure 15.6 come together at low dose rate, and for large fraction numbers they are flatter than for low fraction numbers. This reflects a basic property of this system that recovery occurs both between fractions and during exposure to each fraction, especially at low dose rate. Thus, sparing can be achieved either by lowering the dose rate or by increasing the fraction number, and if sparing is achieved in one way then there is less to achieve in the other.

We can now compare the effectiveness of a single treatment given at low dose rate with many fractions given at high dose rate by external beam. It happens that for the parameters chosen to draw Figure 15.6 the ED_{50} for around 30 fractions at high dose rate (44 Gy) is almost identical with that for a single treatment at 1 cGy/min (indicated by the broken line). If this applied to an actual therapeutic situation and was the same for tumour and normal tissues there would therefore be no radiobiological advantage in the low-dose-rate treatment. A difference in half-time between the tumour and normal tissue will also influence the existence or otherwise of a therapeutic benefit (DeBoer and Lebesque, 1988).

Since continuous low-dose-rate irradiation is the limiting case of treatment with many small dose fractions, one would expect that the low-dose-rate treatment would

232 G.G. Steel

spare late-reacting normal tissues and give a therapeutic advantage for tumours with high α/β ratios (Thames et al., 1982; Thames and Hendry, 1987). This probably is the case, but the similarity of the responses found above between continuous 1 cGy/min and 30 fractions at high dose rate suggests that this advantage will only be obtained at continuous dose rates well below 1 cGy/min.

15.6 Concept of curative zones in implant radiotherapy

The use of interstitial or intracavitary implants leads to non-uniform radiation fields within which the killing effects of irradiation can vary widely. Curves of tumour control probability against dose for external beam radiotherapy are steep and within the radiation field of an implant a similarly steep dose-dependence arises.

Using the Incomplete Repair model it is possible to calculate cell-survival curves for the dose rate that exists at any distance from an implanted source and on the basis of some assumed number of clonogenic cells per cubic centimetre of tissue to determine the distance from the source at which cure can be achieved. This has been done on the basis of the following assumptions: a point source that gives a dose of

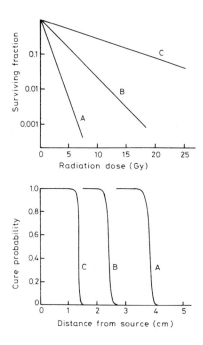

Figure 15.7. The likelihood of cure varies steeply with position around a point radiation source. Survival curves have been calculated for three levels of radiosensitivity at low dose rate (see text). The upper panel shows the survival curves, the lower panel the corresponding tumour-cure curves.

75 Gy in 6 days at a distance of 2 cm; 10^9 clonogenic cells per cm^3. The number of surviving clonogenic cells within spherical shells of thickness 0.1 cm has been calculated, and from a Poisson distribution based on the number of survivors the cure probability has been obtained. Calculations have been done for three hypothetical tumour-cell populations. Using the Incomplete Repair model, we have chosen α to have values that span the range that we have found for human tumour cells (A = 1.0, B = 0.35, C = 0.1 Gy^{-1}). We have assumed a constant α/β ratio of 10 and a constant half-time for recovery of 1 hour.

The resulting survival curves are shown in the top panel of Figure 15.7. These are calculated for the dose rate that exists at the reference radius (about 0.8 cGy/min at 2 cm from the source). The survival curves are almost straight but not quite as flat as if recovery were complete (when the slope would be determined by α alone). The lower panel shows the cure probability within thin shells surrounding the source. These lines are very steep, resulting from the assumption that failure to cure results from the survival of one or more clonogenic cells. Note that in the two panels the three curves come in the opposite order (left to right): sensitive tumour cells (A) can be cured out to a larger radius than insensitive cells (B or C).

These calculations illustrate two conclusions. First, for any particular cell type there will be a critical radius at which tumour control breaks down. Secondly, the radius at which this occurs is strongly dependent upon the low-dose-rate radiosensitivity of the cells. This emphasizes the clinical value of the curves shown in the right-hand panel of Figure 15.2.

15.7 Therapeutic implications of low dose-rate radiobiology

The dose-rate effect impinges on clinical radiotherapy in two respects: in regard to dose adjustments that are required when dose rate is changed, and secondly in relation to the possible existence of a therapeutic benefit from low-dose-rate irradiation.

The experimental data shown in Figure 15.5 indicate that the magnitude of dose adjustment will depend greatly on the normal tissue at risk. There is evidence, supported by the theoretical curves in Figure 15.4, that a significant change in radiosensitivity may result from a relatively small reduction below conventional acute dose rates. Thus, Turesson and Notter (1984) found that when the delivery of each fraction was increased from 4 to 32 minutes, the isoeffect dose for early and late skin damage increased by 10%.

The therapeutic benefit of reducing dose rate depends very much on the relative recovery capacity of the tumour cells and of the limiting normal tissues, both of which can vary widely. There is evidence that the speed of recovery is highly variable and the steepness of the dose-rate effect depends upon this also. The clinical choice is not usually between low-dose-rate treatment and a single high-dose-rate treatment, but between the low dose rate and *fractionated* high dose rate. As indicated in Figure 15.6 (the dashed line), these two treatments may be similarly effective in exploiting cellular recovery. An advantage of continuous low dose-rate irradiation is that it is the most efficient way of delivering radiation dose if recovery is to be maximised and the overall treatment time kept as short as possible.

Acknowledgement

This work was supported in part by NCI grant No. RO1 CA 26059.

References

Curtis, S.B. (1986) Lethal and potentially lethal lesions induced by radiation: a unified repair model. Radiat. Res. 106, 252–270.
DeBoer, R.W. and Lebesque, J.V. (1988) Radiobiological implications of fractionated low dose-rate irradiation. Int. J. Radiat. Oncol. Biol. Phys. 14, 1054–1056.
Down, J.D., Easton, D.F. and Steel, G.G. (1986) Repair in the mouse lung during low dose-rate irradiation. Radiother. Oncol. 6, 29–42.
Fu, K.K., Phillips, T.L., Kane, L.J. and Smith, V. (1975) Tumor and normal tissue response to irradiation in vivo: variation with decreasing dose rates. Radiology 114, 709–716.
Glasgow, G.P., Beetham, K.L. and Mill, W.B. (1983) Dose-rate effects on the survival of normal haemopoietic stem cells of BALB/c mice. Int. J. Radiat. Oncol. 9, 557–563.
Hall, E.J. and Bedford, J.S. (1964) Dose rate: its effect on the survival of HeLa cells irradiated with gamma-rays. Radiat. Res. 22, 305–315.
Kelland, L.R. and Steel, G.G. (1986) Dose-rate effects in the radiation response of four human tumour xenografts. Radiother. Oncol. 7, 259–268.
Mitchell, J.B., Bedford, J.S. and Bailey, S.M. (1979) Dose-rate effects in mammalian cells in culture. Radiat. Res. 79, 537–551.
Steel, G.G., Deacon, J.M., Duchesne, G.M., Horwich, A., Kelland, L.R. and Peacock, J.H. (1987) The dose-rate effect in human tumour cells. Radiother. Oncol. 9, 299–310.
Steel, G.G., Down, J.D., Peacock, J.H. and Stephens, T.C. (1986) Dose-rate effects and the repair of radiation damage. Radiother. Oncol. 5, 321–331.
Steel, G.G., Kelland, L.R. and Peacock, J.H. (1988) The radiobiological basis for low dose-rate radiotherapy, in: Proceedings of the Brachytherapy Working Conference, The Hague, September, 1988.
Stephens, T.C., Eady, J.J., Peacock, J.H. and Steel, G.G. (1987) Split-dose and low dose-rate recovery in four experimental tumour systems. Int. J. Radiat. Biol. 52, 157–170.
Szechter, A. and Schwarz, G. (1977) Dose-rate effects, fractionation and cell survival at lowered temperatures. Radiat. Res. 71, 593–613.
Thames, H.D. (1985) An 'incomplete-repair' model for survival after fractionated and continuous irradiations. Int. J. Radiat. Biol. 47, 319–339.
Thames, H.D. and Hendry, J.H. (1987) Fractionation in Radiotherapy. Taylor and Francis, London.
Thames, H.D., Withers, H.R., Peters, L.J. and Fletcher, G.H. (1982) Changes in early and late radiation responses with altered dose fractionation: implications for dose-survival relationships. Int. J. Radiat. Oncol. Biol. Phys. 8, 219–226.

Turesson, I., Notter, G., Wickstrom, I., Johansson, K.-A. and Eklund, S. (1984) The influence of irradiation time per treatment sessions on acute and late skin reactions: a study on human skin. Radiother. Oncol. 2, 235–245.

Wells, R.L. and Bedford, J.S. (1983) Dose-rate effects in mammalian cells. IV. Repairable and nonrepairable damage in non-cycling C3H 10 T1/2 cells. Radiat. Res. 94, 105–134.

Withers, H.R. (1975) Four Rs of radiotherapy. Adv. Rad. Biol. 5, 241–270.

CHAPTER 16

Clinical aspects of radiation dose rate

ALAN HORWICH

Department of Radiotherapy and Oncology, The Royal Marsden Hospital, Downs Road, Sutton, Surrey SM2 5PT, England

---

16.1 History 237

16.2 Intracavitary radiotherapy 239

16.3 Interstitial radiotherapy 240

16.4 External-beam irradiation 243

16.5 Conclusions 245

16.1 History

At the beginning of this century, radiotherapy was usually administered by single or intermittent exposures to radium and Claudius Regaud (1870–1940) was the first to appreciate the biological effect of protracted treatments. His original observations were on rams' testicles and he noted that protraction of irradiation was able to achieve sterility without the skin damage associated with more acute exposures. While working in the Radium Institute in Paris he applied these ideas to the treatment of human cancer (Regaud, 1922). Clinical studies of dose rate were undertaken by McWhirter (1936) while a recipient of a Cancer Research Campaign (then British Empire Cancer Campaign) grant specifically on this topic. He studied the influence of dose rate from 12 R/hour to 1273 R/hour, using radium moulds on each thigh of 16 volunteers. Treating to between 2000 R and 2300 R given in seven fractions over 7 days, he was not able to detect any difference in acute skin reaction. He did demonstrate the lower dose of 2000 R required for skin tumour control during a 2 hour treatment as opposed to 4400 R required for a 7 day treatment, as reported in detail by Mitchell (1960) (Table 16.1). A dose-rate effect was also noted for the interstitial radiotherapy of oropharyngeal tumours. Both Paterson (1952) and Ellis (1968) produced isoeffect

TABLE 16.1
Dose required for control of small skin tumours treated at a range of dose-rates

Dose rate (cGy/min)	Total dose required (cGy)	Treatment duration (hours)
18.0	1800	1.67
3.7	2250	10
2.0	2880	24
1.13	3300	48.5
0.85	3600	70.3
0.45	4500	169
0.23	4800	336
0.13	4950	600

From Mitchell (1960).

curves in order to supply a proposed dose correction for cases where the dose rate of the implant was found to differ from the standard 0.59 cGy/min (Figure 16.1). This isoeffect plot has been modelled mathematically and used to derive corrections for different dose rates (Kirk et al., 1972; Orton and Ellis, 1973). As described in Chapter 15, isoeffect formulae have also been derived from cell-survival curve equations modified by recovery kinetics (Liversage, 1969; Thames, 1985; Curtis, 1986). The biological effect of dose-rate changes is conceptually complex with rapid repair kinetics and rapid cell proliferation tending to reduce cytotoxicity. In clinical situations where a single low-dose-rate exposure has a reduced overall treatment time compared with fractionated treatment, the effect of rapid repopulation will be less. Redistribution within the cell cycle will tend to increase cytotoxicity by virtue

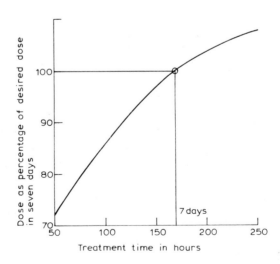

Figure 16.1. Isoeffect total doses for interstitial therapy of oropharyngeal implants. The graph indicates for any chosen treatment time the dose that is equivalent to treatment over 7 days, assumed 100% (Paterson, 1952).

of originally resistant cells progressing to a more sensitive phase. The isoeffect models require consideration of both radiosensitivity and repair kinetics of the tissue under consideration. The magnitude of the calculated dose-rate effect can be illustrated by an example relating to gynaecological brachytherapy for the radical treatment of carcinoma of the cervix, in which two insertions lasting 3.5 days each are compared with 2 insertions lasting 1 day (dose-rate change from approximately 0.75 to 2.7 cGy/min). Using the LPL model (Section 4.2.6) and assuming that α/β is 4 (Section 13.3) for late normal tissue damage, if the half-time of repair of critical normal tissues is 1 hour, the dose correction is from 68 Gy at low dose rate to 42.7 Gy at the higher dose rate. If the half-time is 2 hours, the corresponding isoeffective doses would be 55 and 30.2 Gy.

16.2 Intracavitary radiotherapy

Many factors other than dose rate influence the outcome of intracavitary treatment of gynaecological malignancies, including the dose, fraction time between treatments, and details of additional external beam therapy. Of major importance is the applicator design, in particular as to whether there is rigid fixation. The geometry of the applicator and the distribution of radioactive sources also markedly effect the dose distribution.

The traditional Manchester technique for early carcinoma of the cervix (Paterson, 1963) involved only intracavitary radiotherapy to a total dose at point A of 7500 cGy in two insertions each of approximately 70 hours over a total treatment time of 10 days. During each treatment, the dose rate at point A was approximately 0.9 cGy/min. With the change to a caesium-137 after-loading system, the treatment time for each insertion was reduced to approximately 20 hours, it being considered that better geometry would be maintained during shorter insertions and also that treatments would be more cost effective. A radiobiological experiment was specifically tailored to addressing the question of the appropriate total dose reduction required to compensate for the increased dose rate, the assay being based on mouse tail necrosis (Wilkinson et al., 1980). This experiment suggested that a dose reduction of 33% would be required for increase in dose rate to point A from 0.9 cGy/min to 3.1 cGy/min, i.e., that the dose to point A should be reduced to 5000 cGy. This dose-reduction factor is similar to that predicted on the Thames model (previous Section). For clinical reasons a more modest dose adjustment was evaluated. The increased incidence of bowel damage associated with this change in dose rate would seem to support a dose-rate effect; however, it has been argued that this damage was a consequence of change of technique (Sherrah-Davies, 1985) (Table 16.2). A subsequent trial is investigating dose reductions of 13 and 20% in the treatments at 3.1 cGy/min. A problem may be that if the tumour has a higher α/β ratio than the limiting normal tissue, then as the dose rate is increased the dose reduction required for tumour control becomes less than the dose reduction

TABLE 16.2
Dose rate in intracavitary irradiation (Christie Hospital 1979–1981)

	Isotope	Dose (cGy)	Dose rate to point A (cGy/min)	No. patients	% bowel damage
	Ra	7500	0.9	127	0
Trial	Ra	7500	0.9	33	3
	Cs	7000	3.1	30	10
	Cs	7500	3.1	26	27

From Sherrah-Davies (1985).

required for normal tissue tolerance, and the therapeutic ratio becomes worse.

A contrasting trial at the Institute Gustave Roussy employs preoperative intracavitary radiotherapy for early carcinoma of the cervix, comparing a dose of 6000 cGy in the standard 6 days or the same dose in 3 days, with no change in technique and no total-dose correction. Reports on this trial are expected within the next year or two (D. Chassagne, personal communication).

With the introduction of high dose rate after-loading equipment for the intracavitary treatment of gynaecological malignancies it became necessary to estimate an appropriate fractionation schedule and dose modification. These calculations have been derived from acute cell-survival formulae (Liversage, 1969) and from the isoeffect curve of Ellis (Joslin et al., 1972). Dose rates of 150–300 cGy/min are employed, usually in 4–6 fractions of 600–900 cGy, either weekly or twice per week. Since treatments are usually combined with external beam therapy, the comparison with low dose rate is complex, and a prospective comparative trial has not been performed. It has been suggested that relatively small changes in the high-dose-rate fractionation schedule could have considerable effects on treatment results (Joslin and Sharma, 1984).

16.3 Interstitial radiotherapy

Despite the skill and time required for this technique it has remained popular in clinical radiotherapy because of numerous reports of excellent clinical results. Though this may result from irradiation at low dose rate, it may also be that good anti-tumour effects are obtained because the total dose of radiation is usually administered in approximately one week, thus representing 'accelerated' treatment. The low incidence of normal tissue damage might be related to the small irradiated volume. An example of iridium needle interstitial therapy for a 2 cm squamous carcinoma of the glans penis is illustrated in Figure 16.2. The three-needle single-plane implant to a dose of 65 Gy in 7 days is shown in panel A and the clinical effect 6 months later in panel B. The treated area became hypopigmented with atrophic skin on the ventral surface of the gland. The functional result was good with no impairment of micturition

Dose rate in radiotherapy 241

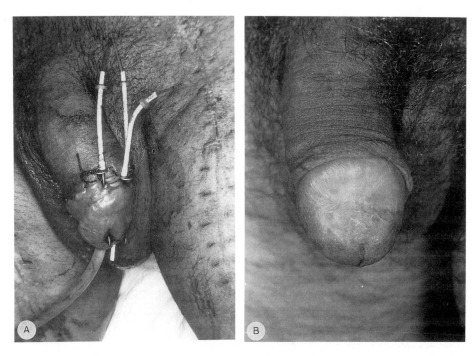

Figure 16.2. (A) Single-plane ^{192}Ir implant for 2 cm diameter carcinoma of glans penis. (B) Clinical result 6 months post-irradiation.

or erection. Figure 16.3A displays a diagrammatic reconstruction of the position of the needles derived from orthogonal radiographs, and the dose rate calculations are based on isodoses shown in panel B. The reference isodose is 85% of the central average dose. Other difficulties which confound analysis of dose rate in this setting are the use of different dosimetry systems including choice of reference isodoses, and also the use of isotopes which may have a different RBE such as iodine-125. Furthermore, the clinical intention has usually been to reproduce a fairly narrow range of dose rate derived from historical practice, usually approximately 0.6 cGy/min at the reference isodose. Retrospective data were reported by Pierquin et al. (1973) and were based on the relatively short half-life of iridium-192 (74.2 days), which meant that partially decayed sources with lower linear activity were often employed. No dose adjustment was made for changes in dose rate which ranged from 0.5 to 1.6 cGy/min. Nevertheless, no clinical dose-rate effects were observed in the analysis which included 110 patients with squamous carcinoma of the skin, 22 patients with carcinoma of the penis, 50 patients with carcinoma of the lower lip and 81 patients with carcinoma of the oropharynx. These data are complemented by reports from Awwad et al. (1974) and Awwad and Burgers (1976) of results of dose correction for increased dose rate in interstitial irradiation of carcinoma of the tongue. Patients with

A

^{192}Iridium implant for carcinoma of penis

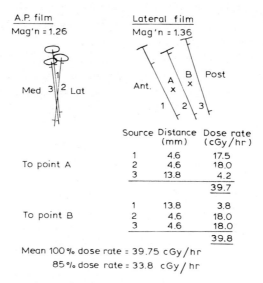

		Source Distance (mm)	Dose rate (cGy/hr)
To point A	1	4.6	17.5
	2	4.6	18.0
	3	13.8	4.2
			39.7
To point B	1	13.8	3.8
	2	4.6	18.0
	3	4.6	18.0
			39.8

Mean 100% dose rate = 39.75 cGy/hr
85% dose rate = 33.8 cGy/hr

^{192}Iridium implant for carcinoma of the penis

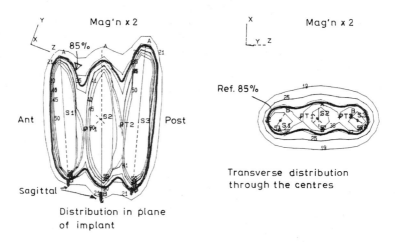

Figure 16.3. (A) Dose-rate calculation for the case shown in Figure 16.2 based on orthogonal radiographs of needle positions. (B) Corresponding isodose distribution.

recurrences had significantly shorter treatment times and consequently lower doses because of the Paterson dose correction.

An exception to the limited range of dose rates employed in interstitial radiotherapy has been iodine-125 where rates as low as 0.1 cGy/min have been prescribed. Early experience suggested that this was insufficient to control early progression of high-grade astrocytomas (Gutin et al., 1981); however, excellent results have been reported in carcinoma of the prostate. Hilaris et al. (1978) reported on 112 patients with T_1 to T_3 carcinoma of the prostate followed to a median of 42 months in whom there were no bowel complications, no treatment-induced impotence and no incidence of urinary incontinence. Others have suggested that the recurrence rate for this technique is high, especially in large or poorly differentiated tumours (Giles and Brady, 1986).

16.4 External-beam irradiation

The clearest radiobiological rationale for low-dose-rate external-beam irradiation is in the use of total-body irradiation prior to bone-marrow transplantation, since the dose-limiting normal tissue is lung and this shows a greater capacity for sublethal damage repair than do bone-marrow stem cells (Peters et al., 1979). In fact the use of low dose rate in this context was not originally based on radiobiological principles but on the requirement for long source-skin distance telecobalt treatment to achieve sufficiently large field sizes to treat the whole body. There is considerable documented support for the sparing of lung by reduced dose rate (Figure 16.3). The risk of interstitial pneumonitis after single-fraction systemic irradiation is lower at a dose rate below 4 cGy/min, and at this dose-rate mortality rises when the dose is increased to 11.5 Gy from 10.5 Gy (Barrett, 1982). Most centres are now using fractionated systemic irradiation at dose rates of 25–50 cGy/min with a total dose split into six fractions of 2 Gy administered over 3 days. A prospective randomised study showed no major differences between a fractionated schedule of 2 Gy per day × 6 and single-fraction low-dose-rate treatment (Thomas et al., 1982). Since the fractionated schedule allows a higher dose, it would be predicted that leukaemia control rates would be improved,

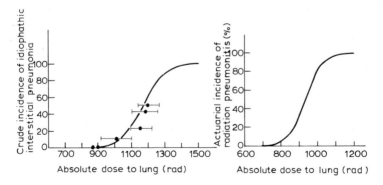

Figure 16.4. Left panel: dose/incidence curve for pneumonitis after low-dose-rate total-body irradiation (Keane et al., 1981). Right panel: dose/incidence curve for pneumonitis after high-dose-rate (40 cGy/min) upper hemi-body irradiation (Van Dyk et al., 1981).

but results from different centres may be distorted because of differences in dosimetry or in the conditioning chemotherapy regimen.

A disadvantage of single low-dose-rate TBI is that early side effects appear during the treatment (Westbrook et al., 1987). In patients treated at approximately 5 cGy/min, nausea is common and vomiting occurs in approximately 50% of patients. Pneumonitis occurs 1–3 months following transplantation and is multifactorial (Neiman et al., 1978; Barrett et al., 1983). Somnolence occurs approximately 2 months after radiotherapy and it resolves after 1 or 2 weeks. Late effects of low-dose-rate, systemic irradiation include cataract, gonadal failure, premature epiphyseal fusion and impairment of pituitary hormone production (Barrett et al., 1987).

The use of low-dose-rate external-beam radiotherapy in other clinical contexts has been more experimental. The influence of skin damage has been studied by Turesson et al. (1984) in patients with breast cancer having direct anterior parasternal fields. Each field was divided into two parts and they were usually irradiated separately at different dose rates to a total dose of 7.9 Gy × 4 over 22 days, 1 fraction per week. One side was treated at a standard dose rate of approximately 200 cGy/min, and the other was treated over 32 minutes in three small fractions. A sparing effect was seen both for acute skin erythema and for late damage, the correction factor being 1.1.

Low-dose-rate external-beam irradiation has also been investigated in the treatment of cancers of the oropharynx. A pilot study was performed in 46 patients (Pierquin et al., 1978) at a dose rate of 1.7 cGy/min. Daily treatment times were 6–9 hours with a 30–45 minute lunch break. A total dose of 65–70 Gy was given at first in a single course of treatment over 9–16 days. However, the severity of acute reactions was such that this was abandoned and further patients were treated in a split course over 5 weeks starting with 7 daily fractions of 6 or 7 Gy over a 10 day period and followed approximately 4 weeks later by a further four similar fractions. Subsequently, a prospective randomised trial was performed in patients with T_{2b} and T_{3a} squamous carcinoma of the oropharynx (Pierquin et al., 1985) comparing low-dose-rate split-course radiotherapy to conventional fractionation (70.7 Gy) administered in 39 1.8-Gy fractions over approximately 7 weeks. The 65 patients in this study have a 2 year

TABLE 16.3
Low-dose-rate external-beam therapy for oropharyngeal cancers[a]

	Low dose rate	Conventional fractionation
Dose	70 Gy	70 Gy
Fractions	12–14	39
Overall time	5 weeks	7 weeks
Patients[b]	32	33
Recurrence rate	16%	61%
Alive NED	44%	24%
Necrosis	5	0

[a] Pierquin et al., 1987.
[b] Minimum follow-up 2 years.

minimum follow-up (Pierquin et al., 1987). The local recurrence rate in 32 patients treated by low-dose-rate irradiation was 16%, whereas with conventional fractionation it was 61% ($P<0.001$), the corresponding survival rate being 44 and 24%, respectively (Table 16.3). Though this appears to confirm the benefits of low-dose-rate irradiation it is noted that the toxicity of this technique was higher, especially when the low dose rate exceeded 2.5 cGy/min.

16.5 Conclusions

It seems clear that some normal tissues are spared by low-dose-rate irradiation. Information on tumour control is much less extensive though low dose rate should improve the therapeutic ratio if the sparing effect in the tumour is poor, if the overall treatment time is short, and if cell-cycle redistribution occurs more extensively. Pierquin's studies on external beam therapy appear to show benefit from low dose rate, however, the 'conventional fractionation' arm has a longer overall treatment time (7 weeks versus 5 weeks) and low dose rate has higher toxicity. Low-dose-rate single-fraction systemic irradiation seeks to exploit differences in sparing between lung and leukaemic cells. This may however, be exploited to a greater extent, using fractionated treatments. Interstitial treatments often produce excellent clinical results but the overall treatment time is short and the irradiated volume is small and it is difficult to dissect these advantages from those that accrue from low dose rate directly.

The current problem in intracavitary irradiation is the appropriate dose reduction to apply when reducing the total insertion time, and valuable data will soon be available from current trials at the Christie Hospital and the Institute Gustave Roussy. It seems likely on the basis of preliminary information from the Christie Hospital that some dose reduction will be required if the dose rate is increased 3-fold and it will be important to establish that this does not compromise tumour control. Clinical benefit of low-dose-rate radiotherapy is apparent in a range of clinical examples, however, it is not clear that equivalent benefits could not be achieved by altered fractionation, possibly associated with more sophisticated external-beam techniques such as conformal therapy.

References

Awwad, H.K. and Burgers, J.M.V. (1976) Studies in dose-time volume relationships in bladder and tongue radium implants. Clin. Radiol. 27, 443–448.

Awwad, H.K., Burgers, J.M.V. and Marcuse, H.R. (1974) The influence of tumour dose specifications on the early clinical results of interstitial tongue implants. Radiology 110, 177–182.

Barrett, A. (1982) Clinical aspects of total body irradiation. J. Eur. Radiother. 3, 159–164.

Barrett, A., Depledge, M.H., Biol, M.I. and Powles, R.L. (1983) Interstitial pneumonitis following bone marrow transplantation after low-dose-rate total-body irradiation. Int. J. Radiat. Oncol. Biol. Phys. 9, 1029–1033.

Barrett, A., Nicholls, J. and Gibson, B. (1987) Late effects of total body irradiation. Radiother. Oncol. 9, 131–135.

Curtis, S.B. (1986) Lethal and potentially lethal lesions induced by radiation – a unified repair model. Radiat. Res. 106, 252–270.

Ellis, F. (1968) The relationship of biological effect to dose-time-fractionation factors in radiotherapy. Curr. Top. Radiat. Res. 4, 357–397.

Giles, G.M. and Brady, L.W. (1986) ^{125}I implantation after lymphadenectomy in early carcinoma of the prostate. Int. J. Radiat. Oncol. Biol. Phys. 12, 2117–2125.

Gutin, P.H., Phillips, T.L., Hosobuchi, Y. et al. (1981) Permanent and removable implants for the brachytherapy of brain tumours. Int. J. Radiat. Oncol. Phys. 7, 1371–1381.

Hilaris, B.S., Whitmore, W.F., Batata, M.A., Barzell, W. and Tokita, N. (1978) Implantation of the prostate: dose-response considerations. Front. Radiat. Ther. Oncol. 12, 82–90.

Joslin, C.A. and Sharma, S.C. (1984) Brachytherapy 1984. Nucleotron Trading BV, The Netherlands.

Joslin, C.A.F., Smith, C.W. and Mallik, A. (1972) The treatment of cervix cancer using high-activity Co sources. Br. J. Radiol. 45, 257–270.

Keane, T.J., Van Dyk, J. and Rider, W.B. (1981) Idiopathic interstitial pneumonia following bone-marrow transplantation: the relationship with total body irradiation. Int. J. Radiat. Biol. Phys. 7, 1365–1370.

Kirk, J., Gray, W.M. and Watson, E.R. (1972) Cumulative radiation effect. II. Continuous radiation therapy-long-lived sources. Clin. Radiol. 23, 93–105.

Liversage, W.E. (1969) A general formula for equating protracted and acute regimes of radiation. Br. J. Radiol. 42, 432–440.

McWhirter, R. (1936) 13th Annual Report of the British Empire Cancer Campaign, pp. 131–144, London.

Mitchell, J.S. (1960) Studies in Radiotherapeutics, Blackwell, Oxford.

Neiman, P., Wasserman, P.B., Wentworth, B.B. et al. (1978) Interstitial pneumonia and cytomegalovirus infection as complications of human marrow transplantation. Transplantation 15, 5.

Orton, C.G. and Ellis, F. (1973) A simplification in the use of the NSD concept in practical radiotherapy. Br. J. Radiol. 46, 529–537.

Paterson, R. (1952) Studies in optimum dosage. Br. J. Radiol. 25, 505–516.

Paterson, R. (1963) The treatment of malignant disease by radiotherapy, 2nd Edn., Williams and Wilkins, Baltimore.

Peters, L.J., Withers, H.R., Cundiff, J.H. and Dicke, K.A. (1979) Radiobiological considerations in the use of total-body irradiation for bone-marrow transplantation. Radiology 131, 243–247.

Pierquin, B., Chassagne, D., Baillet, F. and Paine, C.H. (1973) Clinical observations on the time factors in interstitial radiotherapy using iridium-192. Clin. Radiol. 24, 506–509.

Pierquin, B.M., Mueller, W.K. and Baillet, F. (1978) Low-dose-rate irradiation of advanced head and neck cancers: present status. Int. J. Radiat. Oncol. Biol. Phys. 4, 565–572.

Pierquin, B., Calitchi, E., Mazeron, J.J., Le Bourgeois, J.P. and Leung, S. (1985) A comparison between low-dose-rate radiotherapy and conventionally fractionated irradiation in moderatery extensive cancers of the oropharynx. Int. J. Radiat. Oncol. Biol. Phys. 11, 431–139.

Pierquin, B., Calitchi., Mazeron, J.J., Le Bourgeois, J.P. and Leung, S. (1987) Update on low-dose-rate irradiation for cancers of the oropharynx-May 1986. Int. J. Radiat. Oncol. Biol. Phys. 13, 259–261.

Regaud, C. (1922) Distribution chronologique rationelle d'un traitement de cancer epithelial par les radiations. Comp. Rend. Soc. Biol. 86, 1085–1088.

Sherrah-Davies, E. (1985) Morbidity following low-dose-rate electron therapy for cervical cancer. Clin. Radiol. 36, 131–139.

Thames, H.D. (1985) An 'incomplete-repair' model for survival after fractionated and continuous irradiations. Int. J. Radiat. Biol. 47, 319–339.

Thomas, E.D., Clift, R.A., Hersman, J. et al. (1982) Marrow transplantation for acute non-lymphoblastic leukaemia in first remission using fractionated or single-dose irradiation. Int. J. Radiat. Oncol. Biol. Phys. 8, 817–821.

Turesson, I., Notter, G., Wickstrom, I., Johansson, K.-A. and Eklund, S. (1984) The influence of irradiation time per treatment session on acute and late skin reactions: a study on human skin. Radiother. Oncol. 2, 235–245.

Van Dyk, J., Keane, T.J., Kan, S., Rider, W.D. and Fryer, C.J. (1981) Radiation pneumonitis following large single-dose irradiation: a re-evaluation based on absolute dose to lung. Int. J. Radiat. Oncol. Biol. Phys. 7, 461–467.

Westbrook, C., Glaholm, J. and Barrett, A. (1987) Vomiting associated with whole-body irradiation. Clin. Radiol. 33, 263–266.

Wilkinson, J.M., Hendry, J.H. and Hunter, R.D. (1980) Dose-rate considerations in the introduction of low-dose rate afterloading intracavitary techniques for radiotherapy. Br. J. Radiol. 53, 890–893.

CHAPTER 17

Heavy particles in radiotherapy

JACK F. FOWLER

Department of Human Oncology K4/336, University of Wisconsin Clinical Cancer Center, 600 Highland Avenue, Madison, WI 53792, USA

17.1	Introduction	249
	17.1.1 The types of heavy particle	249
	17.1.2 Rate of energy loss along particle tracks: depth-dose distributions	251
	17.1.3 Slow neutron capture therapy	253
17.2	Radiobiological differences between high LET and low LET radiations	255
	17.2.1 The radiobiological differences	255
	17.2.2 Dependence of RBE on dose per fraction	257
	17.2.3 Rationales for high LET radiotherapy	260
	17.2.4 Clinical results of high LET radiotherapy	260
	17.2.5 Neutron facilities	261
17.3	Physical advantages of heavy-particle beams	262
	17.3.1 Proton and helium ion beams	262
	17.3.2 Heavy-ion/light-ion beams	263
17.4	Conclusions	264

17.1 Introduction

17.1.1 The types of heavy particle

Heavy particles in the context of radiotherapy mean charged or uncharged particles heavier than electrons. Table 17.1 lists the particles we shall discuss. They all require relatively expensive machines such as cyclotrons, synchrotrons or large linear accelerators to produce them, so the cost of treatments is several times that of conventional photon treatments. Nevertheless, advances in accelerator engineering, especially the use of superconducting magnets, is bringing down the size and cost of cyclotrons for neutron production and of ring synchrotrons for proton beams.

TABLE 17.1
Summary of properties of the particles of interest for radiation treatment of cancer

Particle	Mass (amu)	Charge	Physical depth-dose properties	Radiobiological properties
Particle:				
Electrons	1/1850	−1	Finite range; useful for limited depth lesions	Similar to those of photons, i.e. RBE about 1 and OER about 3
Protons	1	+1	Bragg peak; excellent depth-dose distributions; sharp edges.	Similar to those of photons, i.e., RBE about 1 and OER about 3.
Neutrons	1	0	Attenuated like photons; dose falls steadily with depth	High RBE and reasonably low OER; similar to neon ions.
Neutrons (slow) captured by boron	1	0	Poor if thermal neutrons. Reasonable if epithermal neutrons, but they diffuse outside field	Boron capture leads to alpha particle release: high RBE. Depends on boron uptake in tissues.
Negative pi mesons	1/4	−1	Bragg peak at depth in tissue plus pion 'stars' releasing heavy ions which contribute 10–15% of dose in a spread peak	Intermediate, resembling carbon particles: lower RBE and higher OER than fast neutrons or neon ions.
Accelerated nuclei of:				
helium	4	+2	All these ions have a Bragg peak; hence excellent depth-dose distributions, slightly less good with increasing charge (Si and Ar probably too expensive)	Slightly higher RBE and lower OER than photons
carbon	12	+6		Intermediate RBE and OER
neon	20	+10		High RBE and low OER; similar to fast neutrons
silicon	26	+14		Higher RBE and lower OER
argon	40	+18		RBE lower due to overkill

There are two main differences between heavy-particle beams and conventional beams of X or γ-rays or electrons; the biological and the physical difference. At one end of the spectrum are fast neutrons. These have relatively high values of LET (linear energy transfer, a measure of ionising density along the tracks of particles released in tissue), and of RBE (relative biological effectiveness, per unit dose, compared with low LET radiation such as X-rays). However, because neutrons are uncharged they are attenuated in tissue exponentially (as are photons) and in practice have no better penetration than cobalt-60 or 4–6 MeV photon beams from standard radiotherapy linear accelerators, and somewhat worse penumbra.

At the other end of the spectrum of differences from low LET radiation are protons. They provide superbly sharp depth-dose distributions but no radiobiological differences from low LET radiation. They have limited, controllable, range and sharp

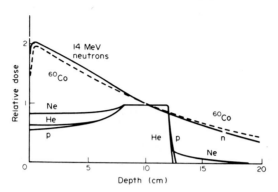

Figure 17.1. Depth-dose distributions of various types of beam in tissue (Tobias et al., 1971).

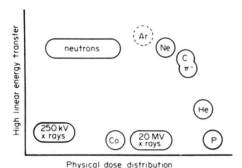

Figure 17.2. Biological advantages of high LET radiation (plotted upward) versus physical depth-dose advantages of the various types of beam (Raju, 1980).

lateral edges to the beam, in which dose falls from 90 to 20% within a few millimetres. Between these extremes come the heavier ions, He, C and Ne, with progressively higher LET and RBE but gradually worsening physical dose distributions (Figure 17.1). Negative pi mesons are like carbon ions both in RBE properties and in physical dose distributions (Figure 17.2).

17.1.2 Rate of energy loss along particle tracks: depth-dose distributions

As a fast charged particle slows in its passage through matter it loses energy more and more rapidly. The rate of energy loss is inversely proportional to the velocity, and proportional to the square of the charge on the ion. The result is a sharp increase in ionisation density (LET) in the so-called Bragg peak, close to the end of each track (Figure 17.3a). The Bragg peak is useful because it deposits more energy per unit volume (i.e., dose) at the end of the particle track than at the beginning. Since the Bragg peak is very sharp, it has to be spread out to cover a useful depth, often 5 cm or more. This is achieved by varying the energy (and thus the range) of the

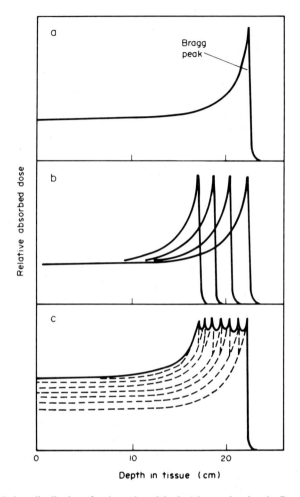

Figure 17.3. Depth-dose distribution of a charged particle (ion) beam, showing the Bragg peak. (a) Single energy; (b) four energies, showing altered ranges; (c) multiple energies, arranged to cover a target or tumour volume at depth (Fowler, 1981).

ion beam either in steps or continuously (Figure 17.3b and c). This is the meaning of 'spread peak' when ion beams are provided for radiotherapy. The LET and RBE may, therefore, be high at the distal edge of the target volume, but are diluted with the lower LET incoming particles at the centre and proximal edge of the spread-out peak region. The dose in the peak region is in general higher than the dose in the incoming track, i.e., in the overlying tissues. This provides the physical advantage of these charged ion beams.

Negative pi mesons have a 'reinforced' Bragg peak. When the pions reach the end of their track, they are attracted into the oppositely charged nuclei of the absorbing

TABLE 17.2
Dose-average LET values (keV/μm) for heavy particles in 10 cm spread peak

Particle	Plateau	Peak region (10 cm deep)		
		proximal	central	distal
Neutrons	75	75	75	75
π^-	6	15	30	60
Helium	5	8	16	30
Carbon	12	30	40	130
Neon	30	70	100	300

From Raju, 1979.

medium. The resulting nuclei have excess mass and energy and quickly disintegrate into 'nuclear stars'. The particles emitted include alpha particles or beryllium nuclei which have ranges of a few cell diameters, i.e., high LET, and they are biologically very effective. Pi mesons, therefore, appear at first sight to be the ideal particles for radiotherapy, but the proportion of dose deposited at high LET is only about 12% of the total dose, depending upon the volume over which the peak is spread. The net effectiveness is no better than that of the carbon ion beam. This is illustrated in Table 17.2. The biologically most effective beams are those of fast neutrons and neon ions.

Fast neutrons interact to release several types of charged particle locally in tissue. Most of the dose comes from the fast protons released which have a range of energies, the fastest giving rise to moderately high LET and the slowest to high LET particles. Their ranges vary from microns to a few millimetres. In addition, there are some disintegration products of the carbon, nitrogen and oxygen nuclei present in tissue, with higher LET and short ranges. Figure 17.4 illustrates the tracks of these and other particles. There is also a few percent of gamma-radiation produced (low LET) which can rise to about 20% of the total dose at 10–15 cm depth in a large field.

17.1.3 Slow neutron capture therapy

Slow neutrons are entirely different because they are produced not as a beam but more like a gas that oozes out of the portal in the side of a nuclear reactor. They are not very biologically effective themselves, but the therapeutic application consists in giving the patient a drug containing boron which should concentrate more in the tumour than in normal tissues; the concentration difference is crucial (Ryabukhin, 1987). Slow neutrons are absorbed into the boron nucleus which then disintegrates into an alpha particle and a lithium nucleus with ranges of a few cell diameters and high LET. The penetration of thermal neutrons, i.e., slowed down to room temperature, is poor in tissue. Half of them are attenuated by 2 cm of unit density tissue; but in Japan they are used to treat nodules of malignant melanoma in the skin (Mishima et al., 1988). Hatanaka (1986) in Japan has reported recent clinical experiences of boron capture therapy for gliomas. Neutrons of slightly higher energy (temperature),

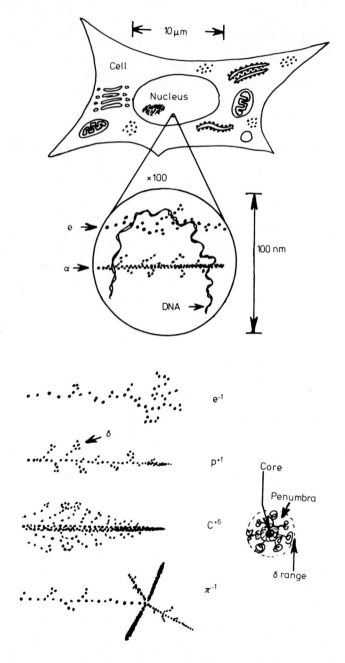

Figure 17.4. Dimensions of mammalian cell and radiation-sensitive sites (∼5 nm) in relation to tracks of some of the particles discussed here (Fowler, 1981).

called epithermal neutrons, have considerably better spreading properties into tissue. They are obtained by filtering out the lower energy neutrons from reactors; sufficient intensity is therefore a problem. In principle, thermal neutrons can be generated in tissue itself by thermalization of an 'intermediate' energy neutron beam of some 50 keV. The maximum dose, however, is still no deeper than about 3 cm (Ryabukhin, 1987).

Although some thermal neutrons are produced at depth in tissue by thermalisation of neutrons produced by photons above 20 MeV from modern radiotherapy accelerators, the proportion of the total dose likely to be contributed by boron capture is low. Interest in slow neutron capture therapy would grow if improved pharmaceuticals were shown to concentrate boron in tumour tissues more specifically.

17.2 Radiobiological differences between high LET and low LET radiations

17.2.1 The radiobiological differences

Figure 17.5 illustrates that as the LET is increased beyond about 30 keV/μm, the RBE increases to a peak at 100–110 keV/μm and then falls. At the same time the oxygen-enhancement ratio (OER) decreases steadily. The reason for both the increase in RBE and the fall in OER is that the higher LET radiation has a greater chance (per unit dose) of depositing a certain minimum energy (about 300 electrons volts, i.e., 10 to 15 ionisations) into each biological 'target volume' of 5 to 10 nm diameter. These biological targets may be pictured as double strands of DNA and histones, 2 or

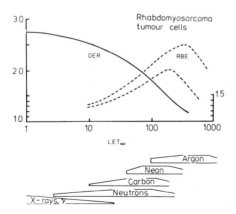

Figure 17.5. Typical changes of RBE and OER with LET. Full line: oxygen enhancement ratio, decreasing but never reaching 1.0. Dotted lines: RBE, peaking about 100–110 keV/μm. Upper curve, hypoxic cells. Lower curve, well-oxygenated cells. At the bottom the approximate distributions of dose in LET are indicated. (Redrawn with permission from Curtis et al., 1982).

256   J.F. Fowler

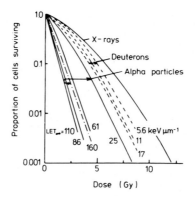

Figure 17.6. Cell-survival curves for human kidney cells in culture exposed to radiation with different LET values as indicated (Barendsen et al., 1963). The dotted lines are for deuterons of three different energies. The dash-dotted line is for alpha particles of the highest LET (lowest energy) used and this is less effective than the alpha particles of LET 110 keV/μm.

3 nm in diameter, with a surrounding water sheath a few nm thick. When the critical amount of energy is deposited within this volume by one track passing through it, one or more double-strand breaks will occur so that the DNA cannot be repaired easily. This type of damage is believed to be what causes the initial slope on survival curves, and it is less dependent upon the presence or absence of oxygen (or on dose rate) than the curved part of the survival curves (see Section 12.5). It is a small proportion of the full effect at low LET, but becomes a much greater proportion as LET is increased, leading to steeper initial slopes, with similar absolute but *relatively* less falling away from the initial slope at higher doses. This effect is illustrated in Figure 17.6. These experiments were done by placing cells plated onto a thin sheet of mylar at chosen distances along the particle tracks such as those in Figure 17.3. These are called track segment experiments (Barendsen et al., 1963). The shoulder disappears and the slope steepens as the LET of the radiation increases, from about 1 keV/μm for X-rays, through 5, 6, 11 and 17 keV/μm for deuteron beams and 25 to 110 keV/μm for progressively slower alpha particles (i.e., at a point along the tracks nearer the Bragg peak). This effect is due to a steepening of the initial slope (the alpha component of the linear quadratic model, see Sections 4.2.3, 12.5) with no significant change in the curvature or beta component. In terms of the Lethal–Potentially-Lethal (LPL) Model (Chapter 4.2.5), a higher proportion of the lethal (unrepairable) lesions (A to C in Fig. 4.5), is caused by high LET radiation, so that the initial slope becomes steeper. This biophysical/biochemical model enables the processes to be pictured reasonably well although the full details are not yet known.

In Figure 17.6 it can be seen that the dose-response curve for the still higher LET of 160 keV/μm is less steep than that of 110 keV/μm. This loss of efficiency is due to 'overkill' in the higher LET track. If more than the requisite 10–15 ionisations

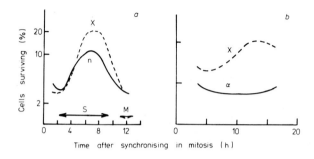

Figure 17.7. (*a*) Chinese hamster V-79 cells irradiated with 7.1 Gy of X-rays or 2.25 Gy of fission neutrons (~1 MeV; Sinclair, 1970). (*b*) Chinese hamster ovary cells irradiated with 9 Gy of X-rays or 2.5 Gy of 4.4 MeV alpha particles (Raju et al., 1975).

are deposited in the target volume, the extra ones are wasted, so that the efficiency per unit dose of the radiation decreases. This factor explains the drop of RBE with increasing LET past the peak of RBE as seen in Figure 17.5.

If we are looking for the range of LET within which the RBE will be highest, and the oxygen enhancement ratio significantly decreased, before the loss of efficiency that occurs well past the peak of RBE, we should consider the range from about 30 to about 300 keV/μm. The effectiveness of various particle beams for high LET radiotherapy can be roughly compared by studying the proportion of dose which each type of beam deposits between 30 and 300 keV/μm (see Fowler, 1981, for these comparisons; also Figure 17.10).

A further difference between low and high LET radiation is that the differences in radiosensitivity that occur between phases of the cell cycle are less marked with high than with low LET radiations, as illustrated in Figure 17.7.

17.2.2 Dependence of RBE on dose per fraction

Figure 17.6 can illustrate how the RBE increases as the dose per fraction decreases. Large doses per fraction would be at the bottom of the diagram and the ratio of X-ray dose to high-LET (110 keV/μm) dose to produce the same cell survival, which is the RBE, is about three: 12 Gy of X-rays divided by 4 Gy of high LET alpha particles. For small doses per fraction, however, near the top of the diagram, the ratio of X-ray to alpha particle (110 keV/μm) doses is about 7. This change is *entirely due to the curvature on the X-ray curve*, and not to any change in efficiency per gray of the high LET at different sizes of dose. This fact makes RBE a potentially misleading index of biological efficiency: a high RBE only indicates the low efficiency of low LET radiation. The effectiveness of low LET radiation varies much more than that of high LET radiation with dose-per-fraction, with the presence of oxygen, sensitizers or protectors, with phase of the cell cycle, and with dose rate.

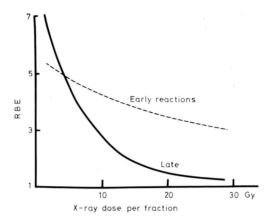

Figure 17.8. The RBE of fast neutrons increases with decreasing dose per fraction. The increase is particularly steep for late reactions at low doses per fraction.

However, until more clinical experience is accumulated with high LET beams, comparisons with the familiar low LET photon and electron beams will continue to be made so that RBE values must be understood. It is emphasised that the changes in RBE seen when biological or physiological conditions are changed are, for a given high LET beam, due to the changes in repair capability of the biological system when irradiated with the low LET, rather than with high LET.

The important point in the present context is that the RBE increases with decreasing dose per fraction in a way which is determined by the shape of the X-ray survival curve. Since the shapes are more curvy for late than for early-reacting tissues (see Chapter 13), the RBE will increase more steeply for late than for early-reacting tissues as dose per fraction is decreased. Figure 17.8 illustrates this point. It has been found clinically that late effects have a higher RBE than acute effects, with an increasing discrepancy as the dose per fraction is decreased. This also was reported clinically. Dr. Catterall at Hammersmith and Dr. Cohen at Fermilab, using neutron doses of about 150 and 180 cGy per fraction, reported fewer unexpected late complications than centres using smaller neutron doses per fraction of about half that size. Figure 17.9 illustrates the same point in terms of schematic survival curves, where it can be seen that the main change of RBE is due to the change of total dose (to produce a given effect) of the low LET radiation, shown shaded; not the high LET radiation. If dose per fraction is changed, larger changes of total dose are necessary for constant late than for constant early reactions, with the low LET radiation. This is the same difference that enables small doses per fraction to be exploited using low LET radiation in hyperfractionated schedules (Horiot et al., 1988; Parsons et al., 1988; see Chapter 13). With high LET radiation such differences are absent or much reduced.

When any fractionated schedule of high LET radiation is used, it will unavoidably cause a similar (rather high) ratio of late to early damage in normal tissues to that

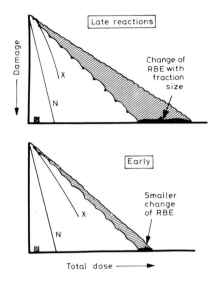

Figure 17.9. The changes of RBE with fraction size illustrated in the previous figure are due mainly to the shoulder on the X-ray dose-response curves. This is illustrated here by a doubling of the dose per fraction (small rectangle in lower left corner) which results in a large change in total X-ray dose to produce the same effect (shown shaded) for late reactions (top); so the RBE has changed substantially. The bottom part shows that the change in total dose, and hence in RBE, is much less for early (or tumour) effects. In this figure the neutron response is assumed to be simply exponential (this is not quite true; as neutron energy increases, a component of low LET causes a slight curvature at the lower end of the neutron dose-response curve).

which would be expected from large doses-per-fraction of X-rays, whether the high LET schedule itself uses low or high doses per fraction. This point has not been well understood but is vital. It means that there is no point in dividing neutron treatments into many small fractions; hyperfractionation will not spare the late damage as it does for low LET treatments.

Of course, there is a proportion of low LET in fast neutron beams, slightly more at higher neutron energies. There are also intermediate situations where high LET treatments are given on 2 days a week and low LET on 3 days. Some types of high LET beam have a significant admixture of low LET all the time, such as pions or carbon ions, and these are diluted examples of the principles just described.

A few laboratory experiments have investigated the possible synergism between low and high LET doses if they are delivered in a certain sequence. None of them reported a large effect and most have reported no significant differences from simple additivity.

17.2.3 Rationales for high LET radiotherapy

These biological differences lead to three rationales for using high LET beams in radiotherapy, whether neutrons or heavy ion beams.
1. Hypoxic cells in tumours are less resistant to high LET than to low LET radiation.
2. Slowly proliferating cells (in G_0 or in long G_1 phase) are less resistant to high LET than to low LET radiation.
3. There is no advantage in multiple small fractions of high LET radiation, so that fewer fractions of high LET than of conventional low LET can be used, with consequent shortening of overall time.

Real differences in radiosensitivity, and hence in RBE, between different types of tumour and normal tissues do occur, but not in any predictable way. They depend on the intrinsic cellular radiosensitivity to small doses of 2 Gy. Ideally, measurements from individual tumour biopsies should be made, so as to select patients for high LET treatment or not (Brock et al., 1986; Peters et al., 1988). It would be desirable to treat tumours with high LET radiation if they had:
a. high intracellular repair (this might be tested by an assay at 2 Gy);
b. poor cell-cycle redistribution;
c. poor reoxygenation during treatment; and
d. A high RBE in an individual 'survival' test,
all of which would lead to more tumour cell kill. Conditions (b) and (c) would be most likely to occur in *slowly proliferating tumours*. Reoxygenation (c) may occur in a majority of tumours but not all; probably more completely in tumours that shrink fast during treatment, although reoxygenation can occur without shrinkage. This theoretical suggestion was supported by the clinical findings of Batterman et al. (1981) that slowly growing lung metastases had higher values of RBE than faster growing metastases. The hypothesis was subsequently tested clinically by using fast neutrons to treat prostate tumours, which grow very slowly and have unusually low values of labelling index. The favourable clinical results obtained by treating locally extensive prostate cancer with fast neutrons support the hypothesis (Wambersie et al., 1986; Errington and Warenius, 1987; Laramore et al., 1985).

The shortening of overall time mentioned as advantage (3) above would of course be most valuable in rapidly proliferating tumours such as those of the head and neck (Fowler, 1988). Instead of 12 treatments in 4 weeks as used by Catterall et al. (1987), 10 treatments are being given in 2 weeks by Skolyszewski et al. (1988) in Poland. Even the 4 weeks used by Catterall and in some other neutron protocols is a useful shortening from the usual 6–7 weeks overall time (Fowler, 1986).

17.2.4 Clinical results of high LET radiotherapy

Clinical conclusions about high LET radiotherapy have been drawn from 15 years'

experience of neutron therapy in over a dozen centres world-wide (Catterall, 1987; Catterall et al., 1987; Duncan, 1987; Duncan et al., 1987; Glaholm and Harmer, 1988; Laramore et al., 1985); from the pion experience at Los Alamos, U.S.A. and SIN at Villigen, Switzerland (on pancreas and bladder), and at TRIUMF, Vancouver, as well as from the heavy-ion beams at Berkeley, U.S.A. (Castro, et al., 1987). The conclusions can be summarised as follows (Fowler, 1985; Wambersie et al., 1986):
1. High LET is the treatment of choice:
   Salivary gland tumours (locally extensive).
2. Advantages shown in the majority of clinical trials:
   Prostate (locally extensive), soft tissue sarcomas.
3. Advantages in some trials but not in others:
   Head and neck, rectum, lung, osteosarcomas, cervix.
4. Disadvantages in most trials:
   Brain, pancreas, bladder.

As mentioned above, clearer clinical trials could be carried out if a method of measuring the RBE at X-ray doses of 2–4 Gy could be introduced to select those patients which showed a high RBE (Brock et al., 1986). Methods of measuring individual human tumours which contain hypoxic cells are still under development (Chapman et al., 1987; Gatenby et al., 1988).

17.2.5 Neutron facilities

Most of the neutron results from which conclusions have so far been drawn were obtained with inadequate neutron beams (Catterall, 1987). Many were of relatively low energy so that their penetration was more like 250–300 kV X-rays than modern high-energy cobalt-60 or linear-accelerator photons; this was a very serious drawback. Many were fixed horizontal or vertical beams. Some were considerable distances from the hospitals. Some of these facilities have now closed and at present (1989) neutron therapy is becoming concentrated in a few centres where new hospital-based high-energy cyclotrons can provide adjustable, isocentric beams with penetration equal to modern linear accelerators. These include Seattle, U.S.A.; Clatterbridge, England; Houston, U.S.A.; Los Angeles, U.S.A.; several centres in Japan and continuing work at Louvain, Belgium and Fermilab, U.S.A. with their stationary but high-energy beams.

It has been suggested that between 10 and 20% of all radiotherapy patients may be found to need high LET radiotherapy (Wambersie et al., 1986). If this percentage is confirmed, it implies that neutron or high LET therapy may deserve a place among other minority radiotherapy techniques such as electron beam therapy, brachytherapy or interstitial therapy. It could mean that one neutron machine is needed for every 5 or 10 high-energy photon machines. The possible reduction in fractionation mentioned above would alter this ratio to one in 10 or 20. Since high LET beams are more expensive than those other techniques, some collaboration between centres would be necessary at the national level.

17.3 Physical advantages of heavy particle beams

17.3.1 Proton and helium ion beams

The improved dose distributions obtained with charged-particle beams, especially protons and helium ions, were mentioned in Section 17.1.2. A great deal of clinical experience has been accumulated using proton beams, especially in the U.S.S.R. and in Boston, U.S.A. and in Japan. Similar results have been obtained with the helium-ion beams at Berkeley, U.S.A. The advantages are purely physical, because of the ability to treat highly localised volumes with millimetre accuracy. There are no radiobiological differences from conventional photon therapy. These clinical results were recently reviewed by Munzenrider et al. (1987) and Tsunemoto et al. (1987). Patients with uveal melanoma have been treated particularly successfully with protons, with retention of vision in 70% of patients with tumours less than 3 mm in diameter and 40% if larger than 3 mm. Enucleation was necessary in only 5.5% of 1006 eyes treated up to the end of 1986. This is claimed to be 'one of the major oncologic and ophthalmologic triumphs of the latter part of the twentieth century' (Munzenrider et al., 1987). Protons with a minimum energy of 60 MeV or preferably 70 MeV are required for this application. Protons of energy 200–250 MeV are required to treat deep-seated cancer.

Patients with chordoma, and chondrosarcoma of the base of the skull are treated with protons (between 25 and 35 of them per year in Boston), and others with the helium ion beam at Berkeley. Others sites are also treated. The clinical successes obtained here and in other centres using protons have already encouraged the development of new proton facilities. Protons are currently used clinically in Switzerland, Japan and Russia. Proton therapy may be re-started at Uppsala, Sweden and started for ocular tumours on the 60 MeV cyclotron at Clatterbridge, England and in Orsay, France. New proton facilities of 200–250 MeV are planned in California, South Africa and Japan.

The proton and helium-ion beams have also been used in the USA to treat arteriovenous malformations with success (Fabrikant et al., 1985). The ability to treat very small target volumes to high doses with excellent sparing of surrounding normal tissues cannot readily be matched with photon beams, even with multiple or moving entry points, although there are currently efforts to try to do this.

17.3.2 Heavy ion/light ion beams

At Berkeley, California, a range of ions from helium to argon is available, including silicon ions. Much radiobiological and clinical work has been done with them (Castro et al., 1987). It appears that neon ions are probably the heaviest that need be considered in radiotherapy. The most useful range of LET is from about 30 to 300 keV/μm. Above this range, overkill reduces the effectiveness of the particles, so that argon ions are less efficient than neon ions; in addition, they are harder to produce at sufficient intensity (Figure 17.10).

Although these particle beams have previously been called 'heavy ions', accelerator engineers can now accelerate ions up to uranium and the ions used in radiotherapy up to neon or argon are now called 'light ions'.

Most of the clinical experience at Berkeley has been with helium and neon ions. The helium beams have given equally good results to the proton results mentioned above for uveal melanomas and tumours in the spine or base of skull. In precision therapy it has been found possible to increase the local dose to the tumour 20–30% above

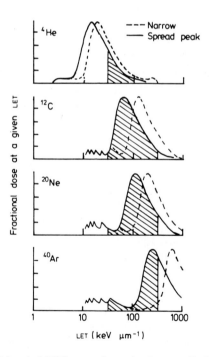

Figure 17.10. Distribution of dose in LET for some heavy-ion beams at Berkeley. Full curves, centre of spread peak. Broken curves, distal edge of spread peak. The most effective particles with respect to high RBE and low dependence on oxygen and phase of the cell cycle, are those delivering the highest proportion of dose in the shaded region from 30 to 300 keV/μm (Raju, 1980; Fowler, 1981). These distributions are only approximate..

that possible with low LET irradiation (Castro et al., 1987). Important development work on the precision of localisation is carried out by the particle beam physicists, and these developments carry over into conventional photon therapy.

The neon or carbon ions, and the pion beams, provide both excellent physical dose distributions and high LET radiobiological advantages (Figure 17.2). New facilities to provide these 'heavy/light' ions for medical use are planned at the NIRS at Chiba, Japan, at Nice in France in collaboration with Louvain, Belgium (EULIMA – European Light Ion Medical Accelerator) and at Berkeley for installation in the Merritt Peralta Hospital in Oakland (LIBRA – Light Ion Biological Research Accelerator). In planning their programs they will be able to draw on the experience of the neutron and pion treatments for high LET insights, and of the proton and helium-ion beam work for physical and localisation developments.

17.4 Conclusions

It would be a particularly important step to be able to have individual tests of RBE (radiosensitivity) and/or of hypoxia in human tumours, so that a selection could be made of those patients most likely to benefit from high LET radiotherapy. This would transform the present somewhat uncertain position about the value of high LET radiation. Such tests are being developed, as mentioned in Section 17.2.3 and Chapter 21. In the meantime, the excellent physical dose distributions from protons and 'light' ions will continue to be used, depending upon the cost of the equipment.

References

Barendsen, G.W., Walter, H.M.D., Fowler, J.F. and Bewley, D.K. (1963) Effects of different ionising radiations on human cells in tissue culture. III. Experiments with cyclotron-accelerated alpha-particles and deuterons. Radiat. Res. 18, 106–119.

Batterman, J.J., Breur, K., Hart, G.A.M. and Van Peperzeel, H.A. (1981) Observations on pulmonary metastases in patients after single doses and multiple fractions of fast neutrons and cobalt-60 gamma rays. Eur. J. Cancer 17, 539–548.

Brock, W.A., Maor, M.H. and Peters, L.J. (1986) Predictors of tumour response to radiotherapy. Radiat. Res. 104 (Suppl.), S290–296.

Catterall, M. (1987) 'Controlled' clinical trials in neutron therapy (editorial). Int. J. Radiat. Oncol. Biol. Phys. 13, 1961–1965.

Catterall, M., Errington, R.D. and Bewley, D.K. (1987) A comparison of clinical and laboratory data on neutron therapy for locally advanced tumours. Int. J. Radiat. Oncol. Biol. Phys. 13, 1783–1791.

Castro, J.R., Phillips, T.L., Petti, P., Collier, J.M., Henderson, S.D., Pitluck, S. and Reimers, M. (1987) Clinical results of charged particle radiotherapy, in: Radiation Research. Proceedings 8th ICRR at Edinburgh, July 1987. (Fielden, E.M., Fowler, J.F., Hendry, J.H. and Scott, D., eds.), pp. 910–915. Taylor and Francis, London.

Chapman, J.D., Matthews, J.H.L. and Urtasun, R.C. (1987) Predictive assays for identifying tumours which might benefit from radiotherapy with sensitizers and/or protectors *in*: Radiation Research: Proceedings 8th ICRR at Edinburgh, July 1987. (Fielden, E.M., Fowler, J.F., Hendry, J.H. and Scott, D., eds.), pp. 756–761, Taylor and Francis, London.

Curtis, S.B., Schilling, W.A., Tenforde, T.S., Crabtree, K.E., Tenforde, S.D., Howard, J. and Lyman, J.T. (1982) Survival of oxygenated and hypoxic tumour cells in the extended-peak regions of heavy charged-particle beams. Radiat. Res. 90, 292–309.

Duncan, W. (1987) Response to a critique of a randomised trial of bladder cancer treated with neutrons. Int. J. Radiat. Oncol. Biol. Phys. 13, 1604–1605.

Duncan, W., Orr, J.A., Arnott, S.J., Jack, W.J.L. and Kerr, G.R. (1987) An evaluation of fast neutron irradiation in the treatment of squamous cell carcinoma in cervical lymph nodes. Int. J. Radiat. Oncol. Biol. Phys. 13, 1793–1796.

Errington, R.D. and Warenius, H.M. (1987) An update of fast neutron therapy results *in*: Radiation Research: Proceedings 8th ICRR at Edinburgh, July 1987. (Fielden, E.M., Fowler, J.F., Hendry, J.H. and Scott, D., eds.), pp. 904–909, Taylor and Francis, London.

Fabrikant, J.I., Lyman, J.T. and Frankel, K.A. (1985) Heavy charged-particle Bragg peak radiosurgery for intracranial vascular disorders. Radiat Res. (Suppl.) S244–258.

Fowler, J.F. (1981) Nuclear particles in cancer treatment. Adam Hilger, Bristol, 178 pp.

Fowler, J.F. (1985) Workshop summary of EORTC high LET therapy group. Strahlentherapie 161, 804–806.

Fowler, J.F. (1986) Potential for increasing the differential response between tumours and normal tissues: can proliferation rate be used? Int. J. Rad. Oncol. Biol. Phys. 12, 641–645.

Fowler, J.F. (1988) What to do with neutrons in radiotherapy: a suggestion. Radiother. Oncol. 3, 233–235.

Gatenby, R.A., Kessler, M.B., Rosenblum, J.S., Cola, L.R., Moldofsky, P.J., Hartz, W.H. and Broder, G.J. (1988) Oxygen distribution in squamous cell carcinoma metastases and its relationship to outcome of radiation therapy. Int. J. Radiat. Biol. Phys. 14, 831–838.

Glaholm, J. and Harmer, C. (1988) Soft-tissue sarcoma: neutrons versus photons for post-operative irradiation. Br. J. Radiol. 61, 829–834.

Hatanaka, H. (1986) Clinical experience of boron neutron capture therapy for gliomas. A comparison with conventional chemo-immuno-radiotherapy, *in*: Boron Neutron Capture Therapy for Tumours, (Hatanaka, H., ed.), pp. 349–369, Nishimura Co., Tokyo.

Horiot, J.C., LeFur, R., Nguyen, T., Schraub, S., Chenal, C., DePauw, M. and Van Glabbeke, M. (1988) Two fractions per day versus a single fraction per day in the radiotherapy of oropharynx trial. Int. J. Radiat. Oncol. Biol. Phys. 15 (Suppl. 1) 178, Abstract.

Laramore, G.E., Krall, J.M., Thomas, F.J., Griffin, T.W., Maor, M.H. and Hendrickson, F.R. (1985) Fast neutron radiotherapy for locally advanced prostate cancer: results of an RTOG randomized study. Int. J. Radiat. Oncol. Biol. Phys. 11, 1621–1626.

Mishima, Y., Ichihashi, M., Hatta, S., Honda, Ch., Sasase, A., Yamamura, K., Kanda, K., Kobayashi, T. and Fukuda, H. (1988) Selective thermal neutron capture therapy of cancer cells using their specific metabolic activity – cure of melanoma prototype, *in*: Progress in Radio-oncology IV, (Karcher, K.H., Kogelnik, H.D., Stadler, B. and Szepesi, T., eds.), pp. 7–11, ICRO, Vienna.

Munzenrider, J.E., Austin-Seymour, M., Gragoudas, E.S., Seddon, J.M., Verhey, L.J., Goitein, M., Gentry, R., Urie, M., Ruotolo, D., Birnbaum, S., Johnson, K., Sisterton, J.M., McNulty, P., Suit, H.D. and Koehler, A.M. (1987) Clinical results of proton beam radiotherapy in Boston, *in*: Radiation Research: Proceedings 8th ICRR at Edinburgh, July 1987. (Fielden, E.M., Fowler, J.F., Hendry, J.H. and Scott, D., eds.), pp. 916–921, Taylor and Francis, London.

Parsons, J.T., Mendenhall, W., Cassisi, N., Isaacs, J.R. and Million, R. (1988) Accelerated hyperfractionation in head and neck cancer. Int. J. Rad. Oncol. Biol. Phys. 14, 649–658.

Peters, L.J., Brock, W.A., Chapman, D.J., Wilson, G.D. and Fowler, J.F. (1988) Response predictors in radiotherapy: a review of research into radiobiologically based assays. Br. J. Radiol. (Suppl. 22), 96–108.

Raju, M.R. (1980) Heavy particle therapy. Academic Press, New York, 500 pp.

Raju, M.R., Tobey, R.A., Jett, J.H. and Walters, R.A. (1975) Age response for line CHO cells exposed to X-irradiation and alpha particles from plutonium. Radiat. Res. 63, 422–433.

Ryabukhin, Y.S. (1987) Problems of neutron capture therapy. *in*: Radiation Research: Proceedings 8th ICRR at Edinburgh, July 1987. (Fielden, E.M., Fowler, J.F., Hendry, J.H. and Scott, D., eds.), pp. 898–903, Taylor and Francis, London.

Sinclair, W.K. (1970) Dependence of radiosensitivity upon cell age *in*: Time and Dose Relationships in Radiation Biology as Applied to Radiotherapy. BNL Rept. 50203 (C57), pp. 97–107.

Skolyszewski, J., Fowler, J.F. and Huczkowski, J. (1988) Short-course neutron therapy for advanced head and neck cancer. Br. J. Radiol. 61, 857–858.

Tobias, C.A., Lyman, J.T. and Lawrence, J.H. (1971) Progress in atomic medicine: Recent advances in nuclear medicine, Vol. 3. (Lawrence, J.H., ed.), pp. 167–218, Grune and Stratton, New York.

Tsunemoto, H., Morita, S., Kawachi, K., Kanai, T., Kawashima, K., Hiraoka, T., Furukawa, S., Kitagawa, T. and Inada, T. (1987) Clinical results of proton therapy in Japan *in*: Radiation Research: Proceedings 8th ICRR at Edinburgh, July 1987. (Fielden, E.M., Fowler, J.F., Hendry, J.H. and Scott, D., eds.), pp. 921–927, Taylor and Francis, London.

Wambersie, A., Bewley, D.K. and Lalanne, C.M. (1986) Prospects for the application of fast neutrons in cancer therapy. Bull. Cancer (Paris) 73, 546–561.

CHAPTER 18

Combined radiotherapy–chemotherapy: principles

G. GORDON STEEL

Radiotherapy Research Unit, The Institute of Cancer Research, Cotswold Road, Sutton, Surrey SM2 5NG, England.

18.1 Exploitable mechanisms in the combined use of chemotherapy and radiotherapy 268

18.2 Spatial co-operation 268

18.3 Simple addition of anti-tumour effects of drugs and radiation 270

18.4 Protection of radiation-induced damage to normal tissues by cytotoxic drug administration 271

18.5 Enhancement of tumour response 272

18.6 The timing of combined radiotherapy-chemotherapy 273

18.7 Overview of drug-radiation combinations 275

Many cancer patients now receive treatment with radiotherapy *and* chemotherapy at some point in their management. This is sometimes but not always as part of a planned protocol of combined modality treatment. Some demonstrable gains have been associated with this form of combination therapy. They are, however, not widespread; along with many patients who have received benefit from such treatment there is also an extensive catalogue of patients who have been harmed by inappropriate combinations of drugs and radiation. The potential benefits of radiotherapy–chemotherapy combinations are clear but the situation is highly complex and the problem of gaining maximum benefit without serious hazard is a difficult one.

18.1 Exploitable mechanisms in the combined use of chemotherapy and radiotherapy

There are a number of conceptually different ways in which chemotherapy can improve the results of radiotherapy (Steel and Peckham, 1979; Steel, 1979):

1. *Spatial co-operation.* An improvement in therapeutic result that is achieved by one agent (drug or radiation) dealing with disease that is spatially missed by the other.

2. *Simple addition of anti-tumour effects.* To administer two effective cytotoxic agents should kill more tumour cells than either alone, provided they do not antagonise one another. For benefit to be obtained in this way it is critically important that the toxicities of drugs and radiation should not greatly overlap; i.e., that chemotherapy does not seriously reduce radiation tolerance or vice versa. Provided full single-agent doses can be maintained in the combination, it is not essential for the anti-tumour effects to add perfectly: A plus any fraction of B is in principle always greater than A alone.

3. *Protection of normal tissues.* Especially the use of drugs that protect against radiation damage to normal tissues, in the absence of similar protection of tumour cells.

4. *Enhancement of tumour response.* The use of combinations that produce a greater anti-tumour response than would have been expected from the response achieved with the agents used separately.

Any one of these mechanisms by itself could give an improved therapeutic strategy compared with radiotherapy or chemotherapy used alone. A particular combination of drugs and radiation may simultaneously exploit more than one mechanism. For instance, if one attempts to achieve enhancement of tumour response (mechanism 4) using agents that have non-overlapping toxicity there maybe benefit from the simple addition of anti-tumour effects (mechanism 2) and the chemotherapy may also deal with disease outside the radiation field (mechanism 1). But to distinguish these processes may help in evaluating the results of combined therapy.

A matter of particular interest is the extent to which the success of drug-radiation combinations depends on interactions between the effects of the two agents. By interaction we mean a situation in which treatment with one agent modifies the response of a tissue (normal or tumour) to the second agent. Mechanisms 1 and 2 above specifically *exclude* interactive effects between the drugs and radiation. On the other hand, protection of normal tissues and enhancement of tumour response *depend* upon interactive effects.

18.2 Spatial co-operation

To demonstrate the exploitability of spatial co-operation in laboratory animal studies

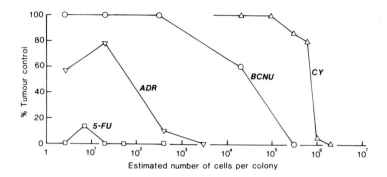

Figure 18.1. The control of a defined metastatic burden by four chemotherapeutic agents. Following an intravenous implantation of Lewis lung tumour cells, sufficient to produce an average of 10–20 lung colonies per mouse, chemotherapy was given after various time intervals and mouse survival scored 60 days later. A separately determined growth curve for lung colonies enabled colony size at the time of treatment to be estimated (abscissa). 5–FU, 5–fluorouracil 150 mg/kg; ADR, adriamycin 15 mg/kg; BCNU, 40 mg/kg; CY, cyclophosphamide 300 mg/kg. From Steel et al. (1976).

is straightforward. As shown in the work of Johnson (1969) and Steel et al. (1978), if one takes mice that have been implanted with tumours at a time when systemic metastases have become established, it is usually possible to cure the primary implant by radiation therapy but the mice will die of their systemic disease. Chemotherapy itself may well eradicate the metastatic seedlings at an early stage but fail to control the primary implant. A combination of the two treatments can yield a high proportion of long-term survivors.

The ability to achieve this in experimental animals depends critically on the effectiveness of chemotherapy. As has been well demonstrated by cell-survival studies on mouse tumours, some drugs given in maximum tolerated dose to the mouse may fail to reduce the surviving fraction of clonogenic tumour cells below 0.1 (i.e., less than one decade cell kill). Other agents may be much more effective, and in favourable situations a maximum-tolerated single dose may produce more than 5 or 6 decades of cell kill. When used in an adjuvant situation, a drug of the first category will fail to eradicate more than 10 single-cell metastatic seedlings and thus be almost completely ineffective. A drug of the second category could deal with up to a thousand 1000-cell metastatic seedlings.

This is well demonstrated by the results shown in Figure 18.1. Mice were injected intravenously with sufficient Lewis lung tumour cells to produce on average 10–20 lung colonies (Steel et al., 1976). The growth curve for lung colonies could be estimated and is expressed as cell number on the abscissa in the figure. Single-dose treatment with maximum-tolerated doses of four different drugs was given at various intervals thereafter, and the mice were kept in order to score the proportion of long-term survivors. Cyclophosphamide was successful in 50% of the mice for colony sizes up to almost 10^6 cells; for BCNU the colony size for 50% control was about $3 \cdot 10^4$

cells; for adriamycin about 600 cells; 5-fluorouracil never achieved 50% control.

The ease of demonstrating spatial co-operation in laboratory animals may be contrasted with the relative difficulty of exploiting it in the clinic (Chapter 19). Despite the fact that it is a common feature of human cancer for patients to present with apparently localised disease but die of widespread metastases, the ability of present-day chemotherapy to deal even with the occult disease is limited. The disease areas in which there is clear evidence for the useful exploitation of spatial co-operation are few: Ewing's sarcoma and some childhood tumours, acute leukaemia and perhaps in osteosarcoma.

18.3 Simple addition of anti-tumour effects of drugs and radiation

This self-evident mechanism in combined modality therapy is based upon the idea that if patients who are receiving radiotherapy can also be given a full course of effective chemotherapy without the need substantially to reduce the doses of drugs or radiation, then the combination may well kill more tumour cells. The target of therapy is disease within the radiation field. The basis for therapeutic advantage is that provided drugs are chosen which have different limiting toxicities than radiation, the toxic effects of drug and radiation are more likely to be independent than are their tumour effects. The tumour effects may well add, the normal tissue effects not.

Table 18.1 illustrates the idea behind this approach for the hypothetical example of treatment of a lung tumour. Radiation produces an incomplete tumour response and is limited (for example) by radiation pneumonitis. Chemotherapy also produces a tumour response but is limited by intestinal or bone marrow damage. Even if the anti-tumour effects of these two treatments are subadditive (++++ instead of the expected +++++) the overall anti-tumour effect may well be greater than either drug or radiation alone. The cost of this advantage is that the patient has to tolerate a wider range of toxic reactions and a critical factor in the reasoning is the assumption that radiation lung damage is not enhanced by the addition of chemotherapy. It is thus vital to select effective anti-tumour drugs that do not exacerbate radiation damage to critical normal tissues within the radiation field.

A considerable amount of laboratory research has been devoted to the study of

TABLE 18.1
Concept of independent toxicity leading to simple addition of anti-tumour effects as a mechanism in combined modality therapy

	Associated toxicity			Response of bronchial tumour
	intestinal	bone marrow	lung	
Radiation	–	–	+++	+++
Drug	+++	+	–	++
Combination	+++	+	+++	++++

enhancement of radiation normal-tissue damage by concurrent chemotherapy. The extent of enhancement depends on the choice of target tissue, the choice of drug, and on the timing between drug and radiation treatments. In some situations full-dose chemotherapy produces no enhancement of radiation damage; in others, enhancement becomes considerable.

The available experimental data on this question have recently been reviewed (Steel, 1988) with the following conclusions:
(i) Of 14 chemotherapeutic agents on which data are available, all substantially enhanced radiation damage to one or more normal tissues. The level of enhancement varied considerably.
(ii) As concluded by Phillips and Fu (1978), enhancement is most severe when the drug on its own has a recognised toxicity to the tissue that is irradiated.
(iii) Most studies have concentrated on drug administration within ±24 hours of irradiation. Where intervals of a week or more were allowed to elapse, there is evidence for less severe enhancement but some enhancement does often persist at this time.

18.4 Protection of radiation-induced damage to normal tissue by cytotoxic drug administration

One normally expects that two poisons will produce more damage than either alone and indeed this usually is the case. However, there are well-documented situations in which certain cytotoxic drugs increase the resistance of normal tissues to radiation or to a second cytotoxic treatment. W.W. Smith observed this with colchicine and the vinca alkaloids over 30 years ago, and more recently the phenomenon has been studied in detail by my colleagues in the Institute of Cancer Research (Millar and Hudspith, 1976; Millar et al., 1978). Cyclophosphamide, cytosine arabinoside, chlorambucil and methotrexate are found to be effective radioprotective agents. An important characteristic of this phenomenon is its dependence upon timing. Maximal radioprotection of animal survival was achieved when cytosine arabinoside was given 2 days before irradiation but the optimum gap for cyclophosphamide was 3 days. A similar protection phenomenon has been found in which a priming treatment with one cytotoxic drug can protect against a large dose of another (Millar et al., 1975; Millar and McElwain, 1978). Studies of the mechanism of this remarkable phenomenon have concentrated upon the bone marrow and intestinal epithelium. In the marrow it has been shown that the most effective of the 'protective' agents, cytosine arabinoside, did not modify stem-cell radiosensitivity; it stimulated enhanced repopulation by surviving stem cells. In the small intestine, microcolony survival experiments have shown that cytosine arabinoside given 12 hours before irradiation greatly increased the survival of intestinal stem cells, perhaps by enhancing the repair of radiation damage.

Protection of normal tissues only leads to therapeutic advantage if tumour tissue is not similarly protected. Investigation of tumour response to a number of normal tissue-sparing combinations, including Ara-C and radiation, has shown no evidence for protection of tumour cells.

18.5 Enhancement of tumour response

Although as indicated above it is reasonable to expect therapeutic benefit from the simple addition of the anti-tumour effects of a drug and radiation, much experimental attention has been given to the possibility of doing even better than this. Is it possible by proper choice of drug and timing to exploit an interactive phenomenon that leads to a greater degree of tumour cell kill than would be expected on the basis of simple addition? There is a large amount of basic data which indicate that some drugs can inhibit the repair of sublethal radiation damage or leave a surviving cell population that is partially synchronised and therefore potentially more sensitive to radiation given at the optimum time interval. There is, however, a conceptual problem in the definition of a 'supra-additive' response (Steel, 1979). When dose-response curves for the individual cytotoxic agents are linear the situation is simple: for each agent doubling the dose gives double the effect and partial doses of the two agents would be expected to combine in a simple additive manner. In most cases, however, the dose-response curves for drugs or radiation are far from linear. For some end-points the response curves are sigmoid, as is the case with cure as an end-point of tumour effect or lethality as an end-point of normal tissue damage, for example. Such responses are so far from linear that addition can give rise to non-sensical results and it should not be attempted. Strongly shouldered or plateau-type response curves similarly make the addition of effects relatively meaningless. In less serious cases where the dose response curves are not far from linear it is possible to calculate using the isobologram approach an *envelope of additivity* which indicates the extent of uncertainty involved in the addition of effects (Steel and Peckham, 1979).

When combined drug-radiation studies on experimental tumours have been analysed by the isobologram approach it is rare to find a sufficiently strong positive interaction to be classified as definitely supra-additive. Moreover, if the effects on critical normal tissues are also supra-additive, then there may be no therapeutic advantage. It would seem unwise, therefore, to seek to demonstrate therapeutic gain in this way. A better approach is as follows: to perform dose-response curves for radiation alone and radiation plus a fixed chemotherapy treatment, documenting tumour response as well as a relevant measure of toxicity. By interpolation along the dose-response curves to identify treatments (drug + radiation and radiation alone) that are equitoxic. If in this situation the combination gives a better tumour response than radiation alone, then a therapeutic gain has been demonstrated.

18.6 The timing of combined radiotherapy–chemotherapy

A well-established method for the study of interactions between pairs of cytotoxic agents is the 'time-line' approach (Vietti et al., 1971). For combined modality work, a dose of radiation is chosen that gives an accurately measurable level of damage (this can be to a tumour or to a normal tissue). Groups of animals are treated with this dose, together with a fixed chemotherapy treatment. Only the timing is varied, ranging from chemotherapy say a few days before radiation to a few days afterwards. Response is measured in each group. The result is a direct indication of the profile of response as a function of timing.

Collections of time-lines for combined modality treatment of transplanted mouse tumours and mouse intestinal epithelium are shown in Figures 18.2 and 18.3 (from Steel, 1988). The data on the intestine have come either from studies using the microcolony survival technique or using early mortality as the end-point. The results

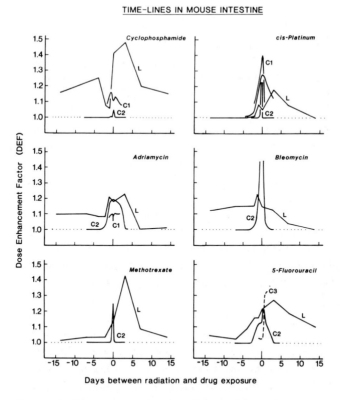

Figure 18.2. Time-lines for enhancement of radiation damage to the mouse intestine by six separate chemotherapeutic agents. Most of these studies (C1, C2, C3) used the microcolony assay; others used lethality after pelvic irradiation as the end-point (L). See Steel (1988) for sources.

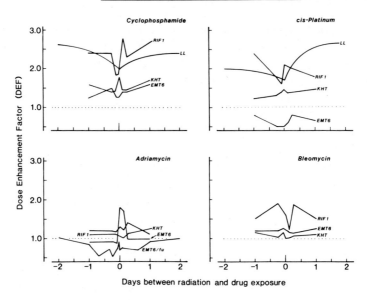

Figure 18.3. Time-lines for enhancement of radiation damage to transplanted mouse tumours by four chemotherapeutic agents. In each case the derivation of *DEF* values is approximate, based on the assumption of linear dose-response curves. See Steel (1988) for sources.

are shown in terms of the dose-enhancement factor (DEF), i.e., the ratio of radiation doses without/with chemotherapy to give a fixed level of damage. When *DEF* = 1.0, the drug has no effect. When it is greater than 1.0, damage is greater than with radiation alone. For instance, when *DEF* = 1.2, it would be necessary to reduce the radiation dose by 17% (i.e., to 1/1.2) to achieve an isoeffect. What this collection of data shows is that studies by different investigators have not agreed well, but some generalisations can be made. Each of the six drugs shows considerable enhancement of radiation damage at short time intervals. The most damaging time interval is either for simultaneous treatment or for drug given a few days after radiation. For longer time intervals between drug and radiation less enhancement is observed: this is especially clear in the case of *cis*-platinum given *before* irradiation.

A collection of time-lines for transplanted mouse tumours is shown in Figure 18.3, for four of the drugs included in Figure 18.2. Studies with a particular combination on different experimental tumours have not agreed well. Much of the data lie well above *DEF* = 1.0; this probably results from the fact that drugs have been chosen that show a good response in these tumour lines and simple addition of anti-tumour effects therefore raises the *DEF*. But the main feature of these data is the lack of evidence for a consistent trend towards maximum tumour response at short time intervals (or at any other interval).

These experimental data do not support the widely held view that to give cytotoxic drugs and radiation close together in time is a good therapeutic strategy. On the contrary, the evidence suggests that this will lead to maximum enhancement of acute normal tissue damage, without a corresponding peak in tumour response. For longer time intervals between drugs and radiation the damage to normal tissues tends to be less, but tumour response may remain high.

18.7 Overview of drug–radiation combinations

As indicated at the start of this review, one of the central questions about the exploitability of chemotherapy–radiotherapy combinations is the extent to which *interaction* between these modalities is necessary for the optimum therapeutic result. We have described two approaches (exploiting spatial co-operation or simple addition) either of which can lead to therapeutic benefit and which do not envisage interaction. The value of both of them has clearly been demonstrated in the experimental literature. In clinical practice there is evidence in a few tumour types for the exploitability of spatial co-operation; it also seems likely that the simple addition of anti-tumour effects of drug and radiation chosen to given independent toxicity has given occasional benefit.

The exploitability of interactive combinations is more in doubt. These have been divided into combinations that protect normal tissues and those that give enhanced tumour response. The existence of the former is experimentally well-demonstrated. The phenomenon of protection (as described above and as distinct from radioprotection by free-radical scavenging agents) occurs with some cytotoxic drugs and not others, and has not been demonstrated in experimental tumours. The effects are not large, involving an effective radiation dose-reduction of only about 10%, but their existence is surprising and their basic mechanism needs further elucidation. The clinical use of this type of protection has been examined with drug–drug combinations. Its application to radiotherapy is limited by its requirement for precise timing of the protector in relation to radiation exposure; it does not work with fractionated radiotherapy.

Interactions between cytotoxic drugs and radiation that lead to enhanced cell killing have been well-demonstrated in some experimental systems, especially in tissue culture. The clearest demonstration is the cell-survival shoulder-reducing property of the cytotoxic antibiotics when given soon before or soon after irradiation. This appears to be a universal property of these drugs and therefore the associated enhancement of toxicity seriously limits the therapeutic benefit that can be expected. Enhanced tumour-cell killing has also occasionally been seen with other drugs but not consistently in different experimental systems. Interactions seen in vitro have often not been reproduced in vivo and interactions seen in one tumour system have often not been confirmed in others (Van Putten, 1979).

In contrast, the increase in damage to normal tissues when some drugs are used with radiation has been well shown. The picture here is more predictable than for the anti-tumour effects, and drugs that enhance the radiation effects on particular normal tissues have been clearly documented. The timing of combined treatment seems to be important, and in general the greater the time interval between treatments, the less the combined toxicity.

The clinically confirmed benefits of combined chemotherapy–radiotherapy have been few. They have been found in a small group of diseases that respond to chemotherapy alone. The moral seems to be that only when a drug or drug combination has the ability to eradicate occult disease or substantially to reduce the size of objectively measurable disease is there likely to be any demonstrable benefit from its use in conjunction with radiotherapy. The risk of increasing damage to normal tissues is considerable; combined modality therapy should therefore not be given without good reason.

The immediate future probably lies in selecting drugs and patients in which a good chemotherapeutic response can be expected, avoiding drugs that seriously enhance radiation damage to normal tissues and keeping drug and radiation treatments far enough apart in time to minimise interactions.

Acknowledgement

This work was supported in part by NCI grant No. RO1 CA 26059

References

Johnson, R.E. (1969) Combined chemotherapy and irradiation in Ewing's sarcoma. Front. Radiat. Ther. Oncol. 4, 195–202.

Millar, J.L., Blackett, N.M. and Hudspith, B.N. (1978) Enhanced post-irradiation recovery of the haemopoietic system in animals pretreated with a variety of cytotoxic agents. Cell Tissue Kinet. 11, 543–553.

Millar, J.L. and Hudspith, B.N. (1976) Sparing effect of cyclophosphamide (NSC-26271) pretreatment in animals lethally treated with γ-radiation. Cancer Treat. Rep. 60, 409–414.

Millar, J.L., Hudspith, B.N. and Blackett, N.M. (1975) Reduced lethality in mice receiving a combined dose of cyclophosphamide and busulphan. Br. J. Cancer 32, 193–198.

Millar, J.L. and McElwain, T.J. (1978) Combinations of cytotoxic agents that have less than expected toxicity on normal tissues in mice, in: Antibiotics and Chemotherapy, (Schönfeld, H. et al., eds.), pp. 271–282, Karger, Basel.

Phillips, T.L. and Fu, K.K. (1978) The interaction of drug and radiation effects on normal tissues. Int. J. Radiat. Oncol. 4, 59–64.

Steel, G.G. (1979) Terminology in the description of drug-radiation interactions. Int. J. Radiat. Oncol. 5, 1145–1150.

Steel, G.G. (1988) The search for therapeutic gain in the combination of radiotherapy and chemotherapy. Radiother. Oncol. 11, 31–35.

Steel, G.G., Adams, K. and Stanley, J. (1976) Size-dependence of the response of Lewis lung tumours to BCNU. Cancer Treat. Rep. 60, 1743–1748.
Steel, G.G., Hill, R.P. and Peckham, M.J. (1978) Combined radiotherapy–chemotherapy of Lewis lung carcinoma. Int. J. Radiat. Oncol. 4, 49–52.
Steel, G.G. and Peckham, M.J. (1979) Exploitable mechanisms in combined radiotherapy–chemotherapy: the concept of additivity. Int. J. Radiat. Oncol. 5, 85–91.
Van Putten, L.M. (1979) Combined modalities in experimental systems, *in*: Radiation Research (Okada, S., Imamura, M., Terasima, T. and Yamaguchi, H., eds.), pp. 815–821, Japanese Association for Radiation Research, Tokyo.
Vietti, T., Eggerding, F. and Valeriote, F. (1971) Combined effect of X-radiation and 5-fluorouracil on survival of transplanted leukemic cells. J. Nat. Cancer Inst. 47, 865–870.

CHAPTER 19

Combined radiotherapy–chemotherapy in clinical practice

ALAN HORWICH

Department of Radiotherapy and Oncology, The Royal Marsden Hospital, Downs Road, Sutton, Surrey SM2 5PT, England

---

19.1	Mechanisms of drug–radiation interaction		279
19.2	Sequencing of radiotherapy and chemotherapy		280
19.3	Clinical objectives		282
	19.3.1	Spatial cooperation	282
	19.3.2	Local cooperation	284
	19.3.3	Both local and spatial cooperation	285
19.4	Conclusions		287

A large number of clinical studies of the combination of radiotherapy and chemotherapy have been performed over the last 15 years and the principles of investigating this complex field have become clear. The challenge to the investigator is to improve the therapeutic ratio of anti-cancer effect to normal tissue toxicity and this requires a thorough understanding of the biological effects of each modality and of how these effects may interact.

19.1 Mechanisms of drug–radiation interaction

Chemotherapeutic agents may interact with radiation to produce cytotoxicity in different ways, some of which may occur concurrently:
1. Increase initial radiation damage to DNA.
2. Modify repair of radiation damage.
3. Change cell-cycle times.

4. Change growth fraction.
5. Reduce tumour stem-cell number.
6. Select drug resistant clones which may have a modified radiosensitivity.

These interactions occur both in tumour and normal cells within the irradiated volume and the biological effect of the interaction depends on the tumour site, target volume and critical normal tissue, the radiation dose and fractionation schedule, timing of drug administration in relation to irradiation, and the details of chemotherapeutic drugs and their dosages.

In clinical practice drugs and radiotherapy have often been combined in schedules which mimic their use as individual modalities of treatment. However, combined modality therapy may require these principles to be re-evaluated. For example, if combined modality therapy is employed in early Hodgkin's disease, the intention is that chemotherapy treats subclinical areas of disease and this reduces the need for extended-field rather than local-field irradiation (Coltman et al., 1982). When 5-fluorouracil is combined with radiotherapy in epidermoid carcinoma of the anal canal, a reduction in radiation dose and a prolongation of treatment time, do not compromise local control (Flam et al., 1983; Cummings et al., 1984). Conversely, when cisplatin is used to increase radiation effects, it may optimally be given as a frequent small dose (e.g., 6 mg/m^2 per day, Schaake-Koning et al., 1986) rather than on the single-modality standard 21 day cycle at 100 mg/m^2.

19.2 Sequencing of radiotherapy and chemotherapy

As detailed in the previous chapter, maximum normal tissue damage usually occurs when drugs and radiation are given simultaneously and this is supported by clinical experience (Horwich et al., 1975; Tefft et al., 1976; Fu et al., 1979; Brooks et al., 1986). However, simultaneous administration also offers a potential for drug interaction with acute radiation damage to the tumour and the clinical result depends upon balance of the effects listed above on tumour and normal tissue.

Separation of the two modalities in time is a logical approach, especially when non-interactive effects on the tumour are sought. For localised tumours the use of radiotherapy before chemotherapy has the advantage of avoiding any delay in effective treatment. However, latent radiation damage may be expressed even when drugs are delayed for some time after radiotherapy and there is evidence that the sequence drug → radiation carries a lower risk of enhancing normal tissue damage (Yarnold et al., 1983). Furthermore, although some patients with localised disease will not respond to drug treatment, these patients can be selected for early change to radiotherapy. Patients who do respond to chemotherapy have the advantage that any subclinical metastatic disease is treated immediately rather than allowing it to progress while the local overt disease is treated. A further rationale for employing chemotherapy before

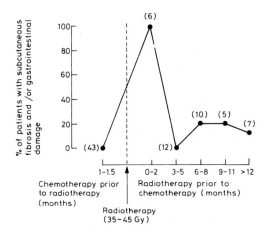

Figure 19.1. Influence of sequence and timing of chemotherapy and radiotherapy on the risk of normal tissue damage in patients treated for advanced testicular non-seminoma (Royal Marsden Hospital, 1976–1981). The values between parentheses represent the number of patients at risk.

radiotherapy is that 'down staging' of the tumour by chemotherapy should increase radiation control rates. Rather surprisingly the clinical evidence for this is lacking, possibly because the earlier treatment could cause accelerated repopulation of tumour stem cells and thus reduce the efficacy of the standard radiotherapy course.

Figure 19.1 illustrates the importance of sequencing on development of normal tissue damage in patients treated with chemotherapy and radiotherapy for metastatic testicular germ-cell tumours (Yarnold et al., 1983). Chemotherapy consisted of a combination of cisplatin, vinblastine and bleomycin (PVB) or cisplatin, etoposide and bleomycin (BEP) and radiotherapy was administered to para-aortic nodes via parallel opposed anterior, posterior portals to a dose of 40–46 Gy in 2 Gy fractions daily. Forty-three patients were treated with a planned sequence of chemotherapy followed by radiotherapy (Peckham et al., 1979). Other patients were treated initially with radiotherapy and then received chemotherapy either as an adjuvant or on relapse. Normal-tissue damage did not occur in patients treated with chemotherapy before radiotherapy.

It is not clear from clinical data how great the time separation should be between chemotherapy and radiotherapy in order to avoid an increase in normal tissue damage. This has been reduced to 7 days in an innovative approach to combined modality therapy termed 'the interdigitated alternating regimen' employed in the treatment of small-cell lung cancer (Arriagada et al., 1985, Tubiana et al., 1988). In this approach short courses of radiotherapy are alternated with chemotherapy. The principles of this approach are that chemotherapy is started early and maintained regularly during the entire induction treatment. Radiotherapy is also given early in the schedule to maximum-tolerated dose and does not interrupt chemotherapy. It is noteworthy that the radiotherapeutic component of this regimen is given in split-course with a long overall treatment time without compromising local control, thus emphasizing the need to define different principles for combined modality than for single-modality therapies.

19.3 Clinical objectives

The clinical objectives of combining chemotherapy and radiotherapy may be categorised as shown in Table 19.1.

19.3.1 Spatial cooperation

This refers to the clinical context where chemotherapy is used to treat sites outside the radiation fields. Since no interaction between chemotherapy and radiotherapy is required, it is usually advantageous to separate the two modalities in time. Clinical examples include early Hodgkin's disease, early aggressive non-Hodgkin's lymphomas and CNS prophylaxis in acute lymphoblastic leukaemia (Figure 19.2). In clinical stage I or II Hodgkin's disease the presentation is usually with cervical lymphadenopathy, sometimes associated with lymphadenopathy at other supradiaphragmatic sites. Approximately one third of patients have occult spread of the disease within the abdomen. Patients presenting with stage I or stage II Hodgkin's disease and poor prognostic features are treated with 3–6 courses of combination chemotherapy prior to radiotherapy to originally involved sites (Horwich et al., 1986). Though this is a logical approach to treatment it has not been clearly demonstrated to achieve a survival advantage compared with the policy of initial radiotherapy alone with salvage chemotherapy for relapse (Horwich and Peckham, 1987). Similar considerations apply to early-stage aggressive histology non-Hodgkin's lymphoma. Results of local radiotherapy are good in stage I presentations where 80–90% of patients remained disease-free

TABLE 19.1
Clinical objectives of combined chemo-radiotherapy

	Disease
Spatial cooperation	Early Hodgkin's disease and non-Hodgkin's lymphomas
	CNS prophylaxis in acute lymphoblastic leukaemia
	Ewing's sarcoma
Local cooperation	Anal canal cancer
	Head and neck cancer
	Rectal cancer
Local and spatial cooperation	Small-cell lung cancer
	Bladder cancer
	Locally advanced breast cancer

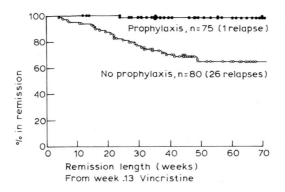

Figure 19.2. Duration of leukaemia-free remission in the CNS. Prophylaxis consisted of craniospinal irradiation and intrathecal methotrexate. MRC Leukaemia Committee (1973).

TABLE 19.2
Stage III Hodgkin's disease: recurrence pattern in 88 patients who relapsed after different initial treatments

Site of recurrence	% recurrence after		
	radiotherapy	chemotherapy	combined chemo–radiotherapy
Local[a]	10	21	5
Distant	51	26	23

[a] Local = site of initial involvement.

but inadequate in patients with stage II disease in whom despite good local control with radiotherapy systemic relapse occurred in some 40–50% of patients. Single-arm studies would suggest that initial combined-modality therapy improves these figures (Miller and Jones, 1983; Horwich and Peckham, 1983). The pattern of cooperation in lymphomas is clearly illustrated by an analysis of 320 patients treated for stage III Hodgkin's disease at the Royal Marsden Hospital (Brada et al., 1989). Sites of recurrence after different initial treatment approaches are shown in Table 19.2. After radiotherapy alone a high proportion of patients relapsed at new sites and the incidence of this was halved when chemotherapy was employed. With chemotherapy alone the incidence of recurrence at an originally involved site was twice as high as when radiotherapy was employed. The combined modality results show that local control was at or below the level achieved by radiotherapy alone; systemic control was at the level achieved by chemotherapy alone. Two large retrospective analyses have suggested that combined radiation and chemotherapy may lead to higher survival in stage III Hodgkin's disease than radiotherapy alone (Mauch et al., 1985; Brada et al., 1989). However, this has not yet been supported by results from a prospective randomised trial.

19.3.2 Local cooperation

Chemotherapy is used to improve probability of local control by radiotherapy attempting to exploit two mechanisms: downstaging and drug–radiation interactions.

Attempt to downstage. Chemotherapy is used initially to reduce the volume and extent of tumour and it is hoped that successful chemotherapy will convert the prognosis after radiotherapy to that of the reduced stage of tumour. The smaller tumour may be more radiocurable since there will be fewer tumour stem cells and better oxygenation, and also since the target volume may be smaller it should be possible to treat to an increased radiation dose. To avoid enhancement of radiation reactions, the modalities can be separated in time. Since it is required that the chemotherapy functions independently, drugs are usually employed in combinations using a regimen shown to be active in the treatment of metastatic disease.

There have been many studies and trials of combined chemotherapy and radiotherapy in advanced head and neck cancer where response rates to combination chemotherapy range from 30–60% (Nervi et al., 1978; Elias et al., 1979; Ensley et al., 1984; Rooney et al., 1985; Marcial et al., 1980; Decker et al., 1983).

A number of randomised studies have recently been completed and have not demonstrated benefit from adjuvant chemotherapy. Taylor et al. (1985) reported a randomised study of 95 patients with head and neck cancer treated with a 2 week course of neoadjuvant methotrexate, followed within 2 weeks by radical radiotherapy to a dose of at least 65 Gy over 7 weeks. The complete remission rate was 88% in the control arm of the study and 78% in those treated with neoadjuvant methotrexate ($p=0.24$). Kun et al. (1986) also performed a prospective randomised study of radiotherapy alone versus induction chemotherapy followed by radiotherapy. The chemotherapy consisted of two courses of bleomycin, cyclophosphamide, methotrexate and 5-fluorouracil (5FU). At completion of radiotherapy there was complete remission in 24 of 43 patients treated with combined modality compared with 30 out of 40 patients treated by radiotherapy with or without surgery. Freedom from local disease at 2 years was also lower after combined modality (35 versus 53%, $p<0.06$). Similarly, the results of induction with 5FU and high-dose cisplatin combinations have not been successful (Martin et al., 1986; Haas et al., 1986) and it has been postulated that this approach may impair the efficacy of radical radiotherapy by virtue of a delay in starting treatment definitive allowing time for chemotherapy-induced acceleration of tumour stem-cell proliferation.

Attempt to exploit interactions. This seeks to exploit molecular interaction between chemotherapeutic and radiation toxicity and thus the two modalities of treatment are administered concomitantly. Since this is associated with enhanced toxicity, it was first explored with single-agent chemotherapy with encouraging results (Lo et al., 1976; Shanta and Krishnamurthi, 1980). Recent reports have not supported the promising early results. Vermund et al. (1985) randomised 222 patients to receive radiotherapy alone or to receive bleomycin 1 hour before each fraction of radiation in a prospective randomised trial in head and neck cancer. The addition of bleomycin significantly increased the morbidity and complication rate; there was no improvement in locoregional control nor in survival. The RTOG have evaluated concomitant radiation and cisplatin chemotherapy (Krisman et al., 1987). Cisplatin was at 100 mg/m^2 by intravenous bolus on days 1, 22 and 43, and radiotherapy was administered daily for 5 days per week to a total dose of 66–73.8 Gy. The complete remission rate was 67% and the regimen was well tolerated.

The use of combination chemotherapy during radiotherapy was recognised to be associated with enhanced radiation toxicity. Fu et al. (1979) reported on a schedule of combined radiotherapy and cyclophosphamide, vincristine and bleomycin. Three of 15 patients had fatal complications but the anti-tumour effect of radiation was felt to be increased. The controversy of sequential versus concomitant combination chemotherapy in the radiotherapy of head and neck cancer has recently been addressed in a multicentre study in 267 patients comparing neoadjuvant and adjuvant VBMF chemotherapy being interspersed between three blocks of radiation therapy. There was no difference in either local control or survival between the 2 arms of the study (SECOG, 1986).

Concomitant radiotherapy and chemotherapy are now widely used in the treatment of carcinomas of the anal canal (Cummings et al., 1984). With the original schedule of 50 Gy over 4 weeks concomitantly with day 1 mitomycin-C 10 mg/m^2 and days 1, 2, 3 and 4, 5-fluorouracil 1000 mg/m^2 per day by continuous infusion, there was high efficacy of treatment (15 of 16 patients remaining tumour-free on follow-up from 24–60 months) but also quite severe acute reactions. This schedule was subsequently modified to a split-course treatment with two blocks of 25 Gy administered in 10 fractions over 2 weeks, repeated 6 weeks from the start of treatment with each block of radiation combined with mitomycin-C and 5-fluorouracil in the same way as previously. For follow-up from 6 months to 24 months, 14 of 14 patients with early-stage disease remained tumour-free (Cummings and Byfield, 1988). From these and other results it was concluded that combined treatment allowed control of early stages of anal carcinoma at relatively low radiation doses, preserving normal function of the anal sphincter.

19.3.3 Both local and spatial cooperation

Over the last decade studies have revealed that carcinoma of the bladder is responsive to chemotherapy (Harker et al., 1985; Sternberg et al., 1988). A combination of methotrexate, vinblastine, adriamycin and cisplatin (M-VAC) produced responses in approximately 75% of patients with metastatic disease and is being explored actively as a neoadjuvant to definitive local treatment (Scher et al., 1988). Although responses to single-agent methotrexate occur in up to 50% of patients (Turner et al., 1977), a prospective randomised trial of neoadjuvant and adjuvant methotrexate in 400 patients with T3M0 carcinoma of the bladder showed absolutely no difference in local control rate, relapse-free survival, or overall survival, compared with local treatment (radiotherapy with or without surgery) (Shearer et al., 1988).

A number of prospective randomised trials have been completed studying combined modality for small-cell lung cancer. Results have been equivocal with approximately equal numbers of trials showing either benefit or lack of benefit from combined modality compared with chemotherapy alone. Toxicity was often severe with concomitant chemotherapy and radiotherapy though this appears to be more effective. Brooks et al. (1986) recorded severe lung toxicity in 5% of patients treated with chemotherapy alone, and in 28% of patients treated with chemotherapy and radiotherapy. Perez et al. (1984) compared chemotherapy with chemotherapy plus thoracic irradiation, the radiotherapy being administered during weeks 5, 8 and 11, interspersed between cycles of chemotherapy. The complete remission rate for combined modality therapy was significantly higher (63 versus 48%), and the 2-year disease-free survival was also higher (28 versus 19%). The total radiation dose was only 40 Gy.

The Cancer and Leukemia Group B compared two concomitant combined-modality schedules, one with radiotherapy administered between weeks 1 and 6 of chemotherapy and the second with the radiotherapy administered between weeks 9 and 14 (Perry et al., 1987). Rather surprisingly, radiation toxicity was much less in the second of these alternatives, though both were more effective than chemotherapy alone. The reduced toxicity with later irradiation would support the idea that chemotherapy may trigger proliferation of normal tissues thus protecting against acute reactions. Alternating radiotherapy and chemotherapy schedules are also being investigated at the Institute Gustave Roussy (Arriagada et al., 1985) and this group report exceptionally high relapse-free survival in non-randomised studies of this approach. Of 63 patients who entered two pilot studies between 1980 and 1985, local control at 2 years was 61% in the first study and 82% in the second with overall relapse-free survival being 32 and 37%, respectively. The first study alternated six cycles of combination chemotherapy (adriamycin, etoposide, cyclophosphamide and methotrexate) with three courses of mediastinal radiotherapy. The second schedule was similar but the radiation dose to the mediastinum was increased from 45 to 55 Gy. Toxicity was acceptable and this approach merits evaluation in a prospective randomised trial.

In locally advanced breast cancer, combined chemotherapy and radiotherapy were compared with radiotherapy alone in a study of 118 patients treated between 1977 and 1980 (Schaake-Koning et al., 1985). The three arms of the study were:
1. Radiotherapy.
2. Radiotherapy followed by 12 cycles of cyclophosphamide, methotrexate, 5-fluorouracil (CMF) and tamoxifen.
3. Two cycles of adriamycin and vincristine alternated with two cycles of CMF followed by radiotherapy, and then by further chemotherapy.

With a median follow-up of just over 5 years there is no improvement in overall survival with the combined modality therapy. Additionally, there was no significant difference in a relapse-free survival.

19.4 Conclusions

It is theoretically attractive to combine chemotherapy with radiation in the treatment of cancer since at least additive effects would be expected. In practice, enhanced radiation toxicity has more commonly been observed than an enhanced anti-tumour effect. Especially disappointing has been the approach of neoadjuvant combination chemotherapy prior to radical local treatment for advanced cancers of the head and neck (Tannock and Browman, 1986). Early studies demonstrated the enhanced toxicity of simultaneous combination chemotherapy and radiation and though this has deterred extensive assessments, early reports of trials in small-cell lung cancer and bladder cancer suggest it to be promising if acute reactions can be controlled.

References

Arriagada, R., Le Chelvalier, T., Baldeyrou, P., Pico, J.L., Ruffie, P., Martin, M., El Bakry, H.M., Duroux, P., Bignon, J., Lenfant, B., Hayat, M., Rouesse, J.G., Sancho-Garnier, H. and Tubiana, M. (1985) Alternating radiotherapy and chemotherapy schedules in small cell lung cancer, limited disease. Int. J. Radiat. Oncol. Biol. Phys. 11, 1461–1467.

Brada, M., Ashley, S., Nicholls, J., Wist, E., Colman, M., McElwain, T.J., Selby, P., Peckham, M.J., Horwich, A. (1989) Stage III Hodgkin's disease – long-term results following chemotherapy, radiotherapy and combined modality therapy. Radiother. Oncol. 14, 185–198

Brooks, B.J., Seifter, E.J., Walsh, T.E., Lichter, A.S., Bunn, P.A., Zabell, A., Johnston-Early, A., Edison, M., Makuch, R.W., Cohen, M.H., Glatstein, E. and Ihde, D.C. (1986) J. Clin. Oncol. 4, 200–209.

Coltman, C.A., Myers, J.W., Montague, E., Fuller, L.A., Curozea, P.N., DePersio, E.J. and Dixon, D.O. (1982) The role of combined radiotherapy and chemotherapy in the primary management of Hodgkin's disease: Southwest Oncology Group studies. in: Malignant Lymphomas (Rosenberg, S.A. and Kaplan, H.S., eds.), pp. 523–535, Academic Press, New York.

Cummings, B.J., Keane, T.J., Thomas, G.M., Harwood, A.R. and Rider, W.D. (1984) Results and toxicity of the treatment of anal canal carcinoma by radiation therapy or radiation therapy and chemotherapy. Cancer 54, 2062–2068.

Cummings, B.J. and Byfield, J.E. (1988) Treatment of cancer of the anal canal. in: Innovations in Radiation Oncology (Withers, H.R. and Peters, L.J., eds.), pp. 91–98, Springer-Verlag, Berlin.

Decker, D.A., Drelichman, A., Jacobs, J., Hoschner, J., Kinzie, J., Loh, J.J.K., Weaver, A. and Al-Sarraf, M. (1983) Adjuvant chemotherapy with cis-diaminodichloroplatinum II and 120-hour infusion 5-fluorouracil in Stage III and IV squamous cell carcinoma of the head and neck. Cancer 51, 1353–1355.

Elias, E.G., Chretien, P.B., Monnard, E., Khan, T., Bouchelle, W.H., Wiernik, P.H., Lipson, S.D., Hande, K.R. and Zenta, T. (1979) Chemotherapy prior to local therapy in advanced squamous cell carcinoma of the head and neck. Cancer 43, 1025–1031.

Ensley, J.R., Jacobs, J.R., Weaver, A. et al. (1984) Correlation between response to cis-platinum-chemotherapy and subsequent radiotherapy in previously untreated patients with advanced squamous cell cancers of the head and neck. Cancer 54, 811–814.

Fu, K.D., Silverberg, I.J., Phillips, T.L. and Friedman, M.A. (1979) Combined radiotherapy and multidrug chemotherapy for advanced head and neck cancer: results of a radiation therapy oncology group pilot study. Cancer Treat. Rep. 63, 351–357.

Flam, S.M., Lovalvo, L.J., Mills, R.J., Ramalko, L.D., Prather, C., Mowry, P.A., Morgan, D.R. and Lau, B.P. (1983) Definitive non-surgical therapy of epithelial malignancies of the anal canal. Cancer 51, 1378–1387.

Harker, W.G., Meyers, F.J., Freiha, F.S., Palmer, J.M., Shortliffe, L.D., Hannigan, J.F., McWhirter, K.M. and Tarti, F.M. (1985) Cisplatin, methotrexate and vinblastine (CMV): an effective chemotherapy regimen for metastatic transitional cell carcinoma of the urinary tract: a Northern California oncology group study. J. Clin. Oncol. 3, 1463–1470.

Hass, C., Anderson, T., Byhardt, R., Cox, J., Duncavage, J., Grossman, T., Hass, J., Libnoch, J., Malin, T., Ritch, P. and Toohill, R. (1986) Randomised neo-adjuvant study of 5-fluorouracil (FU) and *cis*-platinum (DDP) for patients (PTS) with advanced resectable head and neck squamous cancer (ARMNSC). Proceedings of AACR, Vol. 27, p. 185.

Horwich, A., Bloomer, W. and Lokich, J. (1975) Doxorubicin radiotherapy and oesophageal stricture. Lancet ii, 561.

Horwich, A. and Peckham, M.J. (1983) 'Bad risk' non-Hodgkin lymphomas. Sem. Hematol. 20, 35–56.

Horwich, A., Easton, D., Nogueira-Costa, R., Liew, K.H., Colman, M. and Peckham, M.J. (1986) An analysis of prognostic factors in early stage Hodgkin's disease. Radiat. Oncol. 7, 95–106.

Horwich, A. and Peckham, M.J. (1987) Combined chemotherapy and radiotherapy in the management of adult Hodgkin's disease: indications and results, *in*: Hodgkin's Disease (Selby, P. and McElwain, T.J., eds.), pp. 250–268, Blackwell Scientific Publications, Oxford.

Kun, L.E., Toohill, R.J., Holoye, P.Y., Duncavage, J.A., Byhardt, R.W., Ritch, P.S., Grossman, T.W. and Hoffmann, R.G. (1986) A randomised study of adjuvant chemotherapy for cancer of the upper aerodigestive tract. Int. J. Radiat. Oncol. Biol. Phys. 12, 173–178.

Lo, T.C., Wiley, A.L., Ansfield, F.J. et al. (1976) Combined radiation therapy and 5-fluorouracil for advanced squamous cell carcinoma of the oral cavity and oropharynx: a randomised study. Am. J. Roentgenol. 126, 229–235.

Martin, M., Mazeron, J.J., Glaubiger, D. et al. (1986) Neo-adjuvant polychemotherapy of head and neck cancer: preliminary results of a randomised study. Proc. Assoc. 5, 141.

Mauch, P., Goffman, T., Rosenthal, D.S., Cavellos, G.P., Come, S.E. and Hellman, S. (1985) Stage III Hodgkin's disease: improved survival with combined modality therapy as compared with radiation therapy alone. J. Clin. Oncol. 3, 1166–1173.

Miller, T.P. and Jones, S.E. (1983) Initial chemotherapy for clinically localised lymphomas of unfavourable histology. Blood 62, 413–418.

MRC Leukaemia Committee (1983) Treatment of acute lymphoblastic leukaemia: effect of 'prophylactic' therapy against central nervous system leukaemia. Br. Med. J. 2, 381–384.

Nervi, C., Arcangelli, G., Badaracco, G., Cortese, M., Morelli, M. and Starace, G. (1978) The relevance of tumour size and cell kinetics as predictors of radiation response in head and neck cancer. A randomised study on the effect of intra-arterial chemotherapy followed by radiotherapy. Cancer 41, 900–906.

Peckham, M.J., Barrett, A., McElwain, T.J. and Hendry, W.F. (1979) Combined management of malignant teratoma of the testis. Lancet ii, 267–270.

Perry, M.C., Eaton, W.L., Propert, J.K., Ware, J.H., Zimmer, B., Chahinian, A.P., Skarin, A., Carey, R.W., Kreisman, H., Faulkner, C., Comis, R. and Green, M.R. (1987) Chemotherapy with or without radiation therapy in limited small-cell carcinama of the lung. N. Engl. J. Med. 316, 912–918.

Perez, C.A., Einhorn, L., Oldham, R.K., Greco, F.A., Cohen, H.J., Silberman, H., Krauss, S., Hornback, N., Comas, F., Omur, G., Salter, M., Keller, J.W., McLaren, J., Kellermeyer, R., Storaasli, J., Birch, R., Dandy, M., for the Southeastern Cancer Study Group. (1984) Randomised trial of radiotherapy to the thorax in limited small-cell carcinoma of the lung treated with multi-agent chemotherapy and elective brain irradiation: a preliminary report. J. Clin. Oncol. 2, 1200–1208.

Rooney, M., Kish, J., Jacobs, J., Kinzie, J., Weaver, A., Crissman, J. and Al-Sarraf, M. (1985) Improved complete response rate and survival in advanced head and neck cancer after three-course induction therapy with 120-hour 5-FU infusion and cisplatin. Cancer 55, 1123–1128.

Schaake-Koning, C., Van der Linden, E.H., Hart, G. and Engelsman, E. (1985) Adjuvant chemo and hormonal therapy in locally advanced breast cancer: a randomised clinical study. Int. J. Radiat. Oncol. Biol. Phys. 11, 1759–1763.

Schaake-Koning, C., Bartelink, H., Adema, B.H., Schuster-Uitterhoeve, L. and Van Zandwijk, N. (1986) Radiotherapy and cis-diammine dichloroplatinum(II) as a combined treatment modality for inoperable non-small cell lung cancer: a dose-finding study. Int. J. Radiat. Oncol. Biol. Phys. 12, 379–383.

Scher, H.I., Yagoda, A., Herr, H.W., Sternberg, C.N., Bosl, G., Morse, M.J., Sogani, P.C., Watson, R.C., Dershaw, D.D., Reuter, V., Geller, N., Hollander, P.S., Vaughan, E.D., Whitmore, W.F., Jr. and Fair, W.R. (1988) Neoadjuvant M-VAC (methotrexate, vinblastine, doxorubicin and cisplatin) effect on the primary bladder lesion. J. Urol. 139, 461–469.

SECOG Interim Report (1986) A randomised trial of combined multidrug chemotherapy and radiotherapy in advanced squamous cell carcinoma of the head and neck. Eur. J. Surg. Oncol. 12, 289–295.

Shanta, V. and Krishnamurhti, S. (1980) Combined modality oncotherapies. Front. Radiat. Ther. Oncol. 13, 82–101.

Shearer, R.J., Chilvers, C.E.D., Bloom, H.J.G., Bliss, J.M., Horwich, A. and Babiker, A. (1988) Adjuvant chemotherapy in T_3 carcinoma of the bladder. Br. J. Urol. 62, 558–564.

Sternberg, C.N., Yagoda, A., Scher, H.I., Watson, R.C., Herr, H.W., Morse, M.J., Sogani, P.C., Vaughan, E.D., Bander, N., Weiselberg, L.R., Geller, N., Hollander, P.S., Lipperman, R., Fair, W.R. and Whitmore, W.F. (1988) M-VAC (methotrexate, vinblastine, doxorubicin and cisplatin) for advanced transitional cell carcinoma of the urothelium. J. Urol. 139, 461–469.

Tannock, I.F. and Browman, G. (1986) Lack of evidence for a role of chemotherapy in the routine management of locally advanced head and neck cancer. J. Clin. Oncol. 4, 1121–1126.

Taylor, IV, S.G., Applebaum, E., Showell, J.L., Norusis, M., Holinger, L.D., Hutchinson, J.C., Jr., Murthy, A.K. and Caldarelli, D.D. (1985) A randomised trial of adjuvant chemotherapy in head and neck cancer. J. Clin. Oncol. 3, 672–679.

Tefft, M., Lattin, P.B., Jereb, B., Cham, W., Ghavimi, F., Rosen, G., Exelby, P., Marcove, R., Murphy, M.L. and D'Angio, G.J. (1976) Acute and late effects on normal tissues following combined chemo and radio-therapy for childhood rhabdomyosarcoma and Ewing's sarcoma. Cancer 37, 1201–1213.

Tubiana, M., Arriagada, R. and Cosset, J.-M. (1988) Optimising combinations of drugs and radiation. The interdigitated alternating regimen, in: Innovations in Radiation Oncology (Withers, H.R. and Peters, L.J., eds.), pp. 265–276, Springer-Verlag, Berlin.

Turner, A.G., Hendry, W.F., Williams, G.B. et al. (1977) The treatment of advanced bladder cancer with methotrexate. Br. J. Urol. 49, 673–678.

Vermund, H., Kaalhus, O., Winther, F., Trausjo, J., Thorud, E., Harang, R. (1985) Bleomycin and radiation therapy in squamous cell carcinoma of the upper aero-digestive tract: a phase III clinical trial. Int. J. Radiat. Oncol. Biol. Phys. 11, 1877–1886.

Yarnold, J.R., Horwich, A., Duchesne, G., Westbrook, K., Gibbs, J.E. and Peckham, M.J. (1983) Chemotherapy and radiotherapy for advanced testicular nonseminoma. 1. The influence of sequence and timing of drugs and radiation on the appearance of normal tissue damage. Radiother. Oncol. 1, 91–99.

G.G. Steel, G.E. Adams & A. Horwich (Eds.)
The Biological Basis of Radiotherapy, Second Edition
© 1989 Elsevier Science Publishers B.V. (Biomedical Division)

CHAPTER 20

Cellular and tissue effects of hyperthermia and radiation

STANLEY B. FIELD

MRC Cyclotron Unit, Hyperthermia Unit, Hammersmith Hospital, Ducane Road, London W12 OHS, England

---

20.1   Introduction 291

20.2   Rationale for the clinical use of hyperthermia 292

20.3   Biological effects of heat alone or in combination with radiation 293
       20.3.1   Heat alone 294
       20.3.2   Thermotolerance 296
       20.3.3   Step-down sensitization 298

20.4   Interaction between hyperthermia and radiation 298
       20.4.1   Effect of sequence and interval 299
       20.4.2   Re-treatment of previously irradiated tissue 299

20.5   Role of tumour microcirculation and microenvironment 300

20.6   Thermal dose 301

20.1 Introduction

It has been known for more than a century that prolonged fever may lead to regression of malignant disease. However, it was not until the 1960s that a systematic investigation of the anti-cancer effects of hyperthermia began. This included a variety of experimental and clinical studies and also analysis of a vast literature of anecdotal reports. The results confirmed that an increase in temperature by only a few degrees has profound effects on cellular and body functions, and that hyperthermia does have an anti-tumour effect. The biological studies showed that there was a rationale for expecting hyperthermia to have a greater effect on tumours than on normal tissues.

Gradually, the techniques for heating tumours and raising temperatures in situ have been improved and the overall interest and effort in this field has increased dramatically.

Hyperthermia has now been used extensively to treat localised superficial tumours with temperatures in the range of 42–45°C. It has also been used to treat widespread disease, using either whole-body or regional heating at temperatures in the region of 41–42°C. Hyperthermia has an anti-tumour effect if used alone, but appears to be more useful if combined with radiotherapy or chemotherapy.

20.2 Rationale for the clinical use of hyperthermia

There are several reasons why hyperthermia might cause more damage to tumours than to normal tissues. In particular, the vasculature and blood supply in tumours is generally different and inferior to that of normal tissues (Reinhold and Endrich, 1986). Although average blood flow in tumours is not necessarily less than in normal tissues, it is frequently disorganised and heterogeneous, leaving regions of tumours poorly perfused. This has a number of consequences.

1. Some tumours or regions within tumours will have poorer cooling capacity than normal tissues and may thus become hotter in a localised treatment field. There is evidence in man to support this, but the extent to which a temperature differential may occur will vary with tumour, type of treatment and also during the course of a fractionated hyperthermia treatment.
2. Deficiencies in tumour vasculature result in the development of cells which are:
   (a) hypoxic, which (in contrast to X-rays) does not seem to affect markedly their response to hyperthermia.
   (b) at low pH and/or nutrient deficient. Both these factors cause cells to become substantially more sensitive to heat. In addition it is widely believed that tumours have a natural tendency towards anaerobic metabolism and hence low pH (Gullino et al., 1964).
3. Cells in the DNA synthetic phase of the cell cycle are particularly sensitive to heat but relatively resistant to X-rays, so that a combined treatment with hyperthermia and radiotherapy may, in some circumstances, be advantageous.
4. Combining heat with chemotherapeutic drugs may enhance the therapeutic effect either by increasing drug uptake or by enhancing sensitivity to the drugs.
5. It has been suggested that neoplastic cells may be intrinsically more sensitive than the normal cells at risk. However, this possibility remains the subject of discussion and has not been proven.

In summary, hyperthermia is likely to be most effective in poorly perfused regions, which is where radiotherapy and chemotherapy are least effective. A therapeutic gain might, therefore, be obtained by combined treatments. For further discussion of these factors, see Hahn (1982) and Wike-Hooley et al. (1984).

20.3 Biological effects of heat alone or in combination with radiation

Hyperthermia may cause direct cell killing or at lower 'heat doses' may enhance the damage caused by radiation or chemotherapy. In general, temperatures greater than approximately 40°C cause important changes in mammalian cells. However, it is not clear which, amongst these changes, are primarily responsible for cell death and sensitization to other agents. With ionising radiation the principle target is the DNA, and cells die when they attempt to divide. When cells in DNA synthesis are heated, they appear to die as the result of chromosomal injury. However, at other times during the cell cycle, membrane damage is strongly implicated as the primary target, either the plasma membrane or cytoskeleton. It is possible that hyperthermia results in denaturation of a protein as the critical target, possibly a membrane protein, chromosomal protein or repair enzyme (Leeper 1985). Membrane injury causes cells to die and lyse rapidly, i.e., sooner than after equally lethal doses of ionising radiation. Many tissues, especially those that are slowly dividing, respond to hyperthermia far

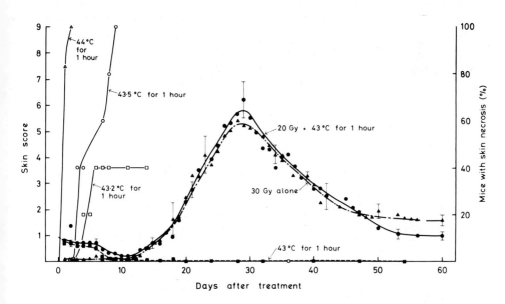

Figure 20.1. The response of the mouse ear to hyperthermia or ionising radiation. Open symbols give the percentage of ears showing necrosis after heat alone (right-hand axis): △, 44°C for 1 hour; o, 43.5°C for 1 hour and □, 43.2°C for 1 hour. Closed symbols give skin reaction using an arbitrary numerical score (left-hand axis). Scores of 1 and 2 indicate degrees of erythema. Scores of 3–9 indicate increasing areas of moist desquamation: ■, hyperthermia alone 43°C for 1 hour; ▲, X-rays alone and ●, X-rays followed by hyperthermia at 43°C for 1 hour. (From Law et al., 1978.)

more quickly than to ionising radiation. Even post-mitotic cells can be rapidly killed by heating.

There are therefore important differences between damage by X-rays and hyperthermia. However, with cells in vitro or with tumours in vivo the differences may not be apparent, because in both these situations the end-points result directly from cell killing, with the mode and timing of cell death hardly affecting the endpoint. It is, however, possible to separate the effects of the two modalities with normal tissues. For example, as illustrated in Figure 20.1, skin shows radiation damage as radio-dermatitis: the injury is enhanced by moderate hyperthermia but remains qualitatively similar to the radiation response in time of appearance and healing (Law et al., 1978). In contrast, severe hyperthermia causes rapid tissue necrosis. The damage appears within 10 days, much earlier than the wave of response that follows irradiation. Similar distinctions have been made with other normal tissues.

20.3.1 Heat alone

In general, the pathology of damage due to hyperthermia is similar to that following a thermal burn, but less severe. Depending on its severity, hyperthermia may be followed by oedema, focal haemorrhage, granulocytic infiltration and even necrosis within the first day or two. Later changes include loss of blood vessels, necrosis, monocyte infiltration and fibrosis. Most observations imply that once the 'acute' response to heat has healed, there are no 'late' effects. Damage to supporting tissues, particularly the vasculature, plays an extremely important role in heat injury, both to tumours and normal tissues. The pathological effects of hyperthermia in various normal tissues have been reviewed by Fajardo (1984).

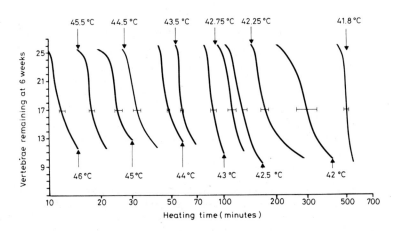

Figure 20.2. Dose-response curves for loss of vertebrae in the tails of young rats. (From Morris and Field, 1985.)

Although it is possible to obtain survival curves after heating in situ, the majority of in vivo studies rely on an assessment of gross tissue response. An example is shown in Figure 20.2 where the probability of causing necrosis in the rat tail is plotted against time of heating at various temperatures. It is seen that at any given temperature, once the time of heating is sufficiently long to reach the threshold of injury, a small further increase in heating time of approximately 20% or an increase in temperature of only 0.5°C will increase the probability of necrosis to 100%. Variations in tissue temperature are impossible to avoid in clinical treatments, and therefore may lead to marked variations in biological response. It is important therefore to monitor temperatures at as many points as possible. On the other hand, if tumours are only slightly more sensitive, or at slightly higher temperatures than the surrounding normal tissues, then hyperthermia should result in a therapeutic advantage.

It is necessary to understand the relationship between temperature and time of heating to produce a given level of response. Such isoeffect curves may be derived from dose-response curves such as those shown in Figure 20.2. An example is given in Figure 20.3 for heat-induced necrosis in the cartilage of the tail of the baby rat. Under normal blood-flow conditions the upper curve was obtained. A transition occurs at 42.5°C, which is fairly typical both for cells and tissues. When the blood supply to the tail was occluded by a clamp, there were two major changes in response. Firstly, the tissue became substantially more sensitive by a factor of approximately 2 in heating time, probably due to reduced pH. Secondly, the transition at 42.5°C was eliminated. This transition is thought to result from the induction of thermotolerance, which is known to be reduced or abolished at low pH (see below).

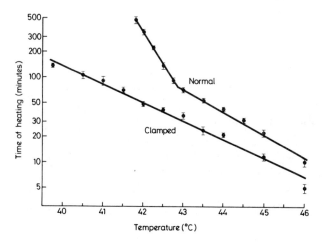

Figure 20.3. Relationships between time of heating and temperature under normal blood-flow conditions to produce a given loss of vertebrae in the tail of a baby rat (upper curve). When the blood supply was clamped during hyperthermia (lower curve) the tissue became substantially more sensitive. (From Morris and Field, 1985.)

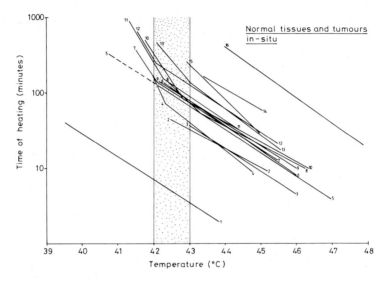

Figure 20.4. Relationship between time of heating and temperature for a given level of damage in a range of normal tissues and tumours in situ. 1, mouse testis weight loss (Hand et al.); 2, rat tumour 9L, heated in vivo, assayed in vitro (Wallen et al.); 3, mouse jejunum LD_{50} (Henle); 4, mouse jejunum, 50% loss of crypts (Hume et al.); 5, mouse sarcoma 180, majority cure (Suit from Crile); 6, baby rat tail, 50% necrosis (Morris et al.); 7, mouse ear skin, 50% necrosis (Law); 8, rat skin epilation (Okumura and Reinhold); 9, baby rat tail, 5% stunting (Morris et al.); 10, baby rat tail (whole tail necrosis) (Morris and Field); 11, mouse tumour C3H/Tif regrowth (Nielsen and Overgaard); 12, mouse tumour F(Sal) (TCD_{50}) (Overgaard and Suit); 13, mouse foot skin epilation (Overgaard and Suit); 14, mouse skin, feet and legs (Robinson et al.); 15, mouse tumour C3H, 50% cures (Robinson et al.); and 16, pig and human skin necrosis and cutaneous burns (Moritz and Henriques). (From Field and Morris, 1983.)

Tumour response (or at least that in some regions of tumours) might be represented by the lower curve in Figure 20.3, whereas normal tissues are more likely to respond as shown in the upper curve. Thus, the maximum differential might be achieved by heating at relatively low temperatures for long times. Unfortunately, this is not very practical clinically.

A summary of in vivo data of the type shown in Figure 20.3 is shown in Figure 20.4. It is seen that the general features of the upper isoeffect curve in Figure 20.3 are retained, the transition occurring between 42 and 43°C. Absolute tissue sensitivity (i.e., the vertical position of the lines) is seen to be extremely tissue-dependent. In general, a change in temperature of 1°C is equivalent to a change in heating time by a factor of 2 at temperatures above the transition and by a factor of 6 below (Field and Morris, 1983).

20.3.2 Thermotolerance

Clinical hyperthermia is normally given in several fractions. A major consideration

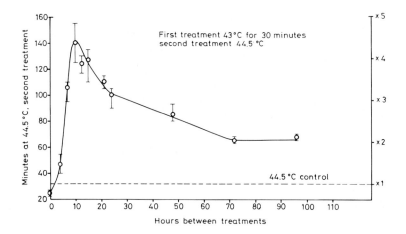

Figure 20.5. Thermotolerance in the rat tail following 43°C for 30 minutes, tested by measuring the time required to cause a given level of necrosis at 44.5°C at various intervals after the initial treatment. The broken line shows the effect of the 44.5° test treatment alone. (From Field and Morris, 1985.)

then becomes the inductance of thermotolerance, i.e., the induction of resistance to subsequent heating. Two types of thermotolerance have been identified, i.e., that which develops during prolonged heating below a critical temperature (about 42°C) and that which develops between individual hyperthermia fractions given at higher temperatures. Thermotolerance is an extremely large effect, but it is transient, the time-course depending on the particular cell type or tissue.

An example of thermotolerance in vivo is shown in Figure 20.5, for necrosis in the rat tail. When treatment at 44.5°C is preceded by a more gentle hyperthermia treatment (which alone appears to cause no change), the tail becomes increasingly resistant to the second treatment. The maximum effect in this case occurred at about 10 hours after the first treatment at which time the duration of heating required to cause a given level of injury was increased by a factor of more than 4. This is followed by decay over several days, the tissue slowly returning towards normal sensitivity.

Almost all cells and tissues show this type of thermotolerance, the maximum extent varying between an increase in heating time of a factor between 2 and 4.5 (Field, 1985).

Both the extent of the maximum thermotolerance and its timing have been shown in vitro and in vivo to be related to the effectiveness of the first treatment. Thus, the greater the effectiveness of the first (or primary) heat dose the greater is the extent of thermotolerance and the longer it takes before the maximum is reached (Nielsen and Overgaard, 1982; Field and Morris, 1985; Dikomey et al., 1988). The time course of thermotolerance in vivo and in vitro is similar, strongly suggesting that it is a cellular, rather than a physiological, phenomenon. Reduced pH causes a reduction in thermotolerance, on which basis it has been suggested that it may be less in some tumours (or regions of tumours) than in normal tissues. However, the experimental studies to date have given no clear indication that tumours have a reduced capacity to develop thermotolerance, and there is no basis for optimism that differences in the development of thermotolerance between normal tissues and tumours may lead to a therapeutic gain (Field, 1985).

The molecular basis for thermotolerance is not well understood, but there are numerous reports that hyperthermia results in the synthesis of a specific set of proteins (heat-stress or heat-shock proteins). There is evidence that thermotolerance is related to one such protein with molecular weight 65–70 kDa (Li and Mivechi, 1986).

The topic of thermotolerance has been reviewed, in detail, by Henle (1987). For a more detailed review of thermotolerance in normal tissues, including the effects of fractionation, the reader is referred to Law (1988).

20.3.3 Step-down sensitization

When cells or tissues are heated to approximately 43°C or above, followed by temperatures of 42°C or below, then the lower temperature becomes more effective than if given alone (Henle, 1980). The effect normally occurs only if the first treatment is above the transition temperature and the second treatment is lower. It is termed 'step-down sensitization' and can be important clinically if there are marked temperature variations during treatment. The time-course is different from that of thermotolerance, step-down sensitization being present immediately after the first heating and decaying far more rapidly.

20.4 Interaction between hyperthermia and radiation

As seen in Figure 20.1, when radiation is combined with a mild heat treatment which alone does not cause any visible damage, the response to radiation may be enhanced. The following list summarises the ways in which radiation responses are influenced by heating:
1. Increased sensitivity to X-rays, i.e., a decrease in D_o.
2. Reduction in the capacity for:
   (i) repair of sublethal damage
   (ii) repair of potentially lethal damage
3. Selectively enhanced effects on the cells in radioresistant phases of the cell cycle (e.g., in late S).

After 'mild hyperthermia' the tissue response to combined treatment is qualitatively similar to the radiation response. It is therefore possible to compute a thermal enhancement ratio (*TER*): the ratio of dose of radiation alone to that with hyperthermia to produce a given level of damage. *TER* values have been measured for a range of normal tissues in different laboratories. It is generally found that the *TER* becomes slightly greater than unity for a 1 hour treatment at 41°C, *TER* values increasing with increasing temperature or time of heating. However, when the results for normal tissues are compared with values for experimental tumours, there does not appear to be a consistently higher *TER* for tumours, as was originally predicted. It is important, therefore, to examine whether the rationale for using hyperthermia alone also applies to hyperthermia when used to enhance the effect of X-rays. The findings are summarised below:

1. Studies in vitro indicate that when heat is used to enhance radiation response, pH is far less important than for direct heat cytotoxicity.
2. It appears that the oxygen enhancement ratio for ionising radiation (about 3 for low LET radiation) does not change significantly for the combination of heat and radiation. Heat enhances radiation injury to hypoxic and oxic cells approximately equally.
3. Only if the tumour becomes hotter than the surrounding normal tissues will the combined treatment give a therapeutic advantage.

Thus the clinical rationale for using heat to enhance radiation damage is weaker than that for heat alone. Other ways must be sought to combine heat with ionising radiation to obtain the advantages of both modalities.

20.4.1 Effect of sequence and interval

It is known from animal studies that the effect of combining heat and radiation is maximal if the two modalities are given simultaneously. As the separation between the two modalities is increased, the enhancing effect decreases. This is true for heat given both before and after irradiation. However, when heat is given after X-rays, the data indicate that the interaction is reduced to zero when the interval is 3–4 hours or greater. When this is so, the two modalities act independently and the heat damage to tumour would be expected to be greater than that to normal tissues for reasons given above.

Heat given 3–4 hours after radiation would therefore be expected to add to the radiation effect, destroying those cells which are resistant to X-rays. It will not enhance the radiation injury so that the radiation dose need not be altered, which is an important advantage. The technique has recently been demonstrated to be clinically effective (Overgaard and Overgaard, 1987).

20.4.2 Re-treatment of previously irradiated tissue

Hyperthermia is often used clinically to treat tumours that have recurred after previous therapy. Most clinicians have reported that such treatment is normally without complications, although a 'recall' effect has been reported for whole-body hyperthermia given after radiotherapy to the central nervous system (Douglas et al., 1981).

Several studies on rodent skin and intestine have shown an increased sensitivity to hyperthermia when heat is given at various times after radiation treatment. The time-course of this increase in heat sensitivity is variable and depends on the prior radiation dose (Law, 1988). Clearly there is an effect of prior radiotherapy and care must be taken in re-treatment, although currently available clinical evidence has so far not shown this to be a problem

20.5 Role of tumour microcirculation and microenvironment

As tumours grow, they incorporate host vasculature and develop new vessels, the proportion of each depending on tumour type, size and site. There are major differences between the vessels in normal tissues and those in most tumours (see review by Reinhold and Endrich, 1986). Tumour vessels tend to be longer and more tortuous and lack smooth muscle. In experimental tumours it has frequently been observed that blood flow is extremely heterogeneous, so that regions exist where perfusion is virtually zero. Also, anaerobic glycolysis is more prevalent in tumours, producing lactic acid which is removed slowly. High interstitial pressure resulting from lack of lymph drainage increases the probability of occlusion. These factors reduce blood flow and removal of lactate and result in a decrease in pH in those areas, which may cause major changes in vascular function and heat response (e.g., Wike-Hooley et al., 1984; Vaupel and Kallinowski, 1987).

Tumour vasculature appears to respond to hyperthermia differently from that of normal tissues. Normal vessels respond by a major increase in blood flow until very high temperatures (46–47°C) are reached after which vascular stasis is induced. In contrast, tumour flow is only marginally increased by hyperthermia with vascular stasis and damage resulting from fairly mild treatments. This important finding, however, has yet to be confirmed in human tumours.

The application of hyperthermia may itself lead to a further reduction in nutrient flow and stasis via several pathways. It is known that the inflammatory response increases sticking of white cells to vessel walls, thus decreasing nutrient flow. High temperatures and low pH cause an increase in erythrocyte rigidity and aggregation and the formation of fibrinogenin gel, all of which decrease effective vascular diameter and cause occlusions. Details of the possible changes can be found in reviews by Jain and Ward-Hartley, 1984; Reinhold and Endrich, 1986; Vaupel and Kallinowski, 1987; Field and Vernon, 1988.

There is, therefore, considerable therapeutic potential for manipulation of blood flow. The potential use of vasoactive agents in hyperthermal treatments has been reviewed by Jain and Ward-Hartley (1984) and Jirtle (1988). Of particular importance to hyperthermia are compounds which selectively reduce flow in tumours, e.g., hydralazine which acts on smooth muscle, therefore increasing flow to normal tissues and possibly 'stealing' blood from the tumour. Administration of hydralazine has been shown in transplanted tumours to decrease blood flow and increase sensitivity to hyperthermia (Horsmann et al., 1988).

20.6 Thermal dose

The definition of thermal dose is difficult. The term 'dose' is itself not very rigidly defined. In radiation biology we are accustomed to using the energy deposited per gm, since this relates clearly and meaningfully to the resulting effect. Pharmacologists use drug concentration or weight, which also relates to effect. With hyperthermia the biological response is primarily dependent on the time at an elevated temperature, not on the deposition of energy (Hahn, 1982).

Dewey et al., (1977) proposed a simple empirical formula, based on in vitro observations:

$$\frac{t_2}{t_1} = R^{T_1 - T_2}$$

as a means of relating treatments with different temperatures (T) and times of heating (t). A review of available data (Field and Morris, 1983) showed that $R = 2$ for $T > 42.5°C$ and $R = 6$ for $T \leq 42.5°C$. Sapareto and Dewey (1984) proposed that 43°C should be used as a reference temperature and that all treatment be described as equivalent minutes of heating at 43°C. This has become known as the Thermal Isoeffect Dose (TID) and by using this formula account can be taken of variations in temperature.

The formula would not apply if there were very large changes in temperature resulting in a significant effect of step-down sensitization or if the time to reach the target temperature was longer than about half an hour, resulting in thermotolerance. Also it must be emphasised that the formula does not account for absolute differences in sensitivity between tissues, nor does it address the problem of varying sensitivity throughout a course of fractionated heat treatments. The use of this isoeffect relationship must therefore be seen as an interim solution to this problem. However, the Dewey formula does provide a practical and reasonable method of comparing hyperthermic treatments under conditions likely to be met in clinical practice (Field, 1987) and the TID is at present the method of choice.

References

Dewey, W.C., Hopwood, L.E., Sapareto, S.A. and Gerweck, L.E. (1977) Cellular responses to combinations

of hyperthermia and radiation. Radiology 123, 463–474.
Dikomey, E., Eickhoff, T. and Jung, H. (1988) Effect of pH on development and decay of thermotolerance in CHO cells using fractionated heating at 43°C. Int. J. Hyperthermia 4, 555–565.
Douglas, M.A., Parks, L.C. and Bebin, J. (1981) Sudden myelopathy secondary to therapeutic total body hyperthermia after spinal-cord irradiation. N. Eng. J. Med. 210, 583–585.
Fajardo, L. (1984) Pathological effects of hyperthermia in normal tissues. Cancer Res. (Suppl.) 44, 4826s–4835s.
Field, S.B. and Vernon, C.C. (1989) Hyperthermia in the treatment of cancer, in 'Treatment of Cancer', 2nd Edn. (Halnan, K. and Sikora, K., eds.), Chapman Hall, London.
Field, S.B. and Morris, C.C. (1983) The relationship between heating time and temperature: its relevance to clinical hyperthermia. Radiother. Oncol. 1, 179–186.
Field, S.B. (1985) Clinical implications of thermotolerance, in: Hyperthermic Oncology, 1984, Vol. 2, (Overgaard, J., ed.), pp. 235–244, Taylor & Francis, London.
Field, S.B. and Morris, C.C. (1985) Experimental studies of thermotolerance in vivo. 1. The baby rat tail model. Int. J. Hyperthermia 1, 235–246.
Field, S.B. (1987) Studies relevant to a means of quantifying the effects of hyperthermia. Int. J. Hyperthermia 3, 291–296.
Gullino, P.M., Clarke, S.H. and Grantham, F.H. (1964) The interstitial fluid of solid tumours. Cancer Res. 24, 780–794.
Hahn, G.M. (1982) Hyperthermia and Cancer, Plenum Press, New York.
Henle, K.J. (1980) Sensitization to hyperthermia below 43°C induced in Chinese hamster ovary cells by step down heating. J. Nat. Cancer Inst. 68, 1033–1036.
Henle, K.J. (1987) Thermotolerance, Vols. I and II, C.R.C. Press.
Horsmann, M.R., Christensen, K.L. and Overgaard, J. (1988) Hydralazine induced enhancement of hyperthermic damage in a C3H mammary carcinoma in vivo. Int. J. Hyperthermia 5, 123–136.
Jain, R.K. and Ward-Hartley, K. (1984) Tumour blood flow characterisation, modifications and role in hyperthermia. IEEE Transact. Sonics Ultrasonics, SU-31, 504–526.
Jirtle, R.L. (1988) Chemical modifications of tumour blood flow. Int. J. Hyperthermia 4, 355–372.
Law, M.P., Ahier, R.G. and Field, S.B. (1978) The response of the mouse ear to heat applied alone or combined with X-rays. Br. J. Radiol. 51, 132–138.
Law, M.P. (1988) The response of normal tissues to hyperthermia. Hyp. Oncol. M. Urano, 1, 121–159. Hypothermic Oncology, 1984, Vol. 1, (Urano, M., ed.), pp. 121–159, Taylor & Francis, London.
Leeper, D.B. (1985) Molecular and cellular mechanisms of hyperthermia alone or combined with other modalities in Hyperthermic Oncology, 1984. Vol. 2, (Overgaard, J., ed.), pp. 9–40, Taylor & Francis, London.
Li, G.C. and Mivechi, N.F. (1986) Thermotolerance in Mammalian Systems, A review, in: Hyperthermia in Cancer Treatment (Anghileri, L.J. and Robert, J. eds.), pp. 59–78, CRC Press, New York.
Morris, C.C. and Field, S.B. (1985) The relationship between heating time and temperature for rat tail necrosis with or without occlusion of the blood supply. Int. J. Radiat. Biol. 47, 41–48.
Nielsen, O.S. and Overgaard, J. (1982) Influence of time and temperature on the kinetics of thermotolerance in L1A2 cells in vitro. Cancer Res. 42, 4190–4196.
Overgaard, J. and Overgaard, M. (1987) Hyperthermia as an adjuvant to radiotherapy in the treatment of malignant melanoma. Int. J. Hyperthermia 3, 483–502.
Reinhold, H.S. and Endrich, B. (1986) Tumour microcirculation as a target for hyperthermia. Int. J. Hyperthermia 2, 111–137.
Sapareto, S.A. and Dewey, W.C. (1984) Thermal dose determination in cancer therapy. Int. J. Radiat. Oncol. Biol. Phys. 10, 787–800.
Vaupel, P. and Kallinowski, F. (1987) Physiological effects of Hyperthermia, in: Recent results in Cancer Research, Vol. 104, pp. 71–109, Springer Verlag, Berlin.

Wike-Hooley, J.L., Haveman, J. and Reinhold, H.S. (1984) The relevance of tumour pH to the treatment of malignant disease. Radiother. Oncol. 2, 343–366.

CHAPTER 21

Prediction of tumour response to treatment

CHARLES S. PARKINS[1] and ALAN HORWICH[2]

[1] Radiotherapy Research Unit, The Institute of Cancer Research, Cotswold Road, Sutton, Surrey SM2 5NG, England and [2] Radiotherapy and Oncology Unit, The Royal Marsden Hospital, Downs Road, Sutton, Surrey SM2 5PT, England

21.1 The concept of predictive testing 305
21.2 Assays of radiosensitivity 306
    21.2.1 Adhesive tumour cell culture system (ATCCS) 306
    21.2.2 Tetrazolium dye reduction (MTT assay) 308
    21.2.3 Micronucleus production 308
21.3 Tumour hypoxia 309
    21.3.1 Direct measurement of hypoxia or tumour vasculature 310
    21.3.2 Tumour metabolic parameters 310
21.4 Tumour cell proliferation 311
    21.4.1 Thymidine analogues and flow cytometry 311
    21.4.2 The Ki67 antibody 313
21.5 Normal-tissue tolerance 314
21.6 Conclusions 314

21.1 The concept of predictive testing

Radiotherapists are often aware of considerable differences in response among patients receiving standard radiotherapy. In current radiotherapeutic practice the prescription is standardised within a hospital for a particular stage and histology of malignant disease, e.g., 64 Gy in 32 fractions over 6.5 weeks for T_3 bladder carcinoma, although this may be modified, for instance in the elderly. There is now considerable interest in the prospect of tailoring radiation treatment more closely to biological factors in the individual. This can be achieved in two ways: either by tailoring the treatment to the properties of the individual tumour, or by adjusting dose on the basis of some individual estimate of normal-tissue tolerance. The research aim is therefore to develop laboratory tests that predict the outcome of radiotherapy independently of known clinical prognostic factors (Peters et al., 1984; Peters et al., 1988).

Predictive testing should be distinguished from prognostic testing: the first aims to predict response to treatment, the second to predict natural history. Clear-cut prognostic factors are those which predict for the relapse outside the radiation field. Examples are erythrocyte sedimentation rate or systemic symptoms in Hodgkin's disease (Horwich et al., 1986), diameter of abdominal nodes in stage 2 seminoma (Gregory and Peckham, 1986) or local nodal involvement in Ca prostate. Prognostic factors usually apply regardless of the modality of local treatment. The essence of predictive testing before radiotherapy is that choice of treatment should be influenced by the result, whether this choice be a different radiotherapy schedule, combined chemotherapy–radiotherapy, or an alternative treatment such as surgery.

Research in this area is currently directed at three main factors that may be predictive: the radiosensitivity of tumour cells, their proliferation rate, and the level of tumour hypoxia.

21.2 Assays of radiosensitivity

The objective here is to obtain information for individual patients on the initial slope of the cell-survival curve. As indicated in Section 12.3, it is believed that the surviving fraction at 2 Gy (SF_2) is a measure of radiosensitivity that correlates to some extent with clinical response to radiotherapy. It can be argued (Section 12.3.2) that SF_2 is a very sensitive determinant of the overall effect of fractionated radiotherapy. This is illustrated in Figure 21.1. If SF_2 ranges from 0.35 to 0.65, the number of cells that survive out of an initial 10^9 cells irradiated with 30 fractions of 2 Gy ranges from 10^{-4} to over 10^3. Similarly, the dose required to leave just 1 surviving cell on average ranges from 40 Gy to nearly 100 Gy.

Can SF_2 be measured for individual patients? The laboratory studies that are reviewed in Chapters 12 and 15 mainly employed the method of Courtenay and Mills (1981). This is a reliable assay that gives relatively high cloning efficiencies with some human tumours and has been used successfully by Tveit et al. (1988) as a chemosensitivity assay. The method is, however, not easily applicable to human biopsy specimens. The following are some more promising approaches.

21.2.1 Adhesive tumour-cell culture system (ATCCS)

Biopsy specimens are disaggregated and plated directly onto plastic tissue-culture dishes (Baker et al., 1986). Plating efficiency is increased by coating the culture dishes

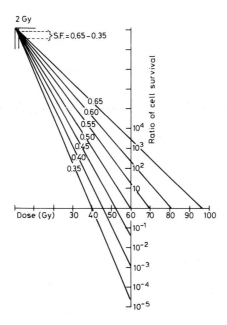

Figure 21.1. The cell kill produced by multi-fraction irradiation depends critically on the cell kill per dose. For an initial population of 10^9 clonogenic cells, the vertical scale shows survival and the horizontal scale is radiation dose (fractions of 2 Gy). Survival is calculated for SF_2 values lying between 0.35 and 0.65 (from Withers, 1986).

with a Cell Adhesive Matrix (CAM, LifeTrac, Irvine, CA) composed of fibrinogen and fibrinopeptides. The medium is supplemented with hormones, transferrin, hydrocortisone, EGF and insulin and cloning efficiencies of around 3% have been achieved in 80% of tumour biopsies. This system has been used to test the sensitivity of human tumour cells both to cytotoxic drugs and to radiation (Ajani et al., 1987; Baker et al., 1988). The results with radiation are consistent with the expected results for in vitro cell lines. Indeed, when the measurements of SF_2 were grouped according to histological type a similar pattern was observed to that shown in Figure 12.3.

The technical details of the assay are briefly as follows. Biopsy specimens are digested to a single suspension using an enzyme cocktail and seeded at 2 to $16 \cdot 10^3$ cells per well on a 24-well culture plate pretreated with CAM. After 24 hours the cells are irradiated with a range of X-ray doses (0–6 Gy) and the surviving cells allowed to grow for a further 13 days. At the end of this time the cells are stained and the integrated optical absorbance (*IA*) is measured using a scanning densitometer. Survival is calculated as the ratio of *IA* values for treated cultures relative to control cultures. Results have agreed well with colony assays on the same cell suspensions. Preliminary results of studies in which the ATCCS is compared with clinical response to radiotherapy are quite promising for the predictive value of this in vitro radiosensitivity test (Peters et al., 1987).

21.2.2 Tetrazolium dye reduction (MTT assay)

Mossman (1983) reported that viable cells could reduce a tetrazolium dye MTT (yellow colour) to an insoluble formazan product (blue crystals). This reaction was studied further by Carmichael et al. (1987a,b) who reported that the assay could be used to estimate cell survival following cytotoxic drug and radiation exposure of human tumour cell lines. The MTT assay is a simple endpoint of mitochondrial function which can readily be automated. The assay has potential as a predictive test because of the short time of about 1 week between seeding the cells and testing response to injury. At this time what is being assayed is not clonal growth but the relative regrowth of surviving cells.

The use of this assay as the basis of a predictive test faces two difficulties that have frustrated many previous attempts (Nissen et al., 1978). First, cell suspensions taken directly from human tumours contain not only malignant cells but also normal connective-tissue cells. When grown in vitro it is frequently found that the normal cells overgrow the tumour cells and a crude measure of cell viability may be unreliable as an assay of tumour cell sensitivity. Secondly, it is well known that cells can undergo one or more cell divisions after irradiation before all their descendents lose reproductive integrity (Section 5.2). If viability is evaluated only a few days after irradiation it is likely that the results will be dominated by doomed cells that will ultimately die.

The current interest in this technique as a predictive test rests on the encouraging data that have come from studies with in vitro cell lines (Carmichael et al., 1987a,b; Wasserman and Twentyman, 1988). It could be that in spite of the drawbacks mentioned above there are tumour types where this simple approach could have predictive value, especially when combined with a selective culture system such as the ATCCS (see above).

21.2.3 Micronucleus production

Micronuclei (MN) are chromosome fragments formed at cell division after treatment of cells by irradiation or other agents that damage the genome. These chromosome fragments are found in the cytoplasm of tumour cells and show a dose-dependent increase in frequency after irradiation. The proportion of cells with micronuclei indicates the loss of reproductive ability and has been found to correlate with clonogenic survival in irradiated cell cultures (Midander and Révész, 1980). These authors found a near-linear dose-effect relationship for MN frequency after both oxic and hypoxic irradiation of Chinese hamster cells and mouse ascites cells, with an estimated oxygen enhancement ratio of 2.4. Similarly, Grote et al. (1981) found a close correlation between MN formation and loss of colony-forming ability in careful studies on Syrian hamster fibroblasts. The clinical usefulness of this assay is supported by the observation that the results correlate in rank order with the TCD_{50} of experimental tumours of widely differing radiosensitivity (Peters et al., 1986). Initial results of MN production in rectal cancers treated with pre-operative irradiation show a good correlation with the outcome of treatment (Streffer et al., 1986).

21.3 Tumour hypoxia

It has long been recognised that hypoxia protects animal tumours from radiation damage and increases the dose required for tumour cure (Chapters 9 and 10). Most of the data in support of this comes from experiments with single exposures or small numbers of fractions, where the dose per fraction was high and the overall treatment time short. Under these conditions there is no doubt that hypoxia is a major cause of radioresistance. However, the animal data also show that as the dose per fraction is reduced and the treatment time increased, hypoxia becomes less important. This is attributed to the phenomenon of reoxygenation (Section 10.6). The role of hypoxia in human tumours is now subject to considerable debate. That most human tumours contain hypoxic cells is generally accepted, although the attempts to detect them using radio-labelled misonidazole have produced variable results (Urtasun et al., 1986). What may be the case, however, is that during conventional fractionated radiotherapy in the clinic reoxygenation is often adequate to reduce the impact of hypoxic cells. This view is supported by the limited success of radiosensitization with misonidazole (Section 10.3).

The view that hypoxia is always important in radiotherapy has therefore now changed to one in which it is believed that hypoxia limits radiotherapy under certain circumstances. These are set out in detail in Chapter 10. In particular:
(i) there may be a minority of tumour types that reoxygenate poorly and within which hypoxia remains a serious problem;
(ii) if treatment is accelerated in order to beat tumour cell repopulation (Section 13.2), the effect of slow reoxygenation may be increased.

It is in the context of such situations that it would be extremely valuable to have methods of detecting tumour hypoxia in individual patients.

An important conceptual problem that all methods face is that what matters radiobiologically is the *hypoxic fraction of clonogenic cells*. Since clonogenic cells may comprise only a small minority of tumour cells (Section 4.1) gross measures of tumour hypoxia may prove to be misleading. For example, as discussed in Section 11.3, a sudden improvement in oxygen transport might lead to a transient increase in oxygen diffusion distance. If the clonogenic hypoxic cells form a thin shell (perhaps only one or two cells thick) at a distance of perhaps 100 μm from blood vessels, then a small increase in diffusion distance might abolish hypoxia in clonogenic cells whilst the total tumour hypoxia, being dominated by a necrotic core, might change very little.

21.3.1 Direct measurement of hypoxia or tumour vasculature

A direct measurement of hypoxia within tumour tissue can be made by use of microelectrodes (Cater, 1964). This is technically difficult, because oxygen electrodes with a diameter of several hundred microns produce severe tissue damage and disturb the micro-circulation and local oxygen consumption. Computer tomography using guided probes allow the pattern of oxygen tension to be mapped more accurately (Gatenby et al., 1985). Further developments that allow accurate detection of cells at low oxygen tensions are needed, especially at the tensions which protect cells from radiation damage (Koch, 1984). An alternative procedure for determining oxygenation status in tumours is to measure the oxyhaemoglobin saturation of individual red blood cells within microvessels (Grunewald and Lubbers, 1976) using cryo-microphotometry. Frequency histograms of the HbO_2 saturation within rat carcinosarcomas have shown a significant proportion of cells with HbO_2 values below 5% saturation. This proportion was reduced significantly when the animals breathed oxygen at 1 or 2 atmospheres pressure (Mueller-Kleiser and Vaupel, 1983). The usefulness of this assay as a predictor is yet to be defined.

One possible indicator of the vascular supply within tumours is the intercapillary distance (ICD). Since the initial observation by Thomlinson and Gray (1955) that necrotic areas form beyond about 100 μm from patent capillaries, it seems likely that regions within tumours where the distances between capillaries are large could have a high proportion of hypoxic cells. Kolstad (1968) reported that the local recurrence rate in cervix carcinomas was higher if the mean ICD was greater than 300 μm. These findings were confirmed by Awwad et al. (1988) and by a study relating vascular density in the stroma of cervix cancer biopsies with the 5-year survival after radiotherapy (Siracka et al., 1982).

21.3.2 Tumour metabolic parameters

The potential use of radiolabelled compounds as markers for metabolic changes within tumours relies on the accurate and specific localisation of the marker. Techniques such as Positron Emission Tomography (PET) help to meet these requirements. ^{15}O has been used in brain tumours for measurement of blood flow and oxygen metabolism and ^{18}F-labelled deoxyglucose (FDG) has been used for measuring glucose metabolism. The oxygen extraction, oxygen metabolic rate and blood flow were lower in tumours than most normal tissues (Ito et al., 1982). Using these techniques it is also possible to determine the relationship between glycolysis and oxidative metabolism in human tumours in vivo. At present, insufficient data are available to determine whether these assays show any predictive ability, but it is likely that the low sensitivity will preclude detection of small populations of hypoxic tumour cells.

Magnetic resonance spectroscopy allows the in vivo levels of phosphorous-containing substrates to be determined non-invasively, both in animals and in man (Okunieff et al., 1986). Characteristic changes in the levels of ATP, ADP, AMP, inorganic phosphate, phosphocreatinine and other metabolites define anaerobic and aerobic metabolism, though how these changes relate to radiobiologically significant hypoxia is yet to be determined.

21.4 Tumour-cell proliferation

As described in Section 13.2, there is a growing realisation that repopulation by surviving clonogenic cells during fractionated radiotherapy could in some cases be a significant cause of failure. Cell proliferation rate is known to vary widely among human tumours (Chapter 6) and thus there is a need to select those patients in whom repopulation is most likely to be a problem. The appropriate response would then be to accelerate treatment in these cases.

21.4.1 Thymidine analogues and flow cytometry

A large body of data exists on cell kinetic parameters obtained using [^{3}H]thymidine labelling and autoradiography (Steel, 1977). Tumour biopsies can be labelled in vitro with thymidine, but the penetration of labelling within small fragments is limited.

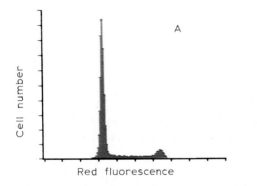 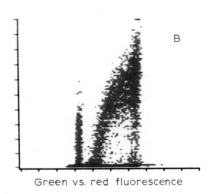

Figure 21.2. Flow-cytometric analysis of BUdR incorporation into a human bladder carcinoma xenograft. The histogram was obtained from a biopsy taken 4 hours after injection of the DNA precursor. The left-hand panel shows the distribution of DNA content, with a large G_1 peak and a smaller G_2 peak. The right-hand panel shows BUdR uptake vertically and DNA content horizontally. The BUdR-labelled cells have moved during the 4 hours period towards G_2 and their distribution within the S-phase region is asymmetric. The relative movement of these cells ($RM = 0.73$) is used to calculate the duration of the S-phase ($T_s = 12.2$ hours) and the potential doubling time (T_{pot}) which was 5.6 days.

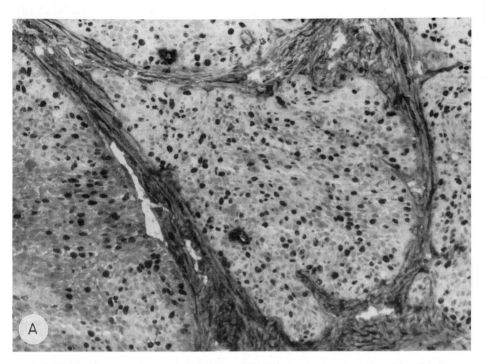

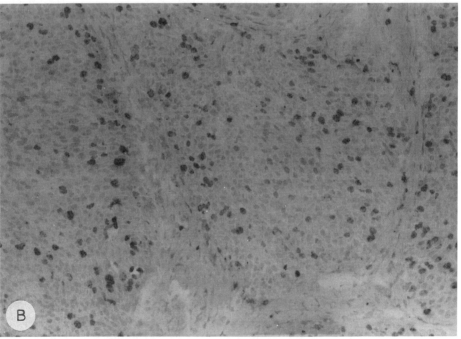

This can be overcome by incubation under high oxygen tension (Steel and Bensted, 1965). Thymidine labelling has been successfully used by a number of investigators, for instance Meyer and Lee (1980) and Silvestrini et al. (1988).

Recently, a monoclonal antibody has been developed that recognises bromo-deoxyuridine (BUdR) or iodo-deoxyuridine (IUdR) in DNA (Gratzner, 1982). Since BUdR and IUdR are analogues of thymidine, they also are taken up by cells that are synthesizing DNA. The advantage of this antibody technique is that BUdR or IUdR are non-toxic and non-radioactive and thus they can more readily be given in vivo to patients. The incorporated BUdR or IUdR can be detected by antibody binding and visualised by immunohistochemical staining of tissue sections or using flow cytometry (FCM) on cell or nuclear suspensions (Dolbeare et al., 1983). This is illustrated in Figures 21.2 and 21.3.

Wilson et al. (1985) demonstrated that sufficient incorporation was achieved after an intravenous injection of 500 mg of BUdR. No side effects have been reported after this dosage, although it is known that sensitization of the skin to sunlight occurs in patients given high doses of the drug as a radiosensitizer. The iodo-substituted precursor (IUdR) is an acceptable alternative to BUdR (Begg et al., 1988) and does not cause radiosensitization.

The FCM provides a fast analysis on a large number of cells. Most tumour cells are aneuploid and the method is usually able to separate the FCM peak for host diploid cells from that for aneuploid tumour cells. If a biopsy is taken 4 to 8 hours after BUdR injection, the relative position of the pulse-labelled S-phase cells indicates the rate of progression of cells through the cell cycle (Begg et al., 1985; White and Meistrich, 1986). The relative movement (RM) of these S-phase cells is used to estimate both T_s and the potential doubling time (T_{pot}, Section 6.3.3). The T_{pot} for a range of human tumours has been found to be surprisingly short, in the range 2 to 20 days (Wilson et al., 1988). It is also possible to obtain ploidy and S-phase indices from paraffin-embedded tissues (Hedley et al., 1983) using flow-cytometry. The estimates are probably less accurate than for the BUdR method but this does allow for retrospective analyses to be performed.

21.4.2 The Ki67 antibody

The Ki67 antibody (Gerdes et al., 1983) is claimed to recognise a nuclear antigen on

---

Figure 21.3. Proliferation markers in sections of human tumours.
(A) Ki67 antigen labelling in a section of human bladder tumour xenograft. Positive nuclei appear darkly stained using an indirect immuno-peroxidase technique. Negatively stained nuclei appear lighter due to the haematoxylin counter stain. The Ki67 labelling index was 31%.
(B) Incorporation of BUdR into the same bladder tumour xenograft. Using a monoclonal antibody specific for BUdR, and an indirect immuno-peroxidase technique as for Ki67, the BUdR labelling index was 19%.

proliferating human cells. It is thus thought to be expressed by cells throughout the cell cycle, but probably not by cells that are out of cycle. Although it is described as staining the growth fraction, this has yet to be confirmed by detailed kinetic studies.

The immuno-histochemical staining procedure is applied to cryostat tumour sections and is simple and fast (Figure 21.3). Ki67 indices for human breast, brain, lung and lymphoid tumours have been reported (McGurrin et al., 1987; Burger et al., 1986; Gatter et al., 1986; Schrape et al., 1987). The values range from virtually zero to 20% in some types of brain tumour or as high as 60% in high-grade breast tumours. In each case the Ki67 index correlated well with the histological grade and with other known prognostic factors. Although there is no firm theoretical basis for regarding the Ki67 index as a measure of T_{pot} or tumour cell repopulation rate, the index is simple to obtain and could prove to be a useful predictive factor.

21.5 Normal-tissue tolerance

It is widely recognised that patients on a standard radiotherapy schedule differ in severity of normal-tissue reaction. The reasons for this are not known but if it were possible to predict for normal-tissue tolerance and to exclude a sensitive sub-group, the radiation dose to the more tolerant patients could be increased, and an improvement in response is to be expected (Lewis, 1987). Experiments on patients with genetically linked disorders have revealed some whose connective-tissue cells or lymphocytes are more radiosensitive than normal (Arlett et al., 1988; Little et al., 1988). The question has been raised whether tumours that arise in radiosensitive patients are also more radiosensitive than usual, but the answer to this is not yet known.

What is now required are detailed studies of the relationship between various measures of normal-tissue sensitivity and the incidence of early and late normal-tissue damage following radiotherapy.

21.6 Conclusions

This is an area of development in radiotherapy which at the present time is at a tantalising stage. There are strong grounds for believing that radiosensitivity, hypoxia and cell proliferation rate vary widely among human tumours and that each of these factors may be related to clinical failure. Assays are available that allow them to be evaluated in the clinical setting. Such information will not be useful unless realistic ways of responding to it in clinical management can be identified. Table 21.1 indicates some of the possible options.

What now are required are careful tests of the predictability of the assays that have been described in this chapter, first to establish a firm correlation with clinical

TABLE 21.1
Modifications to conventional treatment according to results of predictive tests

	Observation	Action
Tumour-cell kinetics	Low proliferative index	No modification of overall time during conventional treatment.
	High proliferative index	Accelerated fractionation
Tumour radiosensitivity	Low tumour sensitivity	Radiation modifiers High LET radiation Alternative modality Hyperfractionation
	High tumour sensitivity	No modification to total or dose per fraction. Decrease total dose?
Normal tissue radiosensitivity	High Low	Decrease total dose (?) Increase total dose

outcome, then to find whether modification of management on the basis of the assays leads to improved results.

References

Ajani, J.A., Baker, F.L., Spitzer, G., Kelly, A., Brock, W., Tomasovic, B., Singletary, S.E., McMurtrey, M. and Plager, C. (1987) Comparison between clinical response and in vitro drug sensitivity of primary human tumours in the adhesive tumour cell culture system. J. Clin. Oncol. 5, 12, 1912–1921.

Arlett, C.F., Green, M.H.L., Priestly, A., Harcourt, S.A. and Mayne, L.V. (1988) Comparative human cellular radiosensitivity. I. The effect of SV40 transformation and immortalisation on the gamma-irradiation survival of skin derived fibroblasts from normal individuals and from ataxia-telangiectasia patients and heterozygotes. Int. J. Radiat. Biol. 54, 911–928.

Awwad, H.K., Naggar, M., Mocktar, N. and Barsoum, M. (1988) Intercapillary distance measurement as an indicator of hypoxia in carcinoma of the cervix uteri. Int. J. Radiat. Oncol. Biol. Phys., in press.

Baker, F.L., Spitzer, G., Ajani, J., Brock, W.A., Lukeman, J., Pathak, S., Tomasovic, B., Theilvoldt, D., Williams, M., Vines, C. and Tofilon, P. (1986) Drug and radiation sensitivity measurements of successful primary monolayer culturing of human tumour cells using cell-adhesive matrix and supplemented medium. Can. Res. 46, 1263–1274.

Baker, F.L., Ajani, J., Spitzer, G., Tomasovic, B.J., Williams, M., Finders, M. and Brock, W.A. (1988) High colony-forming efficiency of primary human tumour cells cultured in the adhesive-tumour-cell culture system: improvements with medium and serum alterations. Int. J. Cell Clon. 6, 95–105.

Begg, A.C., McNally, N.J., Shrieve, D.C. and Karcher, H. (1985) A method to measure duration of DNA synthesis and the potential doubling time from a single sample. Cytometry 6, 620–626.

Begg, A.C., Moonen, L., Hofland, I., Dessing, M. and Barletlink, H. (1988) Human tumour cell kinetics using a monoclonal antibody against iododeoxyuridine: intratumour sampling variations. Radiother. Oncol. 11, 337–347.

Burger, P.C., Shibata, T. and Kleihues, P. (1986) The use of the monoclonal antibody Ki67 in the identification of proliferating cells. Am. J. Surg. Pathol. 10, 611–617.

Carmichael, J., Degraff, W.G., Gazdar, A.F., Minna, J.D. and Mitchell, J.B. (1987a) Evaluation of a tetrazolium based semi-automated colorimetric assay. 1. Assessment of chemosensitivity testing. Cancer Res. 47, 936–942.

Carmichael, J., Degraff, W.G., Gazdar, A.F., Minna, J.D. and Mitchell, J.B. (1987b) Evaluation of a tetrazolium-based semi-automated colorimetric assay. 2. Assessment of radiosensitivity. Cancer Res. 47, 943–946.

Cater, D.B. (1964) Oxygen tensions in neoplastic tissues. Tumori 50, 435–444.

Courtenay, V.D. and Mills, J. (1981) An in vitro colony assay for human tumours grown in immune-suppressed mice and treated in vivo with cytotoxic agents. Br. J. Cancer 37, 261–268.

Dolbeare, F.A., Gratzner, H.G., Pallavincini, M.G. and Gray, J.W. (1983) Flow cytometric measurements of total DNA content and incorporated bromodeoxyuridine. Proc. Natl. Acad. Sci. USA 80, 5573–5577.

Gatenby, R.A., Coia, L.R., Richter, M.P., Katz, H., Moldofsky, P.J., Engstrom, P., Brown, D.Q., Brookland, R. and Broder, G.J. (1985) Oxygen tension in human tumours: in vivo mapping using CT-guided probes. Radiology 156, 211–214.

Gatter, K.C., Dunnill, M.S., Gerdes, J., Stein, H. and Mason, D.Y. (1986) New approach to assessing lung tumours in man. J. Clin. Pathol. 39, 590–593.

Gerdes, J., Schwab, U., Lemke, H. and Stein, H. (1983) Production of a mouse monoclonal antibody reactive with human nuclear antigen associated with cell proliferation. Int. J. Cancer 31, 13–16.

Gratzner, H. (1982) Monoclonal antibody to 5-bromo and 5-iododeoxyuridine: a new reagent for detection of DNA replication. Science 218, 474–475.

Gregory, C. and Peckham, M.J. (1986) Results of radiotherapy for stage 2 testicular seminoma. Radiother. Oncol. 6, 285–292.

Grote, S.J., Joshi, G.P., Revell, S.H. and Shaw, C.A. (1981) Observations of radiation-induced chromosome fragment loss in live mammalian cells in culture and its effect on colony-forming ability. Int. J. Radiat. Biol. 39, 395–408.

Grunewald, W.A. and Lubbers, D.W. (1976) Kryomicrophotometry as a method for analysing the intercapillary HbO_2 saturation of organs under different O_2 supply conditions. Adv. Exp. Med. Biol. 75, 55–64.

Hedley, D.W., Friedlander, M.L. and Taylor, I.W. (1983) Application of DNA flowcytometry to paraffin-embedded archieval material for study of aneuploidy and its clinical significance. Cytometry 6, 327–333.

Horwich, A., Easton, D., Nogueira-Costa, T., Liew, K.H., Colman, M. and Peckham, M.J. (1986) An analysis of prognostic factors in early stage Hodgkin's disease.

Ito, M., Lammertsma, A.A., Wise, R.J.S., Bernardi, S., Frackowiak, R.S.J., Heather, J.D., McKenzie, C.G., Thomas, D.G.T. and Jones, T. (1982) Measurement of regional cerebral blood flow and oxygen utilisation in patients with cerebral tumours, using ^{15}O and positron emission tomography: analytical techniques and preliminary results. Neuroradiology 23, 63–74.

Koch, C.J. (1984) A thin film culturing technique allowing rapid gas-liquid equilibrium (6 seconds) with no toxicity to mammalian cells. Rad. Res. 97, 434–442.

Kolstad, P. (1968) Vascularisation, oxygen tension and local recurrence in cervix cancer. Scan. J. Clin. Lab. Invest. 106, 145–147.

Lewis, P. (1987) Variation in individual sensitivity to ionising radiation, in: Radiation and Health (Jones, R.R. and Southwood, R. eds.), John Wiley & Sons, New York.

Little, J.B., Nove, J., Strong, L.C. and Nichols, W.W. (1988) Survival of human diploid skin fibroblasts from normal individuals after X-irradiation. Int. J. Radiat. Biol. 54, 899–910.

McGurrin, J.F., Doria, M.I., Dawson, P.J., Karrison, T., Stein, H.O. and Franklin, W.A. (1987) Assessment of tumour cell kinetics by immunohistochemistry in carcinoma of breast. Cancer 59, 1744–1750.

Meyer, J.S. and Lee, J.Y. (1980) Relationships of S-phase fraction of breast carcinoma in relapse to duration of remission, estrogen receptor content, therapeutic responsiveness, and duration of survival. Cancer Res. 40, 1890–1896.

Midander, J. and Révész, L. (1980) The frequency of micronuclei as a measure of cell survival in irradiated cell populations. Int. J. Radiat. Biol. 38, 237–241.

Mossman, T. (1983) Rapid colorimetric assay for cellular growth and survival: application to proliferation and cytotoxic assays. J. Immunol. Methods 65, 55–63.
Mueller-Kleiser, W. and Vaupel, P. (1983) Tumour oxygenation under normobaric and hyperbaric conditions. Br. J. Radiol. 56, 559–564.
Nissen, E., Tanneberger, St., Projan, A., Morack, G. and Peek, U. (1978) Recent results of in vitro drug prediction in human tumour chemotherapy. Arch. Geschwulstforsch. 48, 667–672.
Okunieff, P.G., Koutcher, J.A., Gerwick, L., McFarland, E., Hitzig, B., Urano, M., Brady, T., Neuringer, L. and Suit, H.D. (1986) Tumour-size-dependent changes in a murine fibrosarcoma: use of in vivo ^{31}P NMR for non-invasive evaluation of tumour metabolic status. Int. J. Radiat. Biol. Oncol. Phys. 12, 793–799.
Peters, L.J., Hopwood, L.E., Withers, H.R. and Suit, H.D. (1984) Predictive assays of tumour radiocurability. Cancer Treatment Symp. 1, 67–74.
Peters, L.J., Brock, W.A., Johnson, T., Meyn, R.E., Tofilon, P.J. and Milas, L. (1986) Potential methods for predicting tumour radiocurability. Int. J. Radiat. Oncol. Biol. Phys. 12, 439–467.
Peters, L.J., Baker, F.L., Goepfert, H., Campbell, B.H., Rich, T.A. and Brock, W.A. (1987) Prediction of tumour response from radiosensitivity of cultured biopsy specimens, in: Proceedings of the 8th International Congress of Radiation Research (Edinburgh, Scotland), July 19–24, pp. 831–836, Taylor & Francis, London.
Peters, L.J., Brock, W.A., Chapman, J.D., Wilson, G. and Fowler, J.F. (1988) Response predictors in radiotherapy: a review of research into radiobiologically based assays. Br. J. Radiol. (Suppl.) 22, 96–108.
Schrape, S., Jones, D.B. and Wright, D.H. (1987) A comparison of three methods for the determination of the growth fraction in non-Hodgkin's lymphoma. Br. J. Cancer 55, 283–286.
Silvestrini, R., Costa, A., Vereroni, S., Del Bino, G. and Persici, P. (1988) Comparative analysis of different approaches to investigate cell kinetics. Cell Tissue Kinet. 21, 123–131.
Siracka, E., Siracky, J., Pappova, N. and Révész, L. (1982) Vascularisation and radiocurability in cancer of the uterine cervix. Neoplasm 29, 183–188.
Steel, G.G. (1977) Growth Kinetics of Tumours. Oxford University Press, Oxford.
Steel, G.G. and Bensted, J.P.M. (1965) In vitro studies of cell proliferation in tumours. 1. Critical appraisal of methods and theoretical considerations. Eur. J. Cancer 2, 275–279.
Streffer, C., Beuningen, D., Gross, E., Schabronath, J., Eigler, F.W. and Rebman, A. (1986) Predictive assays for the therapy of rectum carcinoma. Radiother. Oncol. 5, 303–310.
Thomlinson, R.H. and Gray, L.H. (1955) The histological structure of some human lung cancers and the possible implication for radiotherapy. Br. J. Cancer 9, 539–549.
Tveit, K.M., Gundersen, J., Hoie, J. and Pihl, A. (1988) Predictive chemosensitivity testing in malignant melanoma: reliable methodology – ineffective drugs. Br. J. Cancer 58, 734–737.
Urtasun, R.C., Chapman, J.D., Raleigh, J.A., Franco, A.J. and Koch, C.J. (1986) Binding of [^{3}H]misonidazole to solid human tumours as a measure of tumour hypoxia. Int. J. Radiat. Oncol. Biol. Phys. 12, 1263–1267.
Wasserman, T.H. and Twentyman, P.R. (1988) Use of a colorimetric (MTT) assay in determining the radiosensitivity of solid murine tumours. Int. J. Radiat. Oncol. Biol. Phys. 15, 699–702.
White, R.A. and Meistrich, M.L. (1986) A comment on 'A method to measure the duration of DNA synthesis and the potential doubling time from a single sample'. Cytometry 7, 486–490.
Wilson, G.D., McNally, N.J., Dunphy, E., Karcher, H. and Pfragner, R. (1985) The labelling index of human and mouse tumours assessed by bromodeoxyuridine staining in vitro and in vivo and flow cytometry. Cytometry 6, 641–647.
Wilson, G.D., McNally, N.J., Dische, S., Saunders, M.I., DesRochers, C., Lewis, A.A. and Bennett, M.H. (1988) Measurement of cell kinetics in human tumours in vivo using bromodeoxyuridine incorporation and flow cytometry. Br. J. Cancer 58, 423–431.

Subject index

Accelerated radiotherapy, 142, 182, 184, 214, 217
Adhesive tumour-cell culture system (ATCCS), 306
Alpha component, 174
Alpha/beta ratio, 95, 167–168, 173, 188, 231
   for human tissues, 193
   table of, 190
Anaemia, radiotherapeutic impact, 136, 138, 147
Ataxia-telangiectasia (AT), 31, 33, 39
   possible consequences of misrepair, 25

BUdR, see Bromodeoxyuridine
Beta parameter, measure of cellular recovery, 173
Biologically effective dose (BED), 189–196
Bioreductive drugs, 155–156
Blood flow, alterations in, 148
Blood pressure, effect on tumour perfusion, 140
Blood vessels, radiation effects, 101, 107
Bragg peak, 252
Brain, time-scale of radiation damage, 111

Bromodeoxyuridine (BUdR), 7, 184, 311, 313
Buthionine sulphoximine (BSO), 35, 124

Carbogen breathing, for radiosensitization, 140
Cell adhesive matrix (CAM) assay, 165
Cell cycle, in tumours, 81
   variation in radiosensitivity, 32
Cell death, after irradiation, 67
   modes of, 91
Cell loss from tumours, 83–84, 184
Cell proliferation in tumours, 80
Cell proliferation, in response to treatment, 87
Cell survival, 46, 47, 66
   assays, 47, 54–55, 164
   clinical correlation, 170
   calculated from tumour regrowth, 119
   calculated for fractionation schedules, 198
   and failure of normal tissues, 61
   and gross response to treatment, 59, 65
   following in vivo irradiation of tumours, 55
   for human tumour cells, 167
   models, 48, 54
   (see also SF_2)

Subject index

Central nervous system (CNS), radiation damage to, 90
CHART, Accelerated radiotherapy, 142, 197–198
Chemosensitization, 157–158
Chemotherapy, cell survival following, 56
    concomitant radiosensitivity, 33
    control of metastatic disease, 269
    classification of agents, 57
    drug resistance, 58
Chemotherapy–radiotherapy, exploitable mechanisms, 268, 275
    clinical objectives, 282–284
    timing of, 273, 280
Chromatin structure, 38
Chromosome aberrations, 9, 24
Clinical radioresponse of tumours, classification, 169
Clonogenic cell surival, see cell survival
Clonogenic cells, concept, 46, 66
    kinetic status, 86, 198
    regrowth of, 59
Clonogenic fraction, 69
CNS syndrome, 91, 111
Conformation of DNA, 38
Contact effect on radiosensitivity, 165
Courtenay assay, 164
CRE formula, 189, 212
Cycle phase-specific drugs, 57
Cysteine, 128–129
Cytotoxic drugs, see Chemotherapy

DNA, charged-particle tracks through, 8–9
DNA damage, 15–17, 34
    biological consequences, 23
DNA strand breakage, clean, blunt, cohesive, 16
    and chromosomal aberrations, 24
    dose–effect relationship, 20
    methods of detection, 18
DNA repair, 36–37
DNA, target for cell killing, 6
DNA transfection, 37
Depth-dose distribution, of charged-particle beam, 252
Descriptive and operational cell kinetics, 77
Dithioerithritol (DTE), 129
Dose per fraction, see Fractionation
Dose-rate effect, 53, 227
    biological mechanisms, 223
    in human tumour cells, 226
    in normal tissues, 229
    models of, 227
Double-strand DNA breaks (see DNA damage)
Dual theory of radiation action, 10–11

Early and late normal-tissue reactions, 89, 185–211
    α/β ratio, 190
    table of parameters, 95
ED_{50}, 231
Electron-affinic radiosensitizers (see Radiosensitizers)
Endothelial cells, radiation effects, 102, 103–105
Enhancement of tumour response, by chemotherapy, 268, 272
Envelope of additivity, 272
Epidermal proliferative unit (EPU), 98
Ethiophos (WR2721), 129
Excision repair of DNA strand breaks, 36
Exonucleases, 21

Fixation of radiation damage, 35
Flexible (F-type) tissues, 73

Flow cytometry, 311
  measurement of T_{pot}, 184
Fluorinated hydrocarbons, 127, 140, 150
Fractionated radiotherapy, historical background, 210
  comparisons of schedules, 197
  dependence on cell kill per dose, 307
  fraction size, 186, 211
Free-radical reactions, 4, 12

Genes, involved in radiosensitivity and repair, 40
Germinal tissue, radiation damage to human, 94
Glutathione (GSH), 35, 124–128
Growth fraction, 82
Growth rate of human tumours, 78–80

Haemoglobin levels, prognostic significance, 136, 146
Haemoglobin saturation curve, modification, 141, 147–148
Haemopoietic tissues, radiation damage to human, 96
Half-times for recovery, 228
Heat, see Hyperthermia
Heavy particles, in radiotherapy, 249–264
  depth-dose distributions, 251
  physical advantages, 262
Hierarchical (H-type tissues), 73, 90–92
High LET component in low LET radiation, 176
High LET radiotherapy, rationales, 260
  clinical results, 260
  early and late reactions, 259
  microdosimetry, 8–9
Hydralazine, 149, 157
Hydrated electron, 3
Hydroxytryptamine (5-HT), 149
Hyperbaric oxygen, 136–137, 146

Hyperfractionation, 182, 187, 201, 214–216
Hyperthermia, 291–303
  combination with radiation, 293, 298
  dose-response curves, 294
  rationale for clinical use, 292
  re-treatment of previously irradiated tissue, 299
  step-down sensitization, 298
  thermal dose, 301
  thermal tolerance, 296–298
  time-temperature plots, 295, 296
Hypofractionation, 213
Hypothermia, 141
Hypoxia in normal tissues, induction, 127
Hypoxia in tumours, impact, 115
  detection, 121–123, 309
  exploitation, 158
  toxicity of bioreductive drugs, 155–156
Hypoxic cell sensitizers (see Radiosensitizers)
Hypoxic fraction of clonogenic cells, 55, 309

Immune-deficient mice, for xenografting, 165
Immune system, radiation effects, 97
Incomplete repair (IR) model, 53, 224–232
Independent toxicity of radiotherapy and chemotherapy, 270
Inherited diseases exhibiting radiosensitivity, 30
Initial DNA damage, 34
Initial slope, see SF_2
Intercapillary distance (ICD), 310
Interstitial radiotherapy, 240–242
  concept of curative zones, 232
  isoeffect curve, 238
Intestine, radiation damage to, 97
Intracavitary radiotherapy, 232, 239

Subject index

Iodo-deoxyuridine (IUdR), 184, 313
Ionisation, by charged particles, 3, 8–9
  see also Linear energy transfer
Isoeffect curves, fractionation, 186–188

K-curve (for oxygen sensitization), 118, 128–129, 147
Ki67 antibody, 313

Labelled mitoses curves on human tumours, 81
Late normal-tissue reactions, 185
Late reactions, α/β ratio, 190
Lethal–potentially lethal damage (LPL) model, 52, 224–228
Linear component of cell killing, 50, 173–174
  nature of, 176
Linear energy transfer (LET), 3, 251
  and OER, RBE, 255
Linear-quadratic model, 49, 187–189, 212
  addition of time factors, 195
  implications for recovery, 173
  parameters for human tumour cells, 168
Local multiply-damaged sites (LMDS), 176
Local tumour control, 60
Low dose-rate radiobiology, therapeutic implications, 226–233
  external beam, 243
  fractionated, 230

Membranes, radiation damage to, 39
Metronidazole sensitization, 125
Micronucleus production, 308
Misonidazole, 125, 130, 136, 151–155
  chemosensitization, 157
  uptake in hypoxic cells, 123, 138, 158
Misrepair, of DNA damage, 35, 52

Mitomycin C, 151, 155
Multiple fractions per day, 214
  intervals between doses, 202
  mucosal reactions, 219
Mutlitarget model, 48
Mutation and survival, relationship between, 7

NSD formula, 189, 195, 212
Neutral filter elution, 20
Neutron therapy, 253, 261
Normal tissue responses to radiation, 72
  prediction of, 314

Overall time, in fractionated radiotherapy, 183–184, 195
Oxygen delivery to tissues, 125, 147
Oxygen effect, 12, 118
  clinical consequences, 135–137
  manipulation of, 141
Oxygen tension, within normal tissues, 116
Oxygen tension, within tumour cords, 117
Oxygen transport, modification, 148
Oxygen, sensitization by normobaric, 126

pH, and hyperthermia, 292
pH, effect on sensitizing efficiency, 152
PLD recovery (see Recovery)
Particle tracks, structure of, 9, 254
Perfluorocarbons (see Fluorinated hydrocarbons)
Peripheral blood counts, radiation effects, 96
Pi mesons, 252
Plasmids, in DNA repair studies, 25, 37
Pneumonitis, after low dose-rate TBI, 243

Positron emission tomography (PET), 310
Potential doubling time (T_{pot}), 83, 184, 313
Potentially lethal damage recovery (PLD), 35, 172
Predictive testing, concept of, 305
  assays of radiosensitivity, 306
  for repopulation rate, 311–313
  possible responses, 315
Prodromal responses, 90
Proliferation, in early- and late-reacting tissues, 183
  in low dose-rate irradiation, 225
  in tumours, 183
Proliferation-dependent drugs, 57
Protection of normal tissues, 268–271
Proton therapy, 262

Q-factor, 51

Radiation chemistry of DNA, 11
Radioprotection, chemical, 128
Radiosensitivity of human tumour cells, 166
  correlation with clinical response, 170
  molecular basis, 29
  variation with oxygen tension, 118
Radiosensitization, by increased oxygen delivery, 125
Radiosensitizers, chemical, 123, 145–162
  combination with radioprotectors, 130
  dual-function, 153
  effect of thiol depletion, 124
  etanidazole (SR-2508), 138, 151
  pimonidazole (Ro 03-8799), 138–139, 151–152
  RSU 1069, 149–158
Radiotherapy–chemotherapy: see Chemotherapy–radiotherapy

RBE, see Releative biological effectiveness
Reassortment or Redistribution, 187, 223
  in neutron therapy, 257
Recombinant DNA technology, 37
Recovery, definition, 35, 223
  during low dose-rate irradiation, 225
  from potentially lethal damage (PLD), 172
  half-times, 224
  in fractionated radiotherapy, 213
  in human tumour cells, 172
  split-dose, from sublethal damage (SLD), 35, 172–175, 224
Regression, rate of tumour, 60
  and clonogenic cell kill, 60
Regrowth delay and cell survival, 71
Rejoining of DNA strand breaks, 35
Relative biological effectiveness (RBE), 250
  dependence on dose per fraction, 257
Relative effectiveness, 191, 194
Reoxygenation, 118, 121, 223
  during fractionated treatment, 122
  in accelerated radiotherapy, 142
  mechanisms and time-scales, 120
Repair inhibitors, effectiveness, 176
Repair of DNA damage, 21–22
  definition, 35
  mechanisms of, 15
  double-strand breaks, 22, 24
  single-strand breaks, 21, 36–37
  unifying theory of repair, 172
  'unstoppable' repair, 52
Repair-saturation models, 50
Repopulation, during and after radiotherapy, 84–85, 183, 196, 213, 223
Restriction endonucleases, 24, 37
Rs of radiobiology, the four, 223

Subject index

SF$_2$, the surviving fraction at 2 Gy, 169–171, 306–307
Silent interval, of tumour growth, 79
Single-strand DNA breaks (see DNA damage)
Skin, radiation damage, 98
   dermal atrophy 110
   time-scale of manifestation, 109
Smooth muscle cells, radiation effects, 106
Spatial co-operation, in combined treatment, 268, 282
S-phase duration, in human tumour cells, 82
Spheroids, multicellular, 165
Split-course radiotherapy, 218
Split-dose recovery, see Recovery (SLD)
Stem cells, tumour, 46
Strandqvist curves, 186
Subpopulations, drug-resistant, 58
Supra-additivity, 272
Survival, see Cell survival
Synchronisation therapy, 82

Target for radiation cell killing, 6
TD_{50} assay, 68
TDF formula, 189, 212
Technique of labelled mitoses, 81
Tetrazolium dye reduction (MTT assay), 308
Thermal isoeffect dose (TID), 301
Thermal enhancement ratio (TER), 298
Thermotolerance, 296–297
Thiols, radioprotection (see also Glutathione), 128

Time factors in fractionated radiotherapy, 195
Time-dose calculations, 194
Time-line studies, 273
   clinical, 281
Tissue-injury unit (TIU), 111
Tissue-rescuing units (TRU), 74, 93
Topoisomerase, type II, 39
Toxicity of drug–radiation combinations, 271
Tumour control probability and cell survival, 70
Tumour growth curves, 79
Tumour growth delay, and cell survival, 61, 68
   and duration of remission, 59
Tumour-bed effect, 60
Tumour-size dependence of chemotherapy, 58

Ultra-soft X-rays, 9–10
Ultraviolet radiation, cellular sensitivity, 33

Vascular effects and normal tissue damage, 101, 109
Vascular insufficiency, leading to hypoxia, 115
Velocity sedimentation of DNA, 18–20
Volume response, of treated tumours, 59
Volume-doubling time, 79

WR-2721 (the radioprotector), 128–130

Xenografts of human tumours, 165, 171
Xrs mutants, 32